T0292808

Persisting Pandemics

Critical Issues in Health and Medicine

Edited by Rima D. Apple, University of Wisconsin–Madison;
Janet Golden, Rutgers University–Camden; and Rana A. Hogarth,
University of Illinois at Urbana–Champaign

Growing criticism of the U.S. healthcare system is coming from consumers, politicians, the media, activists, and healthcare professionals. Critical Issues in Health and Medicine is a collection of books that explores these contemporary dilemmas from a variety of perspectives, among them political, legal, historical, sociological, and comparative, and with attention to crucial dimensions such as race, gender, ethnicity, sexuality, and culture.

For a complete list of titles in the series, please see the last page of the book.

Persisting Pandemics

Syphilis, AIDS, and COVID

Powel H. Kazanjian

Rutgers University Press

New Brunswick, Camden, and Newark, New Jersey

London and Oxford

Rutgers University Press is a department of Rutgers, The State University of New Jersey, one of the leading public research universities in the nation. By publishing worldwide, it furthers the University's mission of dedication to excellence in teaching, scholarship, research, and clinical care.

Library of Congress Cataloging-in-Publication Data

Names: Kazanjian, Powel H., 1953– author.
Title: Persisting pandemics : syphilis, AIDS, and COVID / Powel H. Kazanjian.
Description: New Brunswick : Rutgers University Press, [2025] | Series: Critical issues in health and medicine | Includes bibliographical references and index.
Identifiers: LCCN 2024003512 | ISBN 9781978830677 (paperback ; alk. paper) | ISBN 9781978830684 (hardcover ; alk. paper) | ISBN 9781978830691 (epub) | ISBN 9781978830707 (pdf)
Subjects: MESH: Communicable Disease Control | Syphilis | Acquired Immunodeficiency Syndrome | COVID-19 | Trust—psychology | Health Inequities | Social Determinants of Health
Classification: LCC RA651 | NLM WA 110 | DDC 614.4—dc23/eng/20240624
LC record available at https://lccn.loc.gov/2024003512

A British Cataloging-in-Publication record for this book is available from the British Library.

Cover art: *Hercules Fighting Fury and Discord*, woodcut, c. 1630 by Chistoffel Jegher. Block: 23 5/8 × 14 in. Sheet: 24 1/16 × 14 7/16 in. Courtesy of the Philadelphia Museum of Art: The Muriel and Philip Berman Gift, acquired from the John F. Lewis Collection given to the Pennsylvania Academy of the Fine Arts in 1933 by Mrs. John F. Lewis, with funds contributed by Muriel and Philip Berman, gifts (by exchange) of Lisa Norris Elkins, Bryant W. Langston, Samuel S. White 3rd and Vera White, with additional funds contributed by John Howard McFadden, Jr., Thomas Skelton Harrison, and the Philip H. and A.S.W. Rosenbach Foundation, 1985-52-6.

References to internet websites (URLs) were accurate at the time of writing. Neither the author nor Rutgers University Press is responsible for URLs that may have expired or changed since the manuscript was prepared.

♾ The paper used in this publication meets the requirements of the American National Standard for Information Sciences—Permanence of Paper for Printed Library Materials, ANSI Z39.48-1992.

rutgersuniversitypress.org

To my children, Powel III, Louisa, and Sarine,
and my wife, Sahira

Contents

Persisting Pandemics

Introduction

The Flemish artist Christoffel Jegher's 1620 illustration *Hercules Fighting Fury and Discord* (see front cover) depicts the second of twelve labors of Hercules. In the myth, King Eurystheus of Tiryns called upon the mighty human hero to kill the seven-headed hydra, a naturally appearing poisonous water snake that horrified humans by ravaging them without warning. Jegher captures Hercules's promise as the powerful hero confidently carries out his seemingly triumphant deed. Jegher, however, omits the myth's impending twist: as soon as Hercules clubs off the beast's head, two more appear in its place. The myth implies that unpredictable forces of nature can curtail powerful human efforts to control its harshness.

The myth's theme about the boundaries of the human capacity to conquer unruly natural forces parallels a central theme of this book. The might of Hercules is analogous to the capacity of biomedical programs to eliminate harmful diseases that arise in nature. This book explores the boundaries of biomedicine to control the devastation caused by unexpected, fearsome diseases: syphilis and AIDS. It traces how each epidemic, by striking people during the prime of their lives, burdened families, and threatened communities. Ingenious and powerful human-designed biomedical therapies that formed the basis of public health campaigns offered the promise of subduing and eliminating them within a discrete time frame. Despite human efforts to control these diseases, AIDS and syphilis have challenged biomedical campaigns, exploited economic divides, and, consequently, persisted unevenly in populations. This book explores the impressive accomplishments of biomedicine along with its limitations in the context of human efforts to control syphilis and AIDS.

The shared stories of syphilis and AIDS provide insight into diseases like COVID today. This book traces each epidemic from its origin through March 2023 to gain a better understanding of factors that limit powerful biomedical efforts designed to control epidemics. Promising public health campaigns using innovative therapies for syphilis and AIDS have not succeeded because they have not fully addressed underlying socioeconomic factors that drive disease and interfere with elimination efforts. Powerful biomedical advances are not sufficient to control diseases that ultimately persist unevenly in populations. Despite today's spectacular biomedical progress, which has yielded potent antimicrobials (against, e.g., syphilis and HIV) and effective mRNA vaccines (against COVID), public health measures that employ these products cannot be divorced from broader social, economic, and moral considerations. Efforts that take into consideration social issues and environmental vulnerabilities remain as important today as they did in the nineteenth century, before widespread adoption of the germ theory of disease.

Epidemics like syphilis, AIDS, and COVID, unlike smallpox, do not have discrete endings within targeted timelines, despite well-conceived efforts to end them. They disprove any belief that scientific discoveries have ended the period of acute epidemic diseases that once defined nineteenth-century life (e.g., cholera, yellow fever, typhoid, tuberculosis) and replaced them with chronic cardiovascular diseases and cancers. Today, we cope with a greater array of epidemics than those who lived during the nineteenth century, even though we have the biomedical means to control them. Our cumulative experience with epidemic diseases, together with our attempts to eliminate them, remains a continued component of our existence.

There are several distinctions between AIDS and syphilis. Syphilis has been present substantially longer (over five centuries) than AIDS (four decades). The causal microbes—a spirochete causes syphilis, and a retrovirus causes AIDS—differ. Initially, AIDS was nearly always fatal, while syphilis instead caused chronic symptoms and disability. The treatments differ substantially also. Treatment for syphilis involves an inexpensive one-time shot, whereas AIDS requires costly therapy taken every day for a lifetime. Other differences center on the roles of leadership and the public's response. Activism has played a pivotal role throughout AIDS, but it has not been at the forefront of syphilis. The public health program launched to eliminate AIDS has taken place at the global level, whereas syphilis elimination campaigns are national. Despite these distinctions, the histories of syphilis and AIDS are relevant for diseases like COVID today by providing insight into the power and limitations of biomedicine, unveiling the circumstances where science is trusted and mistrusted, and reinforcing a need for public health programs to encompass socioeconomic as well as biological issues.

Syphilis and AIDS

Syphilis and AIDS were once at the forefront of public attention. These diseases, however, are far from being quiescent today. Syphilis continues to rage globally, and HIV/AIDS persists in its spread, particularly among disadvantaged populations. Both have been recalcitrant to the science-based public health efforts that were designed to eliminate them.

Medical historians have long made comparisons between syphilis and AIDS. In the 1980s, Allan Brandt and Elizabeth Fee focused on their moral framing.[1] The research documented that disease sufferers have historically been viewed as sinners, and that public health measures intended to restore threatened social values failed to achieve disease control.[2] Both historians pointed out that the idiom of pestilence, with its associated blaming and exclusion of sufferers, has compounded the suffering experienced by people who live with these diseases.[3] This book builds upon those comparisons by focusing on how approaches to handling the two epidemics unfolded over time as physicians drew upon the frameworks of knowledge available to them.

The initial responses to these diseases included the social distancing of people considered to have violated moral codes of behavior. As historians note, this moralistic framing persisted in early twentieth-century America.[4] Similarly, persons with AIDS initially encountered discrimination and exclusionary practices in the 1980s.[5] As they did with syphilis, some people invoked AIDS as a legitimation to remove what they considered social evils from society. But these measures, shrouded in moral judgments, did not reduce the spread of disease. Rather, the moralistic framing of public health programs hindered disease control efforts.

New concepts about these diseases based on empiric evidence eventually emerged. By the late nineteenth century, doctors postulated that syphilis was an inflammatory disease.[6] A microbial cause of the inflammation was accepted in the early twentieth century.[7] By 1910, the development of a novel chemotherapeutic agent, Salvarsan, restored health by killing the causative microbe.[8] Subsequently, the treatment of syphilis became known for the spectacular biomedical accomplishments it engendered. HIV/AIDS followed a similar evolution: from a morally framed illness to a condition known for its extraordinary therapeutics.[9] By the 1990s, new understandings of microbial pathogenesis enabled the development of antiretroviral therapy (ART).[10] By 1995, scientific journals lauded these discoveries as triumphs of the biomedical enterprise, and the popular press portrayed them as life-saving miracles.[11]

Scientifically developed treatments for syphilis and AIDS had important public health implications. After the discovery of Salvarsan, public health officers believed it plausible to control syphilis scientifically through diagnostic testing and by the treatment of those individuals identified as having the disease.[12] Nonetheless, a moralistic view of disease persisted. Social hygienic approaches to controlling disease failed to reduce syphilis during World War I and the postwar period.[13] By the 1930s, public health officials sought to eliminate syphilis by optimizing surveillance using widespread testing and by rendering people noncontagious with treatment.[14] By 1946, the availability of simpler, safer, and more effective penicillin treatments and declining rates of disease triggered public health officials to envision a future without syphilis. Likewise, public health experts adopted a strategy of using testing and treatment to eliminate HIV/AIDS in the population.[15] As with syphilis, the campaign to eliminate HIV was based on extending the benefits of treating an individual to the sphere of public health.

Syphilis and AIDS campaigns relied on the idea that therapy could suppress the microbe and interrupt its spread. In this sense, the programs were "scientific," as defined by early twentieth-century public health officials who considered public health programs scientific if they targeted each outbreak to its unique microbial character and ecological mode of spread.[16] Indeed, the programs relied on widespread surveillance using accurate testing and potent treatments to disrupt microbial transmission.

The approaches employed by public health experts to control syphilis and AIDS underscored their trust in biomedicine. A test-and-treat campaign could promptly eradicate a disease like syphilis that had burdened society for centuries, and campaigns could end AIDS as a global threat by maximizing ART distribution. The confidence in these proposals bolstered a mid-twentieth-century narrative that portrayed an unlimited power of biomedicine.[17] The celebration of biomedicine was fueled by a growing confidence in vaccines to control vexing childhood diseases and antibiotics to treat once-lethal infections.[18] The notion that epidemic diseases could be extinguished was reinforced in 1952, when a report in the lay journal *Great Adventures in Medicine* concluded, "It seems likely that in the next few years a combination of antibiotics . . . will furnish a '*cribrum therapeuticum*' from which fewer and fewer microbes will escape."[19]

By the 1950s, society upheld a notion that the modern scientific world would conquer epidemic diseases. Penicillin offered the promise of controlling common conditions like pneumonia and pharyngitis.[20] In the later twentieth century, the public's confidence in biomedicine to manage infectious diseases continued to mount. As historian Nancy Tomes notes, people had also become reassured by the idea that disease-causing microbes could be avoided by protective behaviors that could be learned.[21] This narrative was promoted by the widely publicized promise of biomedicine to eliminate diseases that had burdened societies for centuries.[22]

By the latter part of the twentieth century, one could contemplate an inverted narrative that began with humans victimized by uncontrollable diseases. People were eventually reassured by the idea that medical scientists armed with biomedical products would ultimately subdue epidemics. Science historian Naomi Oereskes has suggested that scientific results are trustworthy because science, by its nature, is a collective enterprise and its findings are verified through methodical vetting and peer reviews.[23] The treatment of AIDS and syphilis add to the notion of trust by delivering irrefutable benefits to individuals and societies.

Despite their rational underpinnings, campaigns against syphilis and AIDS have not reached their goals of eliminating the diseases from populations.[24] The diseases endure unevenly worldwide today, particularly in geographic regions where people are poor, disadvantaged, or marginalized.[25] Higher-income countries have concentrated epidemics of syphilis among specific populations (e.g., men who have sex with men [MSM], transgender women) and regions (low-income inner-city areas). Lower- to middle-income countries (LMICs) continue to have higher endemic rates of syphilis among their general populations.[26] As has been the case with syphilis, the elimination campaign by the Joint United Nations Programme on HIV/AIDS (UNAIDS) also has yet to meet its overall goal because HIV continues to spread in vulnerable environments—in low-income urban centers in the United States and in several LMICs throughout the world.[27] As with syphilis, efforts to eliminate AIDS by differentially allocating treatment have accentuated an unequal distribution of disease in vulnerable environments.

This book explores the multiple reasons why attempts to end syphilis and AIDS have not been attainable. Biologically, the asymptomatic spread of disease threatens accurate public health measures of identification and treatment. Socioeconomic factors, including poverty and migrating populations, create vulnerable environments that impede elimination campaigns.[28] Persistent moralistic framing of disease also discourages people from seeking testing and medical attention.[29] In addition, geopolitical factors (e.g., maintaining elimination programs as a national priority) and effects of concomitant epidemics (e.g., the opioid epidemic) threaten elimination programs.[30] Moreover, there remains the problem of how to tailor global campaign messages to local communities in culturally specific ways.[31] The reasons for failure of elimination campaigns entail more than biological factors and reinforce the need for reforms that address vulnerable social and physical environments.[32]

Why should it matter if campaigns cannot achieve disease elimination if they reduce the burden of disease? One risk is that health workers could become disillusioned if campaigns fall short of their goals. The history of AIDS is replete with campaigns that have overpromised but underperformed. Margaret Heckler, for example, anticipated in 1984 that a vaccine for HIV would be available within three years; in 1998, Bill Clinton predicted that an effective HIV vaccine would be produced within ten years; in 2013 Hilary Clinton envisioned an "AIDS free Generation" within our lifetime. The following year, UNAIDS targeted the elimination of AIDS by 2030, and in 2019, Donald Trump forecasted the elimination of AIDS in the United States before 2029.[33] For syphilis, in 1937 Thomas Parran proposed its eradication within ten years, and in 1961 Leona Baumgartner projected the same. President Kennedy, in 1963, laid out a decade-long goal that syphilis would be eradicated and a human would land on the moon.[34] Specific timelines can certainly galvanize workers and inspire them to achieve goals. But they also create disaffection among workers when a program does not meet its expectations, and engender mistrust in policymakers who set unattainable goals.

Stories of AIDS and syphilis underscore a theme that applies to COVID today: that science will not be sufficient to manage pandemics unless coupled with social programs to rectify the disease's continued spread within vulnerable environments. The necessity for programs to address social issues alters the once-confident narrative of biomedicine as having unlimited powers to end epidemics.[35] AIDS, syphilis, and COVID suggest limitations to that narrative: new epidemics will continue to occur, and they will persist despite scientific interventions that promise to eliminate them. Epidemics and their resulting elimination efforts remain part of our existence, residing in social fault lines among communities that lack privilege and wealth. Science remains powerful in this modified narrative, but no longer unlimited.

Notable episodes that occurred throughout the HIV/AIDS epidemic illustrate how mistrust in science predated COVID. Patient activists during the early phase of the AIDS epidemic viewed medical investigators as misguided when they used placebos to test antivirals in subjects who had the fatal disease, which lacked treatment.[36] In addition, a South African president refused to implement government-sponsored ART based on his denial that HIV caused AIDS.[37] Mistrust was also evidenced by the disregard of the expert opinion that the AIDS virus could not be spread casually, resulting in needless ostracizing of victims.[38]

Moments of overt government inactivity on AIDS and syphilis provide a backdrop to society's mistrust of governmental officials during COVID. Patient-activist groups publicly exposed President Reagan's indifference toward HIV/AIDS and accused federal regulatory agencies of callousness toward AIDS sufferers.[39] In addition, government funding for syphilis elimination programs has been prematurely terminated repeatedly. This insufficiency enabled the continued spread of the epidemic.

The histories of syphilis and AIDS contain notorious events that are pertinent for COVID. There were ethical violations in human experimentation for syphilis, including the U.S. Public Health Service (USPHS) studies in Tuskegee, Alabama, from 1932 to 1972 and in Guatemala from 1946 to 1948, each of which exploited vulnerable populations without their consent.[40] The Tuskegee study left a residue of mistrust in medical scientists and government officials that has negatively impacted the willingness of the public to cooperate with scientifically based recommendations in the case of ensuing epidemics.[41] Adding to this uncomfortable history, an AIDS researcher recently drew criticism from scientists for performing an unethical genetic-editing experiment.[42] Consequently, the sacrifice of research subjects' well-being in order to gain medical knowledge has perpetuated a lasting suspicion that is now part of the legacy of syphilis and AIDS.

The histories of syphilis and AIDS reveal instances where the government has gone too far in restricting the rights of people in the name of public health. During World War I, officials detained sex workers against their will for years to combat syphilis.[43] With AIDS, some alarmed citizens called for instituting compulsory testing and indefinitely quarantining those who tested positive.[44] These restrictive measures demonstrate how control efforts have threatened individual civil liberties. This book will explore these episodes of coercive public health interventions along with others that have contributed to a mistrust of science and government—including ethical lapses in human experimentation and episodes of government inactivity in the face of epidemic spread. A study of syphilis and AIDS, along with the public health programs designed to eliminate them, provides insights into the successes and failures of public health measures used to control COVID.

COVID

Novel biomedical products developed for COVID have been lauded by scientists and society as spectacular breakthroughs.[45] Public health and government officials envisioned that the end of COVID would occur soon after mRNA vaccines were released.[46] But predictions of achieving elimination of the disease in April 2021 were upended by additional surges later in the year. By March 2022, the specter of another surge resurfaced as vaccination rates in industrialized countries remained uneven and LMICs remained undervaccinated.[47] The general population had mixed views regarding the pandemic as of the time this book was completed (March 2023).[48] Most citizens considered the once-fearsome pandemic over and the disease merely a tolerable threat like the common cold that does not require precaution. But to others, particularly those at high risk of severe disease, such as the elderly, medically fragile, or immunocompromised, the fear that a COVID variant could emerge in LMICs and ultimately involve high-income countries seemed plausible. Three years into its course, the threat of another surge that lingers during periods of inactivity has been a defining characteristic of the pandemic. The pandemic persists unevenly in the population, and so does the vigilance individuals adopt to prevent transmission.

A defining lesson from syphilis and AIDS—that effective public health elimination programs must address socioeconomic issues—also applies to COVID. Policy experts have highlighted throughout the pandemic that campaigns to control COVID must include structural interventions aimed at rectifying the socioeconomic issues that create unsafe behaviors.[49] Solutions to these issues have included providing supplemental housing for economically disadvantaged essential workers, which would allow them to safely isolate.[50] Structural strategies must also address how to mass-distribute vaccines to disadvantaged populations living in vulnerable environments such as inner-city areas, including the homeless who live in shelters, crowded jails, or remote Native American Indian Reservations.[51] Because the strategies designed to redress these longstanding socioeconomic issues have not been fully implemented, efforts to handle COVID have accentuated underlying racial and social inequalities.

Mistrust of science has led to noncompliance with key COVID public health guidelines and vaccine acceptance throughout the course of the pandemic. In part, this has emanated directly from government officials and has subsequently jeopardized key public health goals such as social distancing and achieving vaccine coverage.[52] As of March 2023, although three hundred people in the United States who were almost all elderly or medically frail died from

COVID-related conditions daily, overall rates of disease had decreased, mask mandates had been lifted in almost all locales, and the pandemic had been forgotten by most.[53] But others, particularly those at high risk for severe disease, maintained a heightened concern about a recurrent surge and the reimposition of mask recommendations, as happened in April 2021. At that time, when infection rates had declined and the CDC sanctioned not wearing masks, a surprise surge arose in India (the Delta variant) and later South Africa (Omicron). In both places, vaccine rates had been low, and crowding could not be avoided. The uneasy anticipation of another surge makes experts and some citizens skeptical about joining what might be a premature assumption that COVID has ended.

COVID shares a similar narrative with AIDS and syphilis. COVID arrived with a discrete beginning and devastated individuals and societies. Likewise, the arrival of innovative biomedical products offered the prospect of ending the epidemic. But underlying social, economic, and biological issues have challenged any promise that COVID, AIDS and syphilis could end within a specified time frame. Instead, citizens have learned to live with these epidemics, albeit unevenly in the population, along with our efforts to eliminate them. For COVID, this includes enduring repetitive cycles of adopting and relaxing restrictions and the inconveniences of social distancing, particularly among high-risk populations in certain locales (e.g., hospitals). Each epidemic has reached a period of complacency while the disease persists.

Tensions between personal liberty and individualism surfaced again during COVID, as they did during AIDS and syphilis. During the first COVID surge of March 2000, President Trump promoted the risky idea that restrictions based on scientific guidelines unnecessarily infringed on civil liberties. Angry factions, encouraged by the president's rhetoric, publicly flouted recommendations by assembling in large crowds without masks.[54] Meanwhile, some elected officials, like representative Louie Gohmert of Texas, repeatedly disregarded the recommendations of public health officials by refusing to wear masks in meetings held on Capitol Hill.[55]

In the context of COVID, an inclination to place a higher value on individual liberty over the public good has assumed a partisan nature. The tendency to favor the importance of individualism has resonated with the ideologies of conservative Republicans in the United States, to whom rejection of advice to wear masks and adhere to vaccine recommendations has become a symbol of partisan allegiance. This played out during the Sturgis, South Dakota, motorcycle rally of August 2021 and the People's Convoy of Truckers in March 2022. The adoption or rejection of public health policies according to partisan allegiances is not new to COVID. It was also evident during AIDS, when President Reagan ignored the epidemic. In the 1950s, sustained funding to support syphilis control campaigns was reduced by the Eisenhower administration. Although partisan allegiances of public health decisions are not new, today's messages have greater, and instantaneous, dissemination through social media.

Though tensions between personal liberties and public health during COVID have been strained, social-distancing guidelines throughout the pandemic have not been coercive. Historically, the United States has gone much further to prevent spread of disease, such as the mandatory detention of sex workers during World War I and proposals to quarantine those who tested positive for HIV in the 1980s. Public health approaches during COVID in Western democracies have not abolished individual civil rights or deprived people of their livelihoods. This more balanced approach has not been adopted in totalitarian states like China, where three years of harsh "Zero COVID" lockdown rules have led to economic hardship.[56] In the United States, the government has issued temporary COVID restrictions and has granted safety nets (e.g., stimulus packages and assistance with mortgage payments). Today's noncompulsory governmental measures in liberal democracies call for modifying behavior (distancing, mask wearing) to prevent disease spread; they do not abrogate civil liberties.

Indeed, recommendations to follow public health advice, like wearing masks, getting vaccinated, and adopting social-distance measures, are more inconveniences than deprivations of livelihood. Regardless, the imposition of these measures reinforces that we have moved beyond the notion that living with the great nineteenth-century pandemics is over, as some public health officers had speculated.[57] The study of AIDS, syphilis, and COVID reinforces that an obligation to social responsibility, acting out of concern for what prevents harm to others, remains just as important today as it did in the nineteenth century. These diseases, along with others that have appeared, underscore how our cumulative experience with pandemics has numerically expanded since the nineteenth century, even though death rates from infectious diseases have declined overall. To control these infectious diseases, humans must live in solidarity, and with a restored focus on behavior that does not harm others.

The challenge for leaders is to foster solidarity among the factions that have become polarized under the political administrations of several nations, including those of Donald Trump (United States), Jair Bolsonaro (Brazil), and Shri Modi (India). The factions most concerned with honoring their personal freedoms must recognize that liberty is not synonymous with license. They do not have the license to defy scientific guidelines needed to protect the public good. Likewise, the larger sector that is already following guidelines must learn to cooperate with skeptics and work toward a common goal of collectively adhering to scientific advice for the good of the public. Throughout the pandemic, this has not happened. Dialogue between the unvaccinated and vaccinated has stagnated. However, behaving in solidarity is just as essential for public health during COVID today as it was during the 1990s when Treatment Action Group activists collaborated with scientists from whom they had previously been alienated to develop potent HIV drugs.

Stigma continues to pose a threat to public health programs during COVID. Although this trend was less overt during COVID than it had been with syphilis and AIDS, "outsiders" were blamed for spreading COVID to the United States.[58] People of Chinese origin in the United States report feeling stigmatized by the rhetoric of naming the microbe a "Chinese virus."[59] This rhetoric creates unnecessary divides that can only interfere with efforts to foster the solidarity needed to control the pandemic. In addition, some individuals, including President Trump, have also stigmatized those who have worn face masks. Derided as conformists, those following guidelines were set as foes of those who honor personal liberties above all else.[60]

Themes that emerge from the history of syphilis and AIDS have resurfaced during COVID. These include the promise of spectacular biomedical products, the limitation of those products in the realm of public health programs, and the mistrust of science. In addition, AIDS, syphilis, and COVID public health programs must address social and racial disparities, misinformation dissemination, and government indifference. As AIDS has shown, policy experts must assure that biomedical products are allocated equitably on a global scale, thereby avoiding a humanitarian crisis. Additionally, AIDS has shown the need for opposing factions, including those who disagree about public health restrictions, to work together to achieve common goals.

AIDS, syphilis, and COVID show that pandemics and efforts to control them remain part of our existence. As was the case in the pre–germ theory era, epidemics arise suddenly and devastate individuals and society. Today, unlike in the nineteenth century, however, we are reassured that scientific progress offers the potential to tame epidemics and eliminate the uncertainty they introduce into our daily existence. Nonetheless, as this book shows, we continue to live with epidemics.

The material in this book is organized into six chapters.

Chapter 1. "Syphilis: Vanguard of Scientific Medicine." By the early twentieth century, syphilis had come to epitomize the power of biomedicine. The discovery of the microbial cause and groundbreaking chemotherapy allowed a new therapeutic pathway of restoring health. By the 1930s, public health officials launched a "scientific" campaign to eradicate syphilis in the United States using widespread testing and treatment. The promise of syphilis eradication held great political and social appeal. Scientific progress offered the potential to alleviate the burdens syphilis posed for nations during civilian and wartime periods: unemployment, disability, and dependency on the state. The discoveries of treatments for syphilis bolstered a confident narrative of biomedicine and a growing trust in science and technology and their benefits for society. The excitement surrounding the use of these scientific tools contributed to increasing expectations that biomedicine would someday render epidemic diseases obsolete.

Chapter 2. "AIDS: Potential of Biomedicine." The discoveries surrounding AIDS also reinforced a confidence in the powers of scientific medicine. AIDS patients trusted that biomedicine would yield effective therapies, and by 1996 their collaboration with scientists led to the discovery of innovative therapies that reversed the disease's progressively fatal course. But the excessive cost of those therapies prohibited their allocation to LMICs globally. An approach spearheaded by patient advocates lowered drug costs, changed intellectual property laws, and elicited contributions from donor countries. The adjustments proved to equitably distribute the drugs globally. To extend ART to populations, public health campaigns similar in methodology to syphilis elimination programs were implemented in 2014. By the twenty-first century, advancements in treatments for AIDS, like those for syphilis, reinforced a trust that actions based on scientific discoveries would lead to clear-cut benefits for humans.

Chapter 3. "Fate of Elimination Campaigns." Despite their promise, campaigns to eliminate syphilis and AIDS have not reached their goals. Campaigns from the 1960s to the 2000s were centered around testing and treating, but syphilis still rages today. HIV also continues its unabated spread in vulnerable environments. Biomedically based eradication programs that have taken place globally for AIDS and nationally for syphilis have faltered because they have not sufficiently included structural solutions to address underlying social and economic problems that create vulnerable environments. Consequently, AIDS and syphilis persist unevenly in high-risk locales in the United States and globally. Although these epidemics, and public health efforts to eliminate them, remain a part of our experience today, a complacency has developed in the population. These phases—fear, devastation, the promise of biomedicine, the limitations of scientific medicine, and complacency—characterize the pattern of syphilis and AIDS.

Chapter 4. "Legacies of Mistrust: Syphilis and AIDS." The histories of syphilis and AIDS expose the underside of modern medical enterprise. For syphilis, the public became broadly aware of episodes where medical researchers exploited patients by violating ethical human experimentation. AIDS patients have also accused medical scientists of callousness. These episodes left a residue of mistrust of doctors and medicine. The histories of syphilis and AIDS also reveal misguided public health programs that tried to regulate behavior according to societal norms, rather than focusing on scientific approaches. These programs, along with breeches in ethical conduct during human experimentation, show how the histories of AIDS and syphilis entail a long-standing sentiment of scientific mistrust that is relevant for COVID today.

Chapter 5. "COVID: Familiar Patterns Emerge." The trajectory of COVID, like syphilis and AIDS, began with a frightening spread that could ultimately be controlled by spectacular biomedical advances. Nonetheless, public health campaigns to control COVID have not adequately addressed either the underlying social and economic issues that drive the epidemic or the mistrust in science and emphasis on individualism that have challenged cooperation with public health recommendations. As was the case with distributing HIV drugs globally, COVID vaccination efforts unveiled the humanitarian consequences that occur when resource-wealthy countries purchase medical products that LMICs cannot afford. AIDS, syphilis, and COVID show that biomedical and social responses to epidemics must be complementary. These epidemics share a common narrative arc: the promise of biomedicine to eliminate disease tempered by the realization that we must live with them.

Chapter 6. "Vulnerable Environments: Historical Roots." A study of syphilis, AIDS, and COVID shows that elimination campaigns must target environmental structures that determine risky behavior. Public health approaches that take structural issues into consideration at the broader environmental level, rather than solely at the individual level, remain just as relevant today as they were in the pre–germ theory era. Early twentieth-century public health officials hoped to make their campaigns to control diseases more effective and efficient by focusing on the microbe and its interaction with the host, rather than following the earlier approach of focusing on environmental concerns. But such an approach is not sufficient to manage epidemics. Science and microbiology do not displace the need for a comprehensive approach to public health to correct social issues and environmental risks that are not necessarily related to specific pathogens.

Medical historians and public health officials have systematically studied syphilis and AIDS within the context of sexually transmitted diseases. Traditional themes have emerged, including the stigma of the sufferer and the ineffectiveness of public health campaigns that attempt to rectify "social evils" while simultaneously employing scientific public health approaches. This book builds upon these insights and shows how themes derived from sexually transmitted infections (STIs) can apply to epidemics like COVID. Syphilis and AIDS show how doctors have become so confident in biomedical advances that they have relied on them to eliminate diseases at the population level. However, as paralleled by the myth of Hercules's second labor, these campaigns have fallen short of meeting their goals. Consequently, the diseases persist disproportionately in low-income locales and among minorities. This shortcoming has relevance to COVID. Syphilis and AIDS also provide perspective on issues that have surfaced during COVID and that interfere with public health plans—including a mistrust in science and an emphasis on individualism over social obligations. A study of these diseases allows one to appreciate how the human experience of living through multiple pandemics and efforts to control them remains as significant a component of our lives today as it was in the nineteenth century.

Chapter 1

Syphilis

Vanguard of Scientific Medicine

In this chapter, we explore syphilis from its onset in 1495 to the first program designed to eradicate it in the United States. Syphilis receives scant attention in contemporary society, and little active scientific research is being conducted on the disease today. Since the mid-1940s, medical knowledge regarding the causality, diagnostic testing, therapeutics, and strategies to control the disease in the population have not significantly changed. In contrast, during the nineteenth century and the first half of the twentieth century, syphilis has been known for ushering in spectacular biomedical innovations.

This chapter traces how ideas about disease causality, management, and control of syphilis in the population unfolded from the 1400s to the mid-twentieth century. Due to a series of scientific discoveries, the understanding of syphilis evolved over this period as physicians drew from changing frameworks of thinking. As therapeutics evolved, syphilis changed from a disfiguring disease to one that was curable. Once a societal menace, it became eradicable. The evolving knowledge of syphilis and its management created a public narrative that bolstered confidence that biomedicine could conquer not only syphilis but all epidemic diseases.

Initial Outbreak through the Nineteenth Century

Historians have addressed the abrupt appearance of syphilis in Europe in 1495. Alfred Crosby described how the disease arose during France's wartime conquest of Naples, then spread rapidly throughout Europe as King Charles VIII's army disbanded following their return to France.[1] Physicians initially described syphilis as a frightful disease primarily involving the skin, with the onset of solid growths, ulcers, and pustules, sometimes accompanied by disabling joint pains.[2] Physicians speculated on the causes of the disease as it spread rapidly throughout the population.[3] In his 1534 poem *Morbus gallicus*, the Italian physician Girolomo Fracastoro attributed its origins to outsiders—sailors from foreign countries.[4] The Spanish physician Ruy Diaz de Isla wrote in 1542 that syphilis was a new disease encountered in foreign lands by the sailors of Columbus and imported to Europe on their return from their 1492 New World voyage.[5] As the disease spread through Europe, each nation cast blame on the preceding nation, as evidenced by Fracastoro calling syphilis the "French Disease."[6] Placing blame on the outsider had occurred during earlier epidemics, including during the 430 B.C.E. plague, when Athenians blamed Spartans for poisoning the drinking water, and the 1347 Black Death, when some European citizens blamed Jews for poisoning wells.[7]

The legitimacy of the Columbian theory that syphilis was imported to Europe by sailors has been debated among medical historians for decades. Crosby concluded in 1976 that it remained unclear whether the disease was imported by Columbus or whether it had been present in Europe beforehand.[8] More recently, a study using genetic analysis of Northern European human skeletal remains concluded that both venereal and yaws-causing *Treponeme pallidum* strains of syphilis were already present in Northern Europe before Columbus's expedition.[9] Although the results of this study provide compelling evidence to support the pre-Columbian theory, it is beyond the scope of this book to judge whether the study definitively ends debates about the origin of syphilis. The major point is that doctors implicated outsider groups—the blame falling on either North Americans or an outside European nation—for introducing syphilis into Europe.

Fracastoro also believed that syphilis was spread through explicit sexual contact between sexually promiscuous sinners.[10] He observed, "This pestilence . . . was contracted only when two bodies in close contact with each other become extremely heated . . . in sexual intercourse."[11] We can surmise that Fracastoro reached this conclusion from circumstantial observations of skin disorders occurring in those who were diseased. Indeed, Ulrich von Hutten, a German humanist writing at the same time as Fracastoro, articulated this idea. Von Hutten describes the location of skin problems (ulcers, sores, blisters) that "resteth in 'secret places' [of people] who defile themselves . . . especially . . . by copulation [and] . . . intemperate living . . . [and] . . . the more man is given to wantonness the sooner he is infected . . . excepting young children, old men and other(s), which are not given to bodily lust."[12] The location of skin ulcers and blisters in the genital regions of sexually promiscuous individuals led von Hutten to speculate that the disease was contracted through sexual contact.

Syphilis was not the first disease physicians believed to be venereally acquired. In the fourteenth century, the physician Gilbert the Englishman accused those with leprosy of committing sins by having excessive sexual desire, writing, "Lepers search for sexual pleasure more than usual and more than they should."[13] French surgeon Guy de Chauliac wrote of lepers as having "heavy and grievous dreams . . . of sexual excess."[14] Thus, the cause of leprosy in the medieval period was ascribed to a desire for excessive sexual pleasure.[15] Unlike syphilis in the 1500s, however, there was no explicit mention of acquiring leprosy through physical contact during sexual intercourse. Thus, whether doctors understood leprosy to be caused by God's punishment for lust itself or to result from explicit direct sexual contact remains ambiguous.[16]

In addition to speculating that syphilis was spread by direct sexual contact, Fracastoro attributed the spread of contagion to invisible particles that he implied (without definitively stating so) were living. Fracastoro speculated that the imperceptible particles cannot "live . . . quite so long as the hard ones." He also speculated that they replicated, stating, "The original germs . . . generate and propagate other germs precisely like themselves, and these in turn propagate others." Fracastoro, however, also implied that the small particles were inert, stating that they could "evaporate." Though he was not consistent in his depiction of particles as being alive or inert, Fracastoro was clear that "infections [are] originated by small imperceptible notions particles . . . [that are] spread by contagion by direct contact."[17] Fracastoro's conjectures about germs remained speculative, as there was no requirement for empirical proof to make a knowledge claim when he was writing in 1546.

In addition to Fracastoro's ideas, doctors at the time considered syphilis to be a just punishment from God for the sin of sexual excess. Ulrich von Hutten, himself a victim of syphilis, wrote about the shame and humiliation that having a diagnosis of syphilis had caused sufferers. Von Hutten demonstrated contrition by stating that God caused the disease as punishment for what he called his "evil living."[18]

Fracastoro alluded to additional causes of syphilis and their interconnection—astrological, environmental, and humoral predispositions. Thus, Fracastoro postulated a multitude of factors to account for the appearance of a new disease that appeared suddenly and spread quickly. He referred to an excessive phlegmatic humoral predisposition (e.g., an excess of phlegm with cold and wet qualities) that enabled learned physicians to counteract the imbalanced humors by recommending antipathetic qualities by sweating in a

heating chamber.[19] Fracastoro and von Hutten also offered their opinion on therapies that were not based on restoring humoral imbalances. They were troubled by the notable oral and dental toxicities accompanying mercury
ointments, and preferred what they viewed as milder guaiacum treatments.
Von Hutten welcomed treatment with guaiacum because of its origin in the bark
of a tree in North America—a part of the world where he believed the disease
originated.

Physicians' initial understandings of syphilis's sudden appearance in
Europe—for astral, humoral, or moral reasons, or through direct contact—show
how multiple theories of causality can coexist. These understandings of syphilis
as a contagion that spread between persons had its roots in prior epidemics,
such as the Athenian Plague and Black Death. The notion of the disease originating from an altered environment had historical precedence during the
Athenian Plague and Black Death. The idea of disease originating under
the influence of an alignment of certain planets was also rooted in the Black
Death.[20] Thus, the multifactorial explanation—outsider, contagion, environment, and conjunction of stars—provided an explanation to physicians for the
timing of the epidemic and how it spread so quickly, features that overlapped
with the Black Death.[21]

European societies responded to the threat of syphilis by adopting social-
distancing measures. This involved changing customs: the kiss as a customary
greeting gesture was halted, public baths were closed, and public drinking cups
were discarded. These measures changed social relations as people became suspicious of casual contact. Crosby claims that these changes in customs eroded
bonds of respect and trust that bound men and women together.[22] Brothels were
closed in European cities and prostitutes faced punishment by officials.[23] Persons with syphilis were not expelled from society per se, as had been the case
with leprosy, but distanced from within.[24] The extent to which individuals
adopted these measures, and, if so, how they influenced the spread of disease,
remains unknown.

New modes of explaining nature became available to physicians in the
1600s and 1700s. Francis Bacon, in his *Novum Organum* (1620), envisioned a
day when knowledge derived from one's own observations (empiricism) would
provide humans with a better understanding of the world.[25] The writings of
Bacon and eventually John Locke, especially his *Essay Concerning Human
Understanding* (1689), served as a philosophical foundation for new ways of
attaining knowledge through empiricism—that is, the use of one's sensory perceptions to examine nature and of reason to arrive at new knowledge.[26]

Physicians drew upon these influences to expand on clinical descriptions and added pathological descriptions of syphilis based on their observations.

By the late 1600s, the English physician Thomas Sydenham (1624–1689), a contemporary and acquaintance of Locke, objected to traditional medical learning in lecture halls and favored observation at the bedside to advance knowledge.[27] He argued that diseases, including syphilis, should be understood as specific entities based on descriptions of their clinical features, much as people had been doing by categorizing plants based on their distinctive appearances in the field of botany. The source of knowledge would be based entirely on one's own observations, and not through established humoral schemes. Sydenham, unaided by any specialized instruments, described skin manifestations of syphilis that doctors could recognize by their specific visual appearance and their tactile qualities, including the "chancre," a shallow ulcer with hardened, elevated borders.[28]

By the 1750s, physicians used their own observations to expand on Sydenham's clinical descriptions of syphilitic skin manifestations. The French physician Jean Astruc described a chancre with an attendant regional lymph node complex that he termed "condyloma lata."[29] Astruc in the late 1700s described a series of phases that distinguished what he referred to as primary and secondary syphilis according to their time of onset. The English physician Robert Willan elaborated on these descriptions of the skin in the early 1800s. He and other physicians of the time differentiated diseases according to their visible features.[30] Physicians like Benjamin Bell of Scotland, for example, in his work *Treatment of Gonorrhea and lues venera*, used the specific appearances of skin abnormalities to distinguish syphilis from gonorrhea.[31]

The medical historian Claude Quetel has written about the debates during this period over whether venereal diseases like syphilis and gonorrhea were caused by single or multiple illnesses.[32] Undergirding these debates were clinicians' attempts to categorize diseases according to their specific visual and tactile features.[33] Physicians' use of their senses of sight and touch to describe abnormalities underscored how the process of nosology—the means of categorizing diseases and distinguishing them from one another—was emerging in the context of syphilis during the early-modern period. Their ideas of disease specificity were based on clinical descriptions, the foundation for nosology. In the meantime, to locate the anatomic sites for specific diseases in specific internal organs, physicians began to develop the science of pathology.

In 1761, the Italian physician and pathologist Giovanni Morgagni (1682–1771) sought to produce a comprehensive record of disease. In his five-volume book *Of the Seats and Causes of Diseases Investigated through Anatomy*, he provided his descriptions of the morbid anatomy of 640 people.[34] He described the appearance of the diseased organs in an attempt to find and locate an anatomic site of disease (subsequently referred to as "gross" anatomy). For each person, Morgagni noted symptoms and compared his clinical observations with anatomical findings upon examining their bodies postmortem. Having no microscope, his postmortem descriptions contained findings of removed organs that he could discern with the unaided eye. Morgagni observed organs in their gross appearance and posited that diseases originated locally, in specific organs. He described patterns of abnormalities in relation to a person's symptoms.[35] Morgagni, however, was not the first to describe morbid anatomy. The Italian physician Antonio Benivieni and the French physician Theophile Bonet had done so earlier.[36] Morgagni, however, described disease in a significantly greater number of persons and included more information about the clinical symptoms prior to death than either Benivieni or Bonet. In addition, Morgagni also studied a wider scope of diseased organs, including vessels in the brain.

In the 1790s, Morgagni categorized disease based on location within the body and provided evidence for disease localization. He noted visceral abnormalities (soft tumor-like growths) involving various organs on macroscopic examination of removed organs—including the liver, heart, and brain—during postmortem examinations of some people with cutaneous syphilis. He speculated that the gross appearance of these growths, which he described using the term "lues," might be a visceral component of syphilis.[37] Doctors equipped with new instruments would develop this idea further in the nineteenth century.

During the nineteenth century, physicians at the Paris School of Medicine continued to construct new knowledge about syphilis by correlating clinical features of patients with postmortem observations. Ideologically, the Paris School extended what Sydenham and Morgagni had begun earlier. But the Paris School included three innovations: technological aids that enhanced the perception of clinical findings at the bedside, statistical associations correlating clinical and pathological features of diseases, and the new fields of cellular pathology that in the 1840s enhanced previous ideas about diseases.

New ideas about syphilis emerged in the context of the empirical clinical-pathological approach. The new French regime funded large hospitals that became centers of instruction under the authority of a new centralized state. Physicians enhanced their clinical observations by using sensory aids, including stethoscopes, reflex hammers, and percussion techniques. The mission of the Paris School physicians was to extend the scope of clinical inquiry to observation beyond inspecting the surface of the body. The second innovation of the

Paris School involved performing postmortem examinations to locate and provide further insight into the anatomic site of disease.[38] In the autopsy room, new methodologies were developed. Before the 1830s, observations of gross anatomical changes formed the basis of pathological descriptions. In the 1830s, the introduction of compound microscopes and microtome machines allowed the identification of pathological changes at the cellular level.[39] Pathologists could now categorize disease based on new criteria: histological patterns in tissues.

This novel approach enabled a more nuanced characterization of diseases than had been possible beforehand. Specific entities could be sorted into groups.[40] Diseases like syphilis were thought to have clinical and pathological essences, and disease was located as a discrete entity in the body.[41] This sorting process enabled a new avenue for doctors to categorize disease based on clinical, pathological, and histological patterns. This nosology is evident in the expanding number of organ-based diseases (e.g., inflammation, cancer) included in medical textbooks published by the 1840s.[42] By the 1870s, medical texts began to categorize diseases (e.g., pneumonia, gout) based on their clinical criteria and pathological findings.[43] Diseases located in a particular organ such as the lung could be further categorized based on their histopathological patterns, including inflammation (pneumonia) or tumor (lung cancer).[44] Discussions on the prognosis of these diseases were based on observations of patients.

With its multifocal nature and phasic course, however, syphilis was an anomaly for diseases that became defined according to their location within a particular organ. Syphilis in the early nineteenth century was known as a skin disorder.[45] Descriptions of the disease and its course became so detailed that the term "syphilology" was ascribed to the field in the late nineteenth century.[46] In addition, the establishment of a dedicated journal—the *Journal of Dermatology and Syphilology*—in 1870 indicated the emergence of specialization in the context of a single disease.[47] With this scrutiny, physicians began to consider whether syphilis could involve visceral organs, as Morgagni had previously suggested.[48] As physicians gained knowledge about disease and its causality in the nineteenth century, the concept of syphilis changed from that of a skin disease only to one involving visceral organs.

Throughout the nineteenth century, syphilologists noted that involvement of internal organs might occur sometime after the appearance of skin lesions.[49] Confirmation of the theory of visceral involvement in syphilis, however, was confounded by the fact that the internal abnormalities did not occur in every person with syphilis and the pattern of visceral involvement was unpredictable.[50] These variations posed a question: How could clinicians know whether visceral phenomena were related to syphilis? Since antiquity, physicians had considered the ability to prognosticate the course of an illness to be one of their valuable skills.[51] But with syphilis, the unpredictable trajectory of the disease confounded their ability to forecast an outcome.[52]

French physicians addressed the nuances of a multifocal disease in space and time. Jean Louis Alibert and Alpee Cazenave elaborated on the scope of primary and secondary skin eruptions of syphilis in 1829.[53] Phillippe Ricord mapped out its phasic course, where original skin problems (primary disease) might resolve only to have others appear at separate points (secondary disease) after time had lapsed.[54] By the mid-1800s, the British physician Jonathan Hutchinson encountered internal involvement of bone, heart, eye, and central nervous system in some people who had had a previous episode of cutaneous syphilis.[55] He noted that a long period of time elapsed before visceral abnormalities developed, and they did not occur in everybody. Albert Fournier, a French syphilologist, addressed the issue from a statistical standpoint, noting that 65 percent of people with locomotor ataxia—a neurological condition described by Jean-Martin Charcot involving a distinct location in the spinal cord (posterior columns) that caused pain, an unsteady (ataxic) gait, and reduced knee reflexes—had a prior skin condition of syphilis. Fournier speculated that the visceral lesions may have had "a pathogenic connection" to syphilis—either as a direct result of the disease, or as an epiphenomenon he termed "parasyphilis." But the idea of a connection between diseases so different as early cutaneous syphilis and general paresis, separated by years of apparently good health, was difficult for clinicians like Charcot to accept.[56]

Rudolf Virchow, professor of pathology at the University of Würzburg in Germany and the Charite hospital, addressed the question regarding a causal relation between visceral abnormalities and syphilis from a pathological perspective. The field of histopathology had emerged by the 1840s, enabled by the development of the compound microscope in the nineteenth century, dyes that could differentially stain structures within cells, allowing for cellular architecture to be visualized, and machinery to slice tissue into thin specimens suitable for microscopic evaluation.[57] Virchow used these techniques to characterize disease according to cellular changes and to make speculations on disease causality. In 1858, he examined specimens taken from people with a history of primary syphilis who had later died of internal causes. He noted common patterns of cellular damage in visceral organs and skin changes.[58] One pattern was a gumma present in tertiary skin problems; another was a chronic interstitial and perivascular inflammation. These microscopic patterns were present in visceral organs of people who had died of syphilis.[59] Virchow found a unifying scope of syphilis.

Thus, new understandings of syphilis as a multisystem disease of cutaneous and visceral organs were emerging based on statistical correlations (Fournier) and histopathology (Virchow).[60] Virchow and Fournier enlarged the clinical conception of syphilis and helped to develop the concept of what later nineteenth-century textbooks referred to as "constitutional syphilis" or "visceral syphilis," rather than regarding it as a disease isolated to the skin, thus expanding the conception of the disease by its unique spatial and temporal pattern. The idea that syphilis was specific, not localized, and not necessarily progressive was a new idea at that time. By the 1880s, most infectious diseases caused by bacteria were understood to occur in a single anatomic site (e.g., pneumonia) and to progress over time. By the same decade, medical textbooks described syphilis as a multisystemic disorder that could unpredictably result in blindness and paralysis years after the original skin abnormality.[61]

Given the range of manifestations involving skin and internal organs, clinicians began to address another challenge that syphilis posed. By 1879, they noticed that syphilis could mimic a wide variety of noninfectious maladies, including forms of stroke, spinal cord problems, cranial nerve palsies, skin problems, and ophthalmologic disturbances.[62] English physician Jonathan Hutchinson's term "great imitator" was echoed in general medical texts.[63] Since then, the description has become part of the disease's identity—used so often it has become almost a nickname for syphilis.[64]

Throughout the late nineteenth century, physicians debated the etiology of syphilis. Virchow maintained it was inflammation, but what caused these changes? In 1840, the German pathologist Joseph Henle postulated the germ theory of disease: a premise that microbes cause specific disease entities.[65] Fracastoro in the sixteenth century had claimed that germs could be transmitted from one person to another and cause disease.[66] But Fracastoro did not provide empirical evidence, and he made his claim before microscopes became available. In the seventeenth century, Antony van Leeuwenhoek's single-lens microscope provided enough magnification to render visible the bacteria present in scrapings of his mouth, but did not reveal their significance.[67] As methods like the double-lens compound microscope, which was developed in the nineteenth century, improved the capacity to see bacteria, the German physician Theodor Schwann and the French physicist Charles Cagniard-Latour postulated that putrefaction was due to microbes.[68] Henle proposed, based on their findings, that decomposition of organic materials in diseased human tissues was due to living agents. He postulated that microbes caused decomposition of body tissues, inflammation, and human disease. But in 1840, Henle knew that he lacked the technology required to unveil "the secretive lives of invisible organisms." He recognized that "the organisms of the contagium might be too small for our present-day optical methods."[69] He knew he had to await further refinements in technology to prove his theory about germs.[70]

By the 1870s, the introduction of these technologies and methods permitted the experiments to test Henle's germ theory. The Abbe condenser was developed, allowing bacteria to be seen with greater discrimination.[71] Also, aniline dyes first used in German clothing industries allowed different forms of bacteria to be distinguished according to their size, shape, and color.[72] Finally, the development of solidified culture media by Robert Koch allowed bacteria to be isolated from a specimen taken from humans. Solid media were more reliable in generating discrete bacterial colonies than liquid media, in which several species merged. Using these technologies, Koch was able to demonstrate that bacteria were the cause of anthrax in 1878. He used the new equipment to formulate his famous criteria for proof that a specific bacterium is the cause of a specific disease. By showing that bacteria could be isolated in pure culture then reinjected into healthy animals to induce the same disease observed in the human, he claimed that he had proved that distinct bacteria cause specific diseases.[73]

The techniques that Koch used permitted an array of disease-producing organisms to be identified by other European investigators in the next two decades.[74] Isolation of the bacteria that cause gonorrhea (identified in 1879), leprosy (1880), and tuberculosis (1882) encouraged physicians to search for the microbial causes of other diseases.[75] These pursuits resulted in the discoveries of the bacilli that cause cholera (described by Koch in 1883), streptococcus (Fehleisen 1883), typhoid fever (Gafflky 1884), tetanus (Nicolaier 1884), diphtheria (Klebs and Loeffler 1884), plague (Yersin 1894), pneumococcus (Fraenkel 1886), and botulism (van Ermengem 1896).[76] The American neurosurgeon Harvey Cushing wrote about the excitement of discovery during this fertile period. He likened these findings to "new discoveries . . . being announced like corn popping in a can."[77]

By the 1890s, scientists from all over the world invoked the germ theory and used their technology and methodology to identify disease-producing organisms of multiple human ailments.[78] Proofs proposed by Robert Koch to establish causality did not apply to syphilis, as investigators remained unable to identify a microbial cause of syphilis using conventional techniques.[79]

In the absence of a microbial cause for syphilis, multiple theories about causality were debated during the 1880s and 1890s. Medical texts portrayed syphilis as a disease whose cause could be a syphilitic "antecedent"—a poison released by damaged cells of the primary lesion that years later caused tainted blood vessels of distant organs—a "para-syphilitic" phenomenon.[80] Virchow, who was not a proponent of the germ theory, attributed the cause of syphilis to inflammation caused by perturbed internal cellular activities, rather than being triggered by an external microbe. He maintained that germs investigators had visualized in other diseases were adventitious and not causal.[81] Virchow claimed that the true causes of diseases were social, including poverty and poor living conditions.[82]

Debates about whether visceral lesions were separate entities from the primary syphilis skin problem persisted at the turn of the twentieth century. A medical text from 1901 speculated on what "para-syphilis" might be. The text postulated that general paralysis might be the result of a microbe that had not been identified using standard techniques. The yet-to-be-identified microbe causing the initial skin manifestation might then produce a special toxic substance, which could later cause different problems: tabes and general paralysis.[83] Attempts to reconcile how visceral symptoms could be late manifestations of a single microbe remained speculative.

Syphilis continued to pose a challenge to efforts to come up with an ontological definition of disease. A specific disease characterized by variations in space and time remained an enigmatic pattern. Were visceral manifestations due to one cause? Or were they epiphenomena of the original skin manifestation of syphilis? Ideas on how these manifestations may have been linked were developing during the latter part of the nineteenth century. Authors of texts published in 1829, 1848, and 1854 were satisfied that syphilis was a disease of the skin.[84] By 1876, however, texts speculated that abnormalities of the blood may have been a means of causing the ensuing visceral pattern.[85] The German venereologist Eduard Reich wrote in 1887 that damaged blood corpuscles might cause systemic disease and speculated that syphilis might alter the chemistry of the blood.[86] Syphilologist Adolf Lostorfer in 1872 speculated that an abnormal volume of red blood corpuscles might cause systemic disease.[87] Their writings speculated on how the unpredictable course of syphilis could begin as a problem of the skin and culminate in internal organs years later.

In contrast to the evolving ideas about disease causality, treatment of syphilis at the turn of the twentieth century remained static. Texts discussed treatments based on mercury, bismuth, guiacum, and iodides—with no clear assessment of how effective they were for primary and secondary syphilis, and in spite of a hypothesis that mercury and bismuth were ineffective for neurological involvement.[88] By the end of the nineteenth century, mercury treatment, with its attendant toxicities, continued to be used for most cases of syphilis, as had been the situation for centuries.

The waxing and waning temporal course of syphilis confounded physicians who tried to provide a prognosis. Since physicians treated most cases of syphilis with mercury or iodides, despite a lack of agreement that those agents were effective, no sizable pool of untreated cases had existed to study the disease's course. Seeking to clarify the unpredictable course of syphilis and the questionable benefit of mercury, Caesar Boeck, a professor from Oslo, Norway, in 1891 observed the disease's clinical course in the absence of antisyphilitic therapy. Boeck had accrued 2,181 cases when the availability of Salvarsan in 1910 terminated the study. In 1925, Boeck's successor, Edvin Bruusgaard, concluded from Boeck's findings that approximately a third of the original group developed tertiary syphilis over the twenty-year study period.[89] The study was re-evaluated in 1948 by Trygve Gjestland, who reached similar conclusions.[90] Late nineteenth-century physicians, of course, did not have the results of those studies to inform their prognostications.

To recap, by the nineteenth century, new ideas about the cause of syphilis emerged. By the 1840s, Virchow visualized uniform cellular abnormalities in the tissues of skin and multiple internal organ sites to postulate that syphilis was a multifocal disease caused by inflammation.[91] Medical texts by the end of that century had accepted the novel concept of a disease of the skin and blood that involved multiple visceral organs in an unpredictable spatial and temporal pattern.[92] Nonetheless, no new treatments were introduced, and the benefit of mercury remained unestablished. Furthermore, the moral framing persisted, and medical textbooks reflected the persistent moral judgments against syphilis victims.

Causality, Diagnosis, and Therapy: Twentieth Century

By the turn of the twentieth century, medical investigators remained unable to identify a microbial cause for syphilis.[93] By 1903, Elie Metchnikoff and Emile Roux from the Pasteur Institute created an animal model for syphilis by inoculating fluid obtained from human syphilitic chancres into chimpanzees and other apes, who then developed the characteristic chancres of syphilis.[94] But they were unable to demonstrate a causative pathogen.

Investigators from various fields, however, continued a search for a microbial cause by applying techniques that were new to syphilologists. By 1905, Fritz Schaudinn, a German protozoologist, became interested in applying a dye technique—a Giemsa stain—that he had previously used to identify bacterial organisms called spirochetes in the blood of barn owls.[95] Schaudinn worked with dermatologist Erich Hoffman to apply these techniques to fluid taken from human syphilitic chancres. Schaudinn found a threadlike bacterium that had a similar appearance to the treponemes he had observed in his studies of owls (see Figure 1.1).[96] Schaudinn chose the species term *"pallida"* (later *pallidum*)

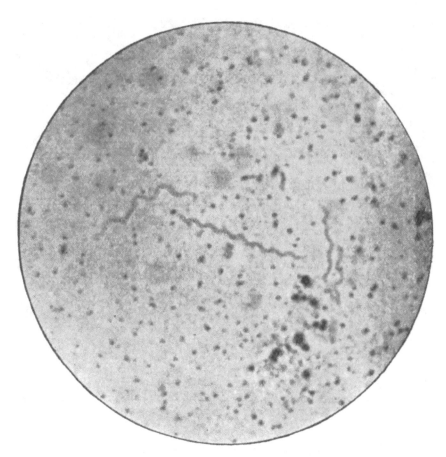

Figure 1.1. Hematoxylin and eosin stain of fluid from an inguinal gland. From Fritz Schaudinn and Erich Hoffmann, "A Preliminary Note upon the Occurrence of Spirochaetes in Syphilitic Lesions and in Papillomata," in *Selected Essays on Syphilis and Small Pox* (London: New Sydenham Society, 1906). Public domain.

based on the pale appearance of the treponeme.[97] The spirochete, although familiar to the Schaudinn, was new to syphilologists.[98]

Due to the challenges inherent in visualizing the pale treponemes, investigators searched for other technologies that could identify treponemes more readily. In 1906, Karl Landsteiner, a pathologist at the University of Vienna, developed darkfield microscopy. Unlike standard compound microscopy, Landsteiner's technique focused light from the condenser outside the objective lens of the microscope so that organisms became visible with diffracted rather than penetrating light. This technique enabled venereologists unfamiliar with the organism to visualize the spirochete clearly as spiraling white threads against a

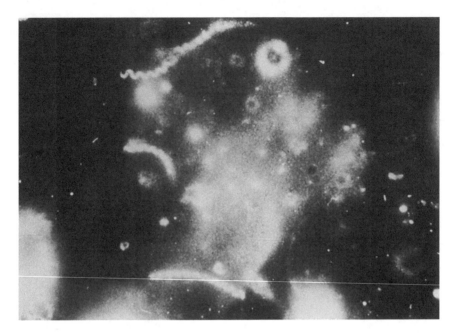

Figure 1.2. Spirochetes portrayed with the use of darkfield microscopy. Darkfield photos were not included in Karl Landsteiner's 1906 paper, Udo Wile's 1909 review, or medical texts of the time. This representation of *Treponema pallidum* is from a recent journal. John Thorne Crissey and David Denenholz, "Darkfield Examination and Allied Procedures," *Clinics in Dermatology* 2, no. 1 (1984): 75. Used with permission of Elsevier, Inc.

dark background (see Figure 1.2).[99] Udo Wile, professor of dermatology and syphilology at the University of Michigan, noted that by 1909, darkfield microscopy had become routinely used in medical practice to diagnose primary and secondary syphilis.[100]

The darkfield examination was useful for detecting syphilis of the skin. But it was not applicable to a person with visceral disease. In addition, uncertainties voiced by physicians about whether multiorgan involvement of syphilis was an epiphenomenon of syphilis or was due to direct invasion remained unsettled. Resolving these questions required new technologies.

A diagnostic blood test held appeal for physicians to establish a precise diagnosis of syphilis. The German bacteriologist August Wasserman developed such a test for syphilis in 1906. Wassermann and his colleagues Albert Neisser and Carl Bruck worked on the application of a new immunological technique, the complement fixation test, that Belgian serologists Jules Bordet and Octave Genou had developed for therapy of pertussis.[101] Wasserman showed that complement was fixed and the serum precipitated (reacted) when blood with antibodies (immune sera) was mixed with liver tissue obtained from humans with visceral syphilis. The test enabled use of a blood test to establish the presence of disease with greater diagnostic precision than clinical suspicion alone. Physicians welcomed the newfound ability to definitively diagnose syphilis given the disease's tendency to imitate other disorders.[102]

The test, however, was not completely accurate. A positive test was not specific for syphilis since the reaction detected antibodies against host tissue substances (soluble fatty acids in human liver tissue) that were released in response to the infection rather than detecting the pathogenic microbe itself.[103] Therefore, conditions other than syphilis could lead to a false positive reaction.[104] In addition, the test did not react in all cases. Despite these limitations, the diagnostic blood test became a tool widely adopted by clinicians and public health officials. Moreover, by 1908, investigators had learned to quantitate the Wasserman reaction by serially diluting patient serum.[105] Physicians came to use this quantitative test as a biological marker to assess treatment outcomes after new therapeutics were invented.

Neither Schaudinn's stain, Wasserman's serology, nor Landsteiner's technique could resolve debates about whether visceral disease was the result of direct microbial invasion or an indirect reaction to an earlier syphilitic skin ulcer. Investigators began to assess new stains to search for organisms contained in tissues of internal organs. Constantin Levaditi of the Pasteur Institute developed a silver stain in 1905 for this purpose.[106] Later, University of Michigan pathologists Aldred Warthin and Allen Starry developed a refined silver stain that identified organisms in the tissue of diseased organs more accurately than Levaditi's stain (see Figure 1.3).[107] On this basis, Warthin favored a single microbe as the cause of syphilitic inflammation in a wide array of organs, including skin, bone, brain, spinal cord, eye, and blood vessels.[108] Warthin and Starry's techniques provided evidence for a unifying microbial cause of the spatial, histopathological, and temporal characteristics of syphilis.

Hideo Noguchi and J. W. Moore of the Rockefeller Institute in New York corroborated the direct involvement of visceral tissue invasion by microbes.[109] Following the work of Warthin and Noguchi, medical texts by the 1910s concluded that the etiology of syphilis was a direct invasion of tissues by microbes, and they ceased using the term "para-syphilis."[110] The visualization of the organism in tissue and a successful animal model provided medical experts evidence to accept a microbial etiology of cutaneous and visceral syphilis.

By this decade, the understanding of syphilis came to represent a unique concept of ontological disease understanding—especially its spatial (multifocal with skin and most visceral organs) and temporal (with a phasic time course

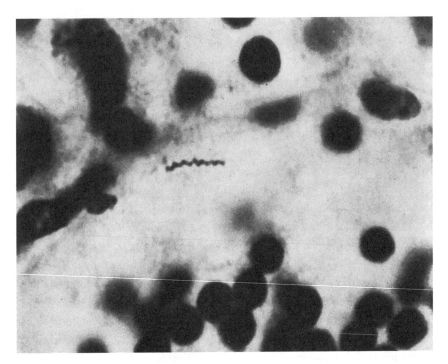

Figure 1.3. Warthin-Starry stain of renal tubule with chronic inflammation. From Aldred Warthin, "The Excretion of *Spirochaeta pallida* through the Kidneys," *Journal of Infectious Diseases* 30, no. 6 (June 1922): 569–591. Public domain.

during which some lesions progressed and others resolved over time) pattern.[111] The Wasserman blood test, together with the darkfield microscope examination of fluid from skin abnormalities, or the Warthin stain of tissue from resected internal organs allowed physicians to diagnose the condition with greater, albeit incomplete, certainty.

By 1910, however, the treatments for syphilis had remained static since the 1500s, when mercury and guiacum had been used. This differed from other infectious diseases because European researchers had been focusing on the therapeutic applications of the germ theory since the 1880s. Louis Pasteur, for example, turned his investigations to vaccination to provide protection from pathogens by the injection of attenuated live germs.[112] Robert Koch applied this strategy to the treatment of tuberculosis, although his attempt at using active immunization with tuberculin failed.[113] Emil von Behring and Shibasaburo Kitasato, students of Koch, demonstrated "passive immunization" as a specific therapy of disease that resulted in the discovery of the diphtheria and tetanus antisera.[114] Late nineteenth-century bacteriologists viewed this as tangible evidence that dramatic cures for infectious disease through antisera (diphtheria, tetanus) or prevention of others using vaccines (rabies) could be attained through the application of the principles of the germ theory of medicine.[115] By the early twentieth century, however, this had not occurred for syphilis, and older therapies continued to be used without conspicuous advantages.

The German bacteriologist Paul Ehrlich in 1910 devised a novel approach to add syphilis to the list of diseases whose treatment was based on the germ theory. Using his background in immune therapies and in differential staining of bacteria at the Koch Institute, Ehrlich developed chemotherapy.[116] Ehrlich believed that every cell (bacterial or human) had an affinity to a particular substance—whether it be an immune response or a reaction to a chemical dye. He reasoned that he could construct a drug with an affinity to microbes, and therefore destroy them without injuring the body tissues where the disease-causing germs resided. The concept of chemotherapy to treat an infection was not new, as quinine—a naturally occurring, nonsynthetic chemical derived from cinchona tree bark—had been used to treat malaria for many centuries. By the eighteenth century it was purified, measured, and dispensed by apothecaries.[117] But Ehrlich's concept of chemotherapy differed from the use of quinine in that chemotherapy involved using a completely synthetic agent that could be chemically modified specifically to kill a disease-causing microbe.[118] In this regard, Ehrlich's discovery was a novel approach.

Ehrlich's rationale for chemotherapy was based on his idea that there is specificity in immunity. He noted that an effective immune response does not occur in all microbes—including syphilis.[119] For microbes that are immune regulated, he hypothesized a side-chain theory of immunity, whereby a host antibody can attach to a specific molecule on a microbe. He used his theory that cells have unique receptors for stains (see Figure 1.4) to develop differential staining—for example, methylene blue, which stains nerve cells only, or carbolfuscin for mycobacteria—and from there to create chemotherapeutics. Ehrlich designed his agent with two components: a nonpoisonous "haptophere" that specifically bound to certain cellular receptors, and a "toxophore," a poison that could not combine with the cell. Ehrlich hypothesized that the toxophore entered the cell through the haptophere after binding occurred.[120] Thus, his synthetic chemotherapeutic agent contained both a dye to specifically recognize a microbial cell and also a poisonous agent that could selectively kill the microbe but not the host cell—a concept he referred to as a "magic bullet."[121]

Ehrlich obtained funding from the state to investigate chemotherapy at his laboratory in Frankfurt, Germany. He first evaluated his idea in an animal model of trypanosomes of African sleeping sickness, for which he used a drug originally synthesized in 1859 by Antoine Béchamp, a French organic chemist. Béchamp

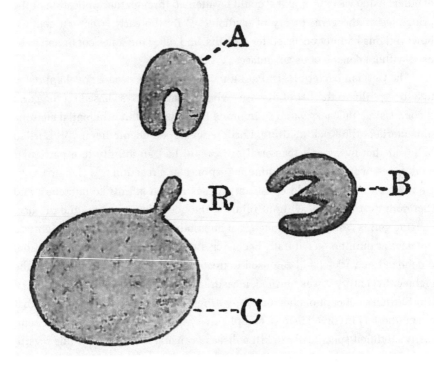

Figure 1.4. Ehrlich's "lock-and-key" theory of cellular action. To quote the caption that accompanied the original illustration, "The cell C has a receptor, R, which will permit it to take up the particle A but not the particle B." From Marguerite Marks, "Paul Ehrlich, The Man and His Work," *McClure's Magazine* 36, no. 2 (1910): 184. Public domain.

caused a reaction between analine and arsenic acid, resulting in a substance he called "Atoxyl," referring to the reduced toxicity of the compound compared with arsenic.[122] Atoxyl was initially used to treat common skin diseases, but in 1905, two British physicians, H. W. Thomas and A. Breinl, discovered that the drug was active against the trypanosomes of sleeping sickness in animals.[123] Ehrlich noted that the drug caused blindness and, together with organic chemist Alfred Bertheim, worked out the structure of Béchamp's Atoxyl, also called "Arsanilic acid." The two chemically modified Arsanilic acid so that it would hit a "bullseye" by killing the microbe without causing toxicity. Ehrlich's stated goal was to use his newly synthesized chemical to be "parisitotrophic" and not "organophilic."[124] In order to discover one drug that was effective and nontoxic (which he numbered "418" and called "arseno-phenyl-glycine"), he assessed over a thousand synthetic compounds on laboratory animals. The Rockefeller Institute, which had an interest in controlling epidemic diseases, provided $10,000 of funding for Ehrlich's work.[125]

After finding a means to treat trypanosomes with arsenicals, Ehrlich expanded his treatment to syphilis after 1906, a time when investigators had identified the organism and created an animal model. Schaudinn at the time believed in the conversion of microbes from one species to another (heterogeneisis), including the conversion of trypanosomes to spirochetes.[126] Ehrlich may have been influenced by Schaudinn's belief in heterogeneisis when he attempted to use the same anti-trypanosomal drug for syphilis, but there is no proof of this. The drug did not work initially in Schaudinn's syphilis model. But Ehrlich reasoned that if he continued to modify the arsenical "toxophore," he would find an effective drug.[127] Eventually, his assistant Sahachiro Hata found that after a single injection of compound "606" into rabbits, spirochetes disappeared from primary scrotal sores and ulcers healed within seventy-two hours without injuring the animal.[128] Ehrlich enthusiastically stated that his 606 "magic bullet" demonstrated *"Therapia sterilisans magna"*—the capacity of one dose to sterilize organisms that caused infection and to cure ulcers.[129]

Based on these animal experiments, Ehrlich requested that several of his colleagues test compound 606 in humans with syphilis.[130] Ehrlich himself did not have a clinical facility, so he provided the compound to physicians who could evaluate the drug. At the time, there were no regulations to mandate that a potentially effective new drug must first be tested in humans before pharmaceutical companies could manufacture it for clinical use.[131] Furthermore, placebo trials were not required by any agency.[132] Ehrlich proceeded from his animal model to use the drug in humans.[133] In essence, he was inviting his colleagues to test the drug's safety and efficacy in clinical practice.

Ehrlich decided to announce the early results of his drug in animals and in humans at a medical conference, the Congress of Internal Medicine, in Wiesbaden, Germany, in April 1910 before asking his colleagues to publish their results in medical journals.[134] At the meeting, Ehrlich described the principles of his discovery, the results of his drug development, the animal experimentation, and his treatment of selected humans. Ehrlich and Hata announced that the drugs healed chancres quickly in animals and humans and eliminated organisms from the chancres. Ehrlich concluded that the drug, which he gave the brand name Salvarsan, surpassed mercury in the effective treatment of primary and secondary syphilis and was not toxic to humans when given at the dose of 0.6 grams per injection. At the time of the convention, Ehrlich had contracted with the chemical factory Hoechst-on-the-Main to patent the drug and have control over its production and distribution.[135]

The medical and lay community responded to Ehrlich's news with jubilation.[136] Newspapers carried the findings with banner headlines, and international scientific periodicals were effusive. Physicians worldwide requested supplies of the medicine.[137] Ehrlich agreed to supply them, just as he had done with his initial group of colleagues, provided that they report their experience in medical journals or at meetings. To meet the demand, the German pharmaceutical company Hoechst Chemical Works manufactured a large-scale supply, and under Ehrlich's guidance, about sixty-five thousand doses were provided without charge to requesting physicians by the end of 1910.[138] At the time, it was legal and ethical for Ehrlich to distribute Salvarsan free of charge to investigators, as there were no obligations to perform controlled trials before a drug could be manufactured and distributed.[139] It remains unknown whether all physicians who received Ehrlich's shipments reported their results.

In September of 1910, Ehrlich presented his work on Salvarsan at another medical conference, the Congress of Doctor of Science and Physicians at Königsberg.[140] Physicians from Germany and all parts of the world attended. Following the presentation of his work at the Wiesbaden conference five months earlier, Ehrlich had reported continued success with Salvarsan's efficacy in treating primary and secondary syphilis. However, he acknowledged that serious side effects could occur, including necrosis at the site of intramuscular injection and drug-associated fevers, and he was cautious.[141] Nonetheless, the medical profession's enthusiastic response to the drug's efficacy overshadowed his vigilance.

In late September 1910, following the Königsberg conference, physicians began to publish their responses to the effectiveness of Salvarsan. An editorial in a urological journal said, "In the over 8,000 cases of syphilis treated, the results have been so striking, in some instances marvelous, that the entire medical world has been aroused and is hailing '606' as an epoch-making discovery in therapeutics. . . . Physicians from every part of the globe have made a pilgrimage to Ehrlich's laboratory and a number have procured 606 for . . . their clinical work." The article mentioned that treatment eliminated the microbe from the skin lesion: "A single injection gives rise to a disappearance of the spirochete, a rapid fading or healing of syphilitic manifestations. . . . Primary lesions are healed within two or three days after an injection. The secondary rash has disappeared in 3 days and large ulcerating gummas [healed with scarring] in 21 to 47 days." The article concluded, "The clinical results . . . furnish conclusive evidence of its great therapeutic efficacy in syphilis. . . . Ehrlich will ever belong in the glory of having opened the door of a new, unexplored chamber in the recesses of the temple of Asclepius."[142]

Similarly, Wilhelm Wechselmann, director of the dermatologic clinic at the Rudolf Virchow Hospital in Berlin, noted the rapid resolution of primary and secondary skin disorders within days after treatment.[143] M. S. Kakels in New

York City reported a study of two patients with internal gummas who responded to Salvarsan and concluded, "What remedy in the whole domain of the pharmacopoeia can accomplish this? [Human]kind truly is indebted to Prof[essor] Paul Ehrlich and owes him a great measure of gratitude."[144] Another article stated, "No previous discovery in medicine has attracted the worldwide attention that has been centered on the marvelous discovery made by Professor Ehrlich. . . . Physicians everywhere are manifesting the deepest interest in the new arsenic that he originated." The article continued, "In eight months following his announcement, over 150 articles have been published on . . . the application of [Ehrlich's] cure. . . . The new drug has been elevated to a prominent position in medicine."[145] Henry Elsner, professor of medicine at Syracuse University, wrote,

> I have never seen a pathologic mass melt away so rapidly. . . . It destroys *Spirochaeta pallida*, and the living contagion of syphilis is removed. . . . 606 favorably affects visible and palpable syphilitic lesions, and removes deep seated gummata. . . . It is more rapid in its effect on specific disease than any other known remedy. . . . It is more valuable than any other remedy in the treatment of specific disease of . . . internal organs. . . . It destroys the living contagion of syphilis, therefore its early use can prevent the spread of syphilis. . . . Ehrlich's ceaseless labors have been rewarded by the discovery of a chemical compound more specific against syphilis than any other yet introduced.[146]

Kakels and Elsner acknowledged a limitation of the therapy in syphilis with visceral involvement. Neurological cases that included "sclerosis," or the hardening of tissue after inflammation, did not respond to Salvarsan. Kakels wrote, "The results are not encouraging in paralytics; cases of tabes and paresis have not been influenced favorably."[147] The article concluded that doctors needed to begin treatment before irreversible sclerotic lesions appeared, and that they should use 606 for cases that had not responded to mercury and for primary and secondary skin causes, but not for neurological cases. Still, these remarks on the limitations of Salvarsan did not detract from doctors' overall celebratory response to the drug. The medical press continued to hail the magic bullet as a triumph of biomedicine.[148]

The narrative reflected the impact on physicians and society of curing a serious, disfiguring disease. Having the power to materially alter the course of a disease like syphilis that had caused suffering to individuals and had vexed societies for centuries evoked an emotional response—the thrill of having a new tool to heal a morbid illness that had been previously incurable.[149] This component is evident in a 1910 article published in the lay journal *McClure's Magazine*; the article states, "By this time, 606 is being deployed in over 100 clinics. Cures with salvarsan have taken place more quickly than with methods practiced hitherto. . . . Every day there are accounts of this drug and its effects in the papers in Europe. It is almost incredible. Ehrlich is overrun by reporters, doctors, and would-be patients. The whole atmosphere is charged with the excitement attending a great discovery."[150]

Ehrlich had reached celebrity status by 1910. The introduction of Salvarsan was taking place during the Progressive Era in a society that was willing to accept the contributions of scientific experts. Society had faith and confidence that the application of rigorous methodology by experts like Ehrlich would improve human lives.[151] The Progressive movement supported the use of new technologies that made lives more convenient and more streamlined. Improvements were occurring in transportation, factories, agricultural machines, and the domestic realm that made the world less unmanageable. These inventions reinforced society's feelings that the developed world was moving in the right direction.[152] In light of progress made possible by scientific expertise, the public celebrated Ehrlich's discovery. His new drug, doctors observed, was more effective than the mercury treatments that had been standard for centuries.

The veneration of Ehrlich continued throughout the next two decades and cemented the portrayal of his discovery as momentous. Popular science writer Paul de Kruif's famous 1926 book *Microbe Hunters* cast Ehrlich as one of twelve valorous medical pioneers. De Kruif gave a heroic version of Ehrlich's discovery, stating how the "step from the laboratory to the patient is dangerous, but must be taken." De Kruif described the applause at the Königsberg conference as "frantic." He dramatized the discovery, writing, "No serum nor vaccine of the modern microbe hunters could come near to the beneficent slaughterings of the magic bullet, compound 606." He sensationalized Ehrlich and his discovery, stating, "[Ehrlich] told of terror of the disease, of sad cases that went to horrible disfiguring death, or to what was worse—the . . . asylums. Such cases were given up to die. One shot of the compound 606 and they were up, they were on their feet. Ehrlich told of healings that could only be called Biblical."[153] The use of religious imagery demonstrates the faith de Kruif had in scientific marvels, accessible not through revelation but by precise, rigorous methodology. In 1933, William Allen Pusey summed up Ehrlich's contributions: "The history of syphilis is a brilliant illustration of what medicine has been able to do in a short period . . . since men have put their minds intensively on the objective study of diseases and their rational explanation. It is a dull man who can contemplate it without a thrill of enthusiasm." Pusey concluded that Ehrlich's "achievements in syphilology can only be described in superlative terms."[154]

Likewise, the lay literature portrayed Ehrlich in a laudatory fashion and Salvarsan as a breakthrough medical advance. An article in *McClure's* said, "Paul Ehrlich has attained world-wide prominence through the discovery of a drug which appears to be a specific and positive cure for syphilis. From all over the world doctors and patients are flocking to him, and the results already attained in the eight months that the drug has been used for human syphilis are almost unexampled in the history of medicine." The author was swept away by the potential Salvarsan represented for scientific medicine, forecasting a "not too distant day when a specific remedy for every germ . . . will be at the service of the medical profession."[155] This quote shows how Ehrlich's discovery helped construct a progressive, triumphant narrative of the limitless powers of biomedicine. Because there was evidence that chemotherapy was effective against one infectious disease, the author inferred, this might be true for all infectious diseases. An article in *Current Literature* summed up the plaudits Ehrlich had been receiving for his discovery, concluding, "Paul Ehrlich has built a renown which seems destined to give him a place beside the medical immortals."[156]

With the adulatory coverage of Ehrlich and Salvarsan, the drug gained widespread use. By the end of 1910, over six hundred experts had used 606 in ten thousand patients, many of whom were cured.[157] In this fervent atmosphere, physicians who received Salvarsan from Ehrlich continued to publish their experience with the drug.

Wilhelm Wechselmann published the largest of these: a two-hundred-page book on his personal experience treating 1,140 patients with syphilis with Salvarsan in 1911. The book provided an overview of the side effects of Salvarsan and the clinical outcome of patients treated over a two-year period. It began with a foreword by Ehrlich, encouraging physicians to continue to report side effects of the drug. Wechselmann reported that primary and secondary skin abnormalities markedly improve or entirely disappeared within forty-eight hours of the patient receiving Salvarsan. He also provided photos of patients before and after treatment to demonstrate the visual improvement (see Figures 1.5 and 1.6). He addressed how visceral syphilis responded to Salvarsan. Some cases that involved bone, larynx, or eye responded. With tabes dorsalis, however, Wechselmann noticed no recovery of neurological function and concluded that damaged nerves could not regenerate in long-standing cases. For most cases, he observed that the Wasserman test turned negative and that spirochetes were eliminated from clinical specimens after treatment. He noted drug-related toxicities, including skin hypersensitivities

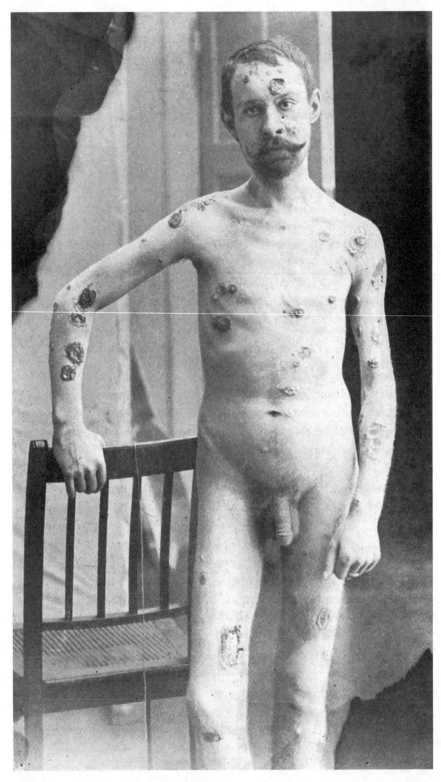

Figure 1.5. Syphilis skin lesions in a patient before treatment with Salvarsan. Wilhelm Wechselmann, *The Treatment of Syphilis with Salvarsan* (New York: Rebman Co., 1911). Public domain.

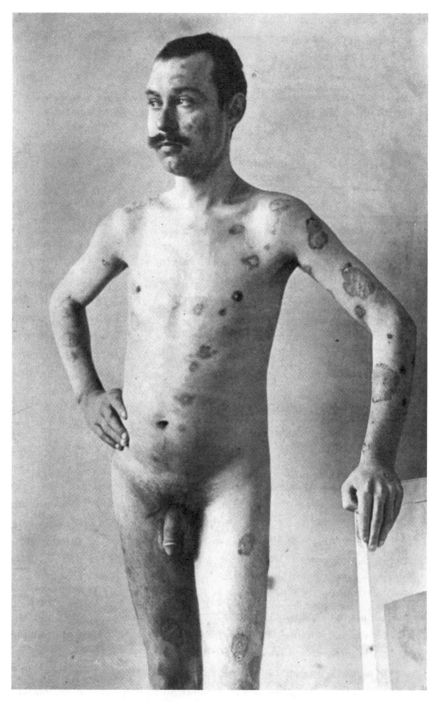

Figure 1.6. Syphilis skin lesions after treatment with Salvarsan. Wechselmann, *The Treatment of Syphilis with Salvarsan*. Public domain.

and Herxheimer reactions (high fevers) with the liberation of endotoxins. He noticed that some cases recurred after treatment, and concluded that for those cases, longer courses of Salvarsan may be necessary. He concluded that "Salvarsan is an extraordinarily potent medium, far superior to the remedies heretofore used and an indispensable agent of specific anti-syphilitic effect. . . . [The drug has] almost magical effects."[158] While noting the drug's limitations (tabes) and side effects, Wechselmann presented it in commendatory terms.

The praise of Ehrlich and his discovery endured. An obituary in 1916 said, "He opened new doors to the unknown, and the whole world at this hour is his debtor."[159] He had received the Nobel Prize for Medicine and other academic honors.[160] The triumphal portrayal of Ehrlich and his innovative discovery has persisted.[161] The use of a diagnostic blood test followed by synthetic chemotherapy to restore health by killing a germ offered an exciting new avenue to control disease. The promise of altering the course of disease using a synthetic chemical was different from most germ-theory-based strategies at the time, which used antisera to counteract the complications of infections. The combination of testing and biomedical therapies represented an innovative approach to accurately diagnosing and then curing an individual through laboratory-based scientific means.[162] With Ehrlich's discovery of Salvarsan for syphilis, biomedicine became the source of understanding, diagnosis, and cure for an illness that was once a menacing disease.

After years of experience with Salvarsan, investigators began reporting that the drug was more harmful than they had hoped. The scope and range of toxicities became more explicitly defined. By 1912, studies had described fevers that could last for three days, headaches, vomiting, marked chills, skin necrosis at the site of injection, temporary drowsiness, renal dysfunction, and skin eruptions.[163] Some deaths occurred, but they were attributable to causes other than syphilis (alcoholism, etc.). By 1917, Salvarsan had been associated with still other side effects, including excessive thirst and sweats.[164] By 1915, medical textbooks reported that Salvarsan had its share of toxicities, which could be mild or severe.[165]

The story of Salvarsan from 1910 to the mid-1940s, when it was replaced by penicillin, provides insight into how physicians evaluated the safety and efficacy of new drugs at a time when there were no regulatory bureaus to provide guidance and no comparative trials to address them. In the United States, the precursor of the FDA began in 1906 with the passage of the Pure Food and Drug Act. The 1938 Food, Drug, and Cosmetic Act required premarket testing for toxicity. But the FDA did not issue a mandate for drugs to be proven safe and effective before marketing until 1962, when the Kefauver-Harris Act required companies to prove a drug's effectiveness to the FDA before marketing it.[166] During the preregulatory period, when Salvarsan was used, wide variations in medical practice reflected the ad hoc fashion by which physicians decided on the proper dose, frequency, and duration of treatment with Salvarsan. During this time, texts show how there were no standards regarding dosage and duration. The drug, for example, was initially intended to be administered in one to two injections.[167] But this course was extended when observers noted that syphilis, even in its early skin forms, could return.[168] In addition, postmortem exams performed on patients treated for syphilis showed evidence of persistent visceral disease.[169] By 1913, texts warned against treating syphilis with one injection and recommended longer courses—every seven days with up to ten doses if there was a clinical response and if the Wasserman reaction converted to negative; others recommended treating for up to two years.[170]

Published reports show marked variation in dosing, schedule, route of administration, and duration of treatment. Doses per injection ranged from 0.3 grams to 0.9 grams if no side effects occurred.[171] Modes of administration varied from subcutaneous intramuscular shots to intravenous ones (to avoid pain and necrosis). By 1915, a new, less toxic synthetic compound, neoarsphenamine, had replaced Salvarsan; physicians could give it at higher doses (1.5 grams), but it also caused side effects at these dosages.[172] Some reports recommended a one- to two-year duration of therapy since doctors observed recurrences eight to twelve weeks after treatment with Salvarsan (five out of twenty-seven cases).[173] Clearly, Ehrlich's enticing concept of sterilizing syphilis with one dose of Salvarsan—*Therapia sterilisans magna*—was unattainable in practice.

Physicians also interpreted a decline in Wasserman serology as an indicator of drug efficacy and to guide the duration of Salvarsan.[174] Some reports recommended the combination of Wasserman results with an assessment of clinical responses to guide duration of therapy.[175] By 1921, one medical text recommended repeating the Wasserman every six months to one year following initial treatment, then retreating if it turned positive again.[176] Notwithstanding these variations in physician practices, the Wasserman was the first biomarker to be used to confirm the efficacy of treatment of an infectious disease and to guide treatment duration.

Several physicians reported poor response of Salvarsan to tertiary disease, particularly with neurosyphilis. Some papers reported that there was no improvement following treatment of paresis or locomotor ataxia (possibly because Salvarsan did not penetrate into brain tissue).[177] Other sources noted that the response was poor overall, but that a few individuals with early tabes might have regained minimal neurologic function after treatment.[178] Because patients with neurological disease did not respond to therapy, texts continued to recommend using potassium iodide for those conditions, a treatment they had been recommending since the 1850s, owing to the ineffectiveness of mercury.[179]

Right from the start, reports showed that Salvarsan, and the newer formulation, neo-Salvarsan, was neither effective nor harmless in all patients. It was never the magic bullet Ehrlich had hoped for. These well-documented limitations, however, were overshadowed by the euphoric atmosphere surrounding the successful treatment of primary and secondary cases of syphilis. In addition, the Salvarsan-related side effects may have seemed milder to physicians at the time, relative to the toxicities of mercury.

Public Health Potential and Proposals to Eliminate Syphilis

Public health experts employed the same biomedical tools to eliminate syphilis in the population—Wasserman testing and Salvarsan—that they had used to treat individuals. Scientifically oriented public health programs based on germ-theory ideas had roots early in the twentieth century. By 1902, Charles Chapin, superintendent of the Providence, Rhode Island, Department of Public Health, advocated for a scientific public health to replace older, sanitarian approaches to eliminating filth.[180] He advocated for tailoring the public health response of each outbreak to its unique microbial character and ecological mode of spread by disrupting the interaction between a pathogenic microbe and its human host.[181] Chapin argued that a microbiologic understanding of the true nature of disease would permit greater discrimination in public health and lead to more rational, customized practices that targeted specific infections (e.g., vaccination [smallpox], cleaning water [cholera], or killing rats [plague]) than previous "indiscriminate sanitation practices."[182]

Other public health experts also argued for downplaying broad environmental sanitation and turning instead to the bacteriology laboratory to handle epidemics. Hibbert Hill of the London School of Tropical Hygiene in 1913 deemphasized older "blanket measures . . . [including] . . . general sanitation" and proposed to substitute the microbiology laboratory to determine the specific source of infection and "abolish or block . . . [its] . . . route of causing disease, in individuals."[183] William Sedgwick, a bacteriologist from Massachusetts Institute of Technology and president of the American Public Health Association, noted that microbiology laboratories, as a means for public health, provided methods to prevent infections by identifying organisms and ways to destroy them or nullify their toxins.[184] As historian Amy Fairchild has pointed out, the American public health profession's mission shifted in the early twentieth century. The profession jettisoned its social mission (identified with housing, sanitation, and labor reform) in favor of science-based bacteriology and the laboratory.[185]

In 1913, Milton Rosenau, a professor of public health at Harvard University, wrote the first edition of his text on public health, *Preventive Medicine and Hygiene*. For the urban epidemics of the day, he promoted a customized approach utilizing the bacteriology laboratory to prevent contact between the pathogen and the human host. He argued that each disease should have its own strategy based on microbiological testing combined with scientific knowledge about how a specific disease is transmitted. Rosenau included a chapter on syphilis. He advocated for a scientific approach using Wasserman testing to identify cases (surveillance), followed by treatment of all positives to make the person noninfectious. He noted, "The use of Salvarsan early in syphilis will prevent the further spread of the infection" by eliminating the organism from chancres.[186]

Rosenau's emphasis on scientific means did not negate a need to address socioeconomic factors that predisposed a person to syphilis. Rosenau wrote, "It has been my object to give . . . the scientific basis upon which the prevention of disease . . . must rest. . . . The capable health officer now possesses facts concerning infections which permit their prevention. . . . Many of these problems are complicated with economic and social difficulties, which are given due consideration, for preventive medicine has become a basic factor in sociology."[187] Rosenau did not elaborate on these socioeconomic "difficulties" or provide specifics about how they should be rectified.

Nonetheless, he considered it his responsibility to address the moral aspect of syphilis. His views reflected the social hygiene movement of the time. He said, "As a danger to the public health, as a peril to the family, and as a menace to the vitality . . . and physical progress of the race, . . . venereal diseases are justly regarded as the greatest of modern plagues, and their prophylaxis the most pressing problem of preventive medicine that confronts us [today]." Rosenau stated that syphilis was among the "greatest of modern plagues" because of its threat to individuals, families, and nations (it weakened military and labor forces), and its burden to society (by causing chronic disability).[188]

Rosenau addressed a paradox he perceived of how a devastating disease like syphilis could persist even though it was completely treatable and preventable by scientific means. He wrote, "There are many striking things about syphilis, but nothing so striking as its persistence in spite of knowledge complete enough to stamp it out. . . . It is preventable, even curable—yet scarcely another disease equals it in the extent and intensity of its ravages." He opined "that it is much more difficult to control a disease transmitted directly from man to man than a

disease transmitted by an intermediate host, or one in which the infective principle is transferred through our environment . . . [because] . . . the control of man
requires the consent of the governed."[189] Rosenau implied that it was easier for
a public health officer to engineer a supply of uncontaminated water than to
persuade sexually promiscuous people to restrain their behavior.

Rosenau addressed the burden that chronic disability from syphilis had on
society. He stated, "The [sequelae of] late manifestations . . . cause great economic loss. About one-fifth of all the insane in our asylums are cases of general
paresis; 90 per cent of these give the Wassermann reaction." Given the unre-
sponsiveness of neurological involvement to treatment, Roseneau wrote, "When
death does not ensue, the results can be more tragic." He did not conceal his
moral judgments, stating, "Chancres of the mouth and on the tonsils result . . .
from 'perverted practices.'"[190]

Thus, Rosenau did not divorce his scientific imperative from broader moral,
social, and economic realms. He advocated the use of education to "keep the
mind clean, away from the sex subject," and the need for continence to preserve
virility not by sexual promiscuity but by chastity. He believed that sexual lust
was controllable. He maintained that carnal lust could be "cooled and quelled
by hard physical work, and attention to personal hygiene—one of the great
advantages of athletic sports for young people."[191] These arguments for self-
regulating conduct to purify the mind and avert dangerous behavior were typi-
cal for social hygienists.

Early twentieth-century public health experts like Rosenau believed that
they should not abandon their moralistic judgments about syphilis while pursuing control of the disease through scientific, laboratory-based medicine. Venereal disease branches were added to public health departments in the 1910s, even
while syphilis came to be considered a controllable disease through scientific
means.[192] Rosenau's comments show that even after the introduction of scientific public health movements to eliminate syphilis, public health officers
continued to understand the disease as a problem of an individual's character
and personal shortcomings. As historians have pointed out, older moral and
social views of syphilis persisted during World War I and the postwar era, when
scientific means of handling the illness were available.[193]

During this period, as Allan Brandt, John Parascandola, and Scott Stern
have discussed, the U.S. government initiated a coercive public health program. This involved closures of brothels and mandatory detention of thousands of female sex workers without due process between the 1910s and 1960s.
The workers were detained in reformatories, where they were subjected to
invasive examinations and forced treatments with arsenic. The goal of the

government-sponsored plan, known as the "American Plan," was to protect the public and simultaneously purge "social evil" from society.[194] This is an example of the government overreaching in the name of science by revoking the rights of those who were perceived to threaten the greater good. These approaches—using sentiment and morals as deterrents to sexual activity, and using coercive measures that rescinded people's livelihood—had no impact on the burden of syphilis.

The earliest twentieth-century syphilis control program, undertaken during World War I, used a test-and-treat strategy. The U.S. secretary of war, Newton Baker, initiated a campaign in 1918 to control the disease, which he believed could diminish America's military force. Congress, prompted by the need to keep the military healthy for duty, passed the Chamberlain–Kahn Act in 1918, which created the Division of Venereal Disease (VD) Control in the U.S. Public Health Service (USPHS) and appropriated funds ($1 million per year for 1919 and 1920) to subsidize state bureaus for control of these diseases.[195] The elements of this program included widespread laboratory testing, reporting of cases, tracing of contacts, and provision of Salvarsan.[196] It also established a public health education program run by sexual hygienists that targeted sexual morality—eliminating promiscuity and restoring chastity.[197]

Rosenau's fourth edition of *Preventive Medicine and Hygiene*, published in 1921, continued to conflate scientific hygiene and moral reform. This version emphasized the scientific control of pathogen transmission but also sought to regulate individual sexual behavioral choices by moral persuasion.[198] Rosenau as a health official was committed to social reform in the name of science.[199] His text reflects how the moralistic framing of public health persisted in the early twentieth century. At that point, social hygienists used syphilis as a justification for removing what they considered social evils from society and, in the process, to restore threatened Victorian values.[200]

The government began to curtail funds to control syphilis shortly after 1920, during Warren Harding's presidency. Lamenting the withdrawn funding in 1926, Thomas Parran, a USPHS officer who had been appointed chief of the Division of VD Control, remarked that "the enthusiasm [to control syphilis] that had gone up like a rocket came down like a stick." Parran pointed out that when treatment was provided, the disease's attack rate had declined, but when funding was terminated, it relapsed. In regard to syphilis in the United States after World War I, he wrote, "No further thought was given to syphilis, and the first national public health effort came to an untimely end."[201] Parran lamented that syphilis had receded from public consciousness following the war, a trend that would recur.

As Brandt and Parascandola have noted, social hygiene approaches together with moralistic means of controlling disease did not reduce the incidence of syphilis during the postwar period.[202] The relationship between social reform and scientific hygiene became disaggregated as Parran recognized that the social hygienists' attempts to control syphilis through moral persuasion were unsuccessful. Instead, he focused on what he termed a "scientific" approach to eliminating the disease in the population. Parran had become familiar with this approach, as his early training after obtaining his medical degree from Georgetown University in 1915 was in scientific public health efforts. He had previously worked in Joseph Kinyoun's Hygienic Laboratory in Washington, DC. Furthermore, in 1916 the USPHS had assigned him as an officer to investigate outbreaks of diarrhea, build privies, and oversee the construction of sanitary water supplies in rural America before he became chief of the USPHS Department of VD in 1926.[203]

Parran, who became surgeon general of the United States during the 1930s, spearheaded a scientific campaign to eliminate syphilis that sought to remove moral judgments. He based his campaign on widespread surveillance, Salvarsan treatment, reporting to public health departments, contact tracing, and partner notification.[204] The campaigns he rolled out relied on voluntary testing, and they used magazines, newspapers, and radio to inform citizens of the need for these steps and to reduce the stigma preventing people from being tested.

At the time Parran initiated his national eradication plan, syphilis had been causing serious problems of disability. The costs of its long-term effects (e.g., commitment to a public institution because of blindness or insanity, and absenteeism or inability to complete tasks among those who had relief jobs created by President Roosevelt's Works Progress Association) were conspicuous nationwide during the Great Depression.[205] In addition to the premature withdrawal of government funding, Parran cited the resurgence of syphilis in America as resulting from the ineffective, moralistic way in which sexual hygienists approached the disease during and after World War I.[206]

Instead, Parran proposed a scientifically oriented plan based on a treatment-as-prevention principle (see Figure 1.7). He explained, "Treatment of all cases must be required in the public health interest to the point where each case becomes noninfectious." Concluding that treatment provided a "duty to the community," he reasoned that the "non-infectiousness of the patient is achieved by a few doses of arsphenamine. . . . From the public health standpoint, . . . it means that one link in the chain of infection has been broken." Parran based his premise on the observation that shortly following treatment, spirochetes from clinical specimens were eliminated, thereby sterilizing genital chancres.

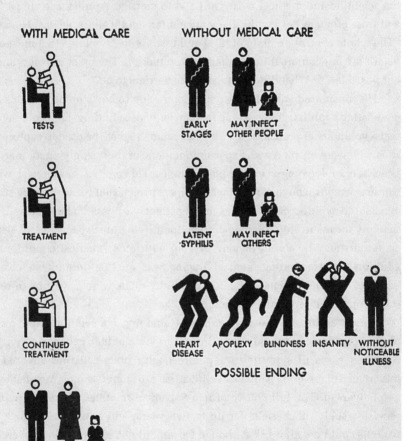

Figure 1.7. A depiction of the treatment-as-prevention strategy in action. Thomas Parran, *Shadow on the Land: Syphilis* (New York: Reynal and Hitchcock, 1937). Used with permission of Harcourt Brace.

The contribution to prevention was greatest, he stressed, when syphilis was treated in primary and secondary stages—that is, when the disease was most infectious.[207] Parran surmised that treatment of infected persons would reduce transmission.

Parran proposed what he termed a "find-and-treat" strategy to maximize surveillance and retain people in a clinic so they could complete their series of shots. Parran employed these biomedical tools as the backbone for his strategy to eliminate syphilis. Regarding testing, he used the Wasserman serology to identify as many cases as possible. He emphasized that even though doctors had the scientific and medical means at hand to manage syphilis, carrying a find-and-treat program out would likely encounter significant problems. He wrote, "The whole control program of 'find and treat' is so . . . simple that most of its details are much more difficult than they sound. . . . The practice is less simple but possible."[208] What did he envision the barriers to be?

He considered surveillance and case tracing to be "stumbling blocks" to eradicating syphilis. To overcome the barrier of case finding, he recommended that a voluntary approach called a "Wasserman dragnet" be used to capture persons who were hospitalized, expectant mothers, or those applying for marriage licenses or undergoing exams for life insurance. This process, he believed, would capture persons who may not otherwise have been tested because of the stigma attached to syphilis. Screening as many patients as possible, he reasoned, was the only means to stop the epidemic by identifying unsuspected cases—since symptoms may be absent or may overlap with other medical conditions. In addition to case finding, contact tracing was another formidable obstacle because, due to associated stigma, some individuals were unwilling to reveal the identity of their sexual contacts.[209]

Parran addressed the importance of attaining cooperation from private physicians. Physicians could be reluctant to violate their patients' privacy by reporting cases of syphilis to a public health officer. Parran stressed the importance of retaining patients in clinical care to complete their treatment with neo-Salvarsan. The full course of neo-Salvarsan treatment could be painful, require weekly office visits for up to two years, and entail an expense that patients could not afford.[210] Although Parran did not address how to overcome these obstacles, he did identify the hurdles he believed needed to be surmounted to eliminate syphilis: patient identification, clinic retention, and partner tracing.

Parran advocated to remove an overly moralistic attitude that would compel people to conceal their disease and avoid seeking treatment. He insisted that Americans must think of syphilis as a dangerous communicable disease, just as they had done with typhoid, diphtheria, and tuberculosis.[211] Parran attempted to transform the syphilis discourse to better align with the scientific public health campaigns he had become familiar with as a USPHS officer investigating earlier diarrheal outbreaks. He addressed the public in popular magazines to remove the moral framing of syphilis that he knew persisted in the 1930s.[212] The persisting bias was exemplified in a 1936 medical text by William Osler. Henry Christian, chairman of internal medicine at the Peter Bent Brigham Hospital in Boston, wrote in his chapter on syphilis, "The social evil remains a great blot upon our civilization. . . . Personal purity is prophylaxis which we, as physicians, are especially bound to advocate. . . . He [the patient] should practice . . . means by which . . . carnal concupiscence may be cooled or quelled, hard work of body and hard work of mind."[213] This is just one example. The moral framing of syphilis was echoed in other medical texts of the era.[214]

In articles in the lay press, Parran battled the suppression of discussions of syphilis in households and schools.[215] He stated that elimination would not be possible unless there was awareness of the disease and its consequences, fostered through public discussions.[216] Parran believed that the inability to openly address issues of sexuality placed people at risk for venereal diseases. He advocated for breaking the silence about syphilis.[217] He championed the need for stringent reporting requirements in popular magazines.[218] He sought to counteract resistance to reporting by educating providers to cooperate with public health officials, encouraging individuals to be tested and treated, and asking the public to think of syphilis scientifically. He wrote, "[The] equation of what is needed: teamwork of government, professions, industry, citizens + money for drugs and facilities + trained personnel for finding and treating cases = eradication of syphilis." He stated that syphilis had become a rare disease in Sweden, where a similar program had been caried out.[219]

Parran identified logistical issues that might confound his campaign to eliminate syphilis. He acknowledged that too few people completed a full course of treatment because it could be prolonged and require several visits to the office. During the Great Depression, when many people were unable to afford the long-term treatments, Parran argued that it was the government's responsibility to provide money to retain them in care, create free treatment clinics, and staff the clinics with knowledgeable physicians. The state, he argued, had previously assumed responsibility to rectify factors that led to the spread of other epidemics (e.g., sanitary measures for cholera, purifying water and milk for typhoid fever). Parran argued the state should do the same for syphilis. Parran was determined to raise the priority of eradicating syphilis on the national agenda, and to provoke the significant effort and resources that would be needed to fight it.

Parran insisted that citizens in the United States had a right to treatment, regardless of their ability to pay, and they had an obligation to take treatment. He considered a centralized, government-funded plan as essential to retain patients so they could receive the full treatment course.[220]

Parran noted social issues that he believed enabled the spread of syphilis. These included the problems of displaced populations, urbanization, poverty, and income inequality that led to prostitution and an environment vulnerable to the spread of syphilis.[221] Moreover, he acknowledged that these social issues might interfere with his efforts to eradicate syphilis.[222] However, he did not propose any specific measures to ameliorate these factors. Nonetheless, the response of the public and medical community to Parran's open discourse was positive.[223]

After portraying syphilis publicly as a national problem, Parran lobbied for federal funding of an eradication campaign. Public expenditures to fight syphilis would, Parran claimed, save the nation money by preventing the expense of managing the disease's chronic, disabling complications.[224] There was, he noted, precedence for allocating state-provided funds to disrupt the spread of other epidemics, like cholera and typhoid fever. He argued that the state should likewise support measures to fight what he termed America's "most pressing" health problem.[225] To that end, Parran organized a USPHS-sponsored national conference on VD control in Washington, DC. On December 28, 1936, more than nine hundred delegates (e.g., city health officers and public health nurses) from thirty states supported the allocation of federal funds to support an anti-VD campaign.[226] Parran thought that arousing public interest was key to extracting the tax dollars needed to "stamp out" syphilis.[227] A receptive President Franklin D. Roosevelt responded in a message sent to the conference: "The Federal Government is deeply interested in reducing the disastrous results of venereal disease."[228] In turn, Roosevelt supported shifting federal funds that had gone to the states to the prevention of VD, thereby reducing the amount spent on the consequences of the disease.

With the advocacy of the surgeon general, the backing of the president, and the raising of public awareness, the federal government subsidized a national anti-VD program with the LaFollette-Bulwinkle bill.[229] Passed and signed into law by President Roosevelt on May 25, 1938, the bill, known as the National VD Control Act, raised the federal appropriation to treating these diseases from $80,000 a year in 1936 to $3,080,000 in 1938, with another $10 million to be split over the next two years.[230] Congress authorized the USPHS to administer the grant by allocating funds to state boards in response to summaries of each state's VD control activities.[231] The legislation also authorized 10 percent of the

$8 million that had become available through Title VI of the 1936 Social Security Act to be channeled to state boards to establish a comprehensive anti-VD program, to set up diagnostic and treatment facilities, to train necessary personnel, and to carry out testing and treatment.[232]

Parran was confident that his scientific approach to ending syphilis—an approach involving public awareness, a shift from moral framing, and funding— would solve the "eradication equation." He believed he could overcome obstacles to his program by educating the public to stop stigmatizing the disease and by obtaining a central program of funding that ensured widespread testing and treatment facilities. Parran predicted that if doctors worked in cooperation with public health officials, the "whole program will make syphilis a rare disease." Parran forecasted, "Eradication [in the United States] will take place in a generation, within 10 years."[233] His reliance on the potency of Salvarsan to render an individual noninfectious enabled him to proceed with his elimination campaign despite the lack of an effective vaccine, the biomedical tool that was typically used in the 1930s for disease prevention (e.g., prevention of diphtheria, rabies, plague, and pneumococcus).[234]

In addition to its public health promise, Parran's scientific campaign held political appeal. As touched on above, the burden of untreated syphilis for American society was considerable during the Great Depression. Syphilis tied up the workforce (young men were unable to work due to the disease's chronic complications), decreased industrial efficiency, and consumed taxpayer money to provide institutional homes for the blind, insane, or paralyzed.[235] Undoubtedly, it threatened the chance of victory in wars by sidelining soldiers. Parran made his proposal when syphilis consumed tax dollars to fund state support of disabled individuals. Parran addressed the burden of the disease on individuals and the country (through absenteeism, lost wages due to inability to work, premature deaths, loss of productivity).[236] As Parran realized, the prospect of controlling syphilis held promise to strengthen the economy by maximizing the workforce and mitigating the burden on taxpayers to house people with chronic syphilis-related disabilities, and to strengthen the nation by having a healthy, battle-ready military. Parran's campaign raised hopes that it would reduce dependency, spending, and disability during civilian times and during wartime (see Figure 1.8).

Syphilis was added to a growing list of diseases that public health departments could control through pathogen-specific "scientific" means by interrupting the spread of a pathogen by its host. Parran's program used the microbiology laboratory to devise a customized "find and treat" approach to interrupt the point of contact between the microbe that caused syphilis and the human host.

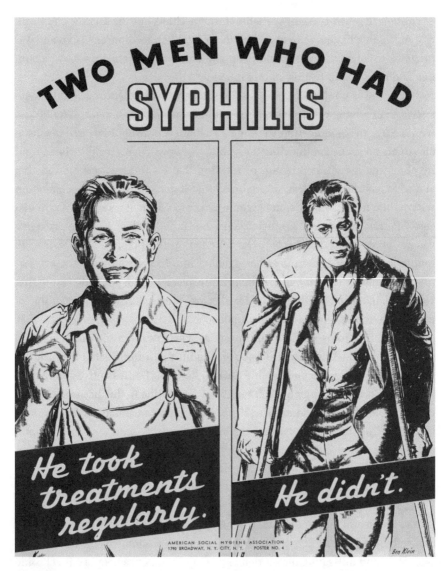

Figure 1.8. Undated poster (1930s) from the American Social Hygiene Association. It illustrates Parran's points about the socioeconomic benefits of destigmatizing syphilis and administering treatment: absenteeism is diminished, enabling a healthy workforce. Used with permission of the National Archives and Records Administration.

His program therefore could be classified as a scientific public health campaign, as defined by Chapin, Hill, and Rosenau. Parran's key premise that treatment rendered an individual noninfectious was supported by observations that organisms from sores following treatment were no longer visible and by the fact that the quantitative Wasserman test declined posttreatment.[237] Parran used widespread voluntary testing to optimize surveillance and render noncontagious a significant number of people through treatment and contact identification. The lay press celebrated Parran's scientific proposals to end syphilis within ten years and thereby to remove the disease's burden from society.[238] Medical and public health journals (Chapin and Rosenau in the 1900s) and lay press (Ehrlich in the 1910s and Parran in the 1930s) promoted the appeal of controlling disease through scientific means.

Thus, by the time the Unites States entered World War II, in 1941, Surgeon General Thomas Parran had begun a campaign to eliminate syphilis through purely scientific means, rather than reverting to a morality-based agenda.[239] From the perspective of an individual disease sufferer, the expectation of what the doctor could provide had evolved. By the 1940s, people with syphilis likely still felt a sense of remorse for having contracted the disease, which has never escaped its moral framing. But they could expect their doctors to offer something different from treatment with mercury or guiacum, which had been used with questionable benefit since the 1500s. Instead, the prospect of curability with Salvarsan, and the ability to materially alter the course of disease, became part of how patients viewed the disease. The public's confidence in the ability of a scientific approach to eliminate syphilis was revitalized in 1943, when doctors reported that new antibiotic penicillin was more effective and less toxic than neo-Salvarsan against primary and secondary syphilis.[240]

As it had done for Salvarsan, the public raved about penicillin as a spectacular new drug. But unlike Salvarsan, it was a naturally occurring compound, and it was effective against other infections besides syphilis. Indeed, by the time penicillin had been used to treat syphilis in 1943 and licensed in 1945, it had already been heralded as a wonder drug for its use for nonsyphilitic infections.[241] The first successful report of humans treated with penicillin was published in 1941.[242] Shortly later, additional reports published in the medical literature exalted penicillin, which was given as two injections daily, for treating injury-associated infections in soldiers during World War II.[243] *Newsweek* reported that the "precious dust" was "the most glamorous drug ever invented."[244] *Time* considered it the "greatest therapeutic drug of all time."[245] As they had done with Salvarsan, newspapers invoked religious imagery to celebrate the benefits of "the miracle drug that comes from mold . . . [and that] . . . is the answer to the prayers of every medical man since the world began."[246] Articles in the medical literature reported on the successful treatment with penicillin of pneumococcal pneumonia, "with infrequent adverse reactions" in people who failed to respond to antisera.[247]

It is possible that the timing of penicillin's widespread clinical use during wartime was responsible for these effusive accounts. Science historian Daniel Kevles argues that during World War II, there was widespread confidence that the nation's success in armed combat had been, to a considerable degree, a product of its scientific and technological prowess.[248] Thus, the enthusiasm regarding penicillin that was expressed in lay and medical journals could be viewed within the overall context of the reliance on the powers of technology prevalent during World War II and the postwar era. In this analogy, a successful outcome (cure of infection or victory at war) occurs when powerful products of technology (penicillin or weapons of war) are used to defeat the enemy (bacteria or Japan).

The first treatments of syphilis with penicillin began during shortly after doctors used penicillin to treat pneumonia and the infection of battle wounds in World War II. In 1943, John F. Mahoney, director of the VD Research Laboratory in Staten Island, New York, used penicillin to successfully treat syphilis skin manifestations, and the confidence in the drug as a cure for syphilis was quickly heralded in the lay press.[249] Investigators reported the successful treatment of four patients with primary syphilis by a single injection of penicillin.[250] This was clearly more convenient and less costly than giving the alternative, neo-Salvarsan, which during the 1930s was administered weekly for eighteen months and only discontinued when the Wasserman test turned negative.[251] One to two shots of a less toxic dose of penicillin, in comparison, avoided the problems of lengthy clinic retention and vexing side effects. Medical texts by the late 1940s had listed penicillin as the drug of choice for all forms of syphilis, and physicians no longer used Salvarsan or iodides.

Doctors and the lay press exalted penicillin as a pathway to end syphilis. An article published in 1952 titled "End of Syphilis in Sight?" claimed that it would not be long before medical students would have to consult textbooks to obtain information about the disease.[252] In an article titled "A New Magic Bullet Ends an Old Disease," reporter John Pfeiffer predicted that syphilis would be relegated to a thing of the past. Pfeiffer claimed that the results of the "one shot magic bullet" were so dramatic they would once have been thought of as "science fiction," and that cures were no longer "day dreams."[253] With penicillin, people no longer required lengthy treatment with neo-Salvarsan, which texts published in the early 1940s continued to recommend.[254] Sufferers could complete the therapy with one dose of long-acting bicillin, a modified penicillin molecule, and not risk being contagious to others if they dropped out of treatment. In addition, prompt treatment of syphilis would prevent devastating neurological sequela, thereby reducing the need for long-term-care facilities to manage syphilis-related disabilities.[255] Medical researchers and the press in the 1950s began to envision how a syphilis-free future might appear.

Penicillin replaced Salvarsan as the treatment of choice for all forms of syphilis.[256] Textbooks published in the late 1940s and 1950s touted penicillin as the preferred treatment for primary and secondary syphilis.[257] Its ease of use also made penicillin ideal for public health campaigns. However, the effectiveness of penicillin against advanced phases of syphilis, including vascular and neurological disease, was, like the effectiveness of Salvarsan, questionable. Medical texts from the 1940s to the 1960s noted that people with syphilitic aortitis, paresis, and locomotor ataxia had questionable responses to penicillin.[258] This incomplete response in the late, tertiary stage of the disease reaffirmed previous public health recommendations to diagnose and treat syphilis as early as possible to ensure the best chance of recovery.

Conclusion

The ways of understanding and managing syphilis changed with the introduction of science. By the end of the nineteenth century, some older notions of disease causality were discarded (humoral, astral), while others persisted (moral, blaming the marginalized). Science, then, did not replace older views of the disease; it altered them in such a way that older beliefs could exist alongside newer scientific understandings. Science also redefined the public's perception of syphilis from being uncontrollable to a disease that could be tamed. This prospect exhilarated physicians, who previously had had no capacity to materially alter the disease's course. Public health officials believed that they now had the tools to end the "scourge" of society. Confidence in the powers of science was, in fact, so strong that people envisioned an end to syphilis within ten years. Scientific medicine promised to remove the burden of a disease that had menaced society for centuries.

The mid-twentieth century confidence in society's ability to control syphilis provides insight into the evolving narrative of scientific medicine. The popular portrayal of triumphant scientific advances bolstered a linear narrative of biomedicine that was taking place in early to mid-twentieth-century society.[259] By the mid-twentieth century, the groundbreaking scientific understandings of disease causality and therapy that were highly touted in medical journals and heralded in the public press led to a narrative of syphilis as conquerable. The same narrative also propelled a linear, triumphant story of biomedicine. Syphilis, once dismissed as a disease of moral depravity by health departments, became the exemplar of the seemingly limitless promise of modern medicine to overcome uncontrollable disease.[260]

The belief in the potential for scientific medical discoveries to improve human life in the realm of contagious diseases had started in the late nineteenth century. At the time, physicians began to speculate that microbes were the cause of specific diseases. Ehrlich introduced the possibility of using therapeutics to restore health by killing a microbe with chemically modified compounds. In 1909, Ehrlich believed in the potential of Salvarsan to cure syphilis without causing the horrific side effects of mercury. Chapin, Ehrlich, and Rosenau had grown confident that insights gained in the laboratory would transform medicine and public health into fields governed by empirical, laboratory-derived evidence. Parran's vision that chemotherapy could not only heal the individual but also eliminate syphilis from the population bolstered this confident narrative of scientific progress. Syphilis helped both construct and reinforce a triumphant narrative of biomedicine that reached its apogee in the mid-twentieth century with the promise of eliminating all epidemic diseases. It also provides insights into times when science is trusted—when science-based actions deliver their promise of making people healthier.

The progressive narrative of biomedicine that thrived during 1950s, however, did not go uncontested. At the time, René Dubos, a microbiologist at the Rockefeller Institute, saw no convincing reason to believe that epidemics would cease to occur. They would continue to happen despite efforts to the contrary, he claimed, because environmental changes due to human activities would usher in new, unexpected infectious diseases. He saw no reason to doubt that humans would continue to change the environment through their habits and customs in ways that would cause unforeseen consequences, as had happened in the past. New, untoward ramifications, he predicted, would be unleased as civilization unfolded (e.g., 1916 polio epidemic paradoxically followed general sanitation and water-purification efforts in the early twentieth-century sanitary movement).[261] Dubos challenged the Enlightenment's view of human dominion over nature and claimed that any attempt to manipulate the environment would trade one problem for another.

Dubos did not address syphilis, but his arguments are applicable to its 1495 origins. One can consider syphilis a disease of civilization and globalization. Population mobility, resulting from overseas exploration, war, or both, led to migration of populations and opportunities for contact between disease and the uninfected. The displacement of populations during times of travel and war led to loneliness and stress that may have eroded existing bonds of fidelity. Growing urbanization at trading ports, and new, unequally distributed wealth led to the growth of the sex industry. Looking back with a modern perspective at how the epidemic spread removes the moral judgment and instead calls for an examination of what made society vulnerable to syphilis. Notwithstanding these arguments and Dubos's critique in the 1950s, syphilis bolstered a progressive narrative of biomedicine at a time when a counternarrative was developing. How AIDS would affect this powerful story in the ensuing decades, as well as its counternarrative, is the subject of the following chapter.

Chapter 2

AIDS

Potential of Biomedicine

This chapter covers AIDS from its appearance in 1981, through the first organized program designed to eliminate it in 2013, and beyond. We will explore the overlapping narratives of syphilis and AIDS—from the unexpected appearance of each one as a frightening disease, to its devastation on society, to the potential for eliminating it through innovative biomedical achievements. Although the appearance of AIDS shattered the belief that infectious diseases were conquered, the discovery of spectacular life-prolonging therapies to treat it received significant attention. The results were dramatic, visibly restoring health to individuals who had become emaciated. The accomplishments of drug development and allocation were applauded in scientific journals and the lay press. With the discovery that antiretroviral therapy (ART) could render an individual noninfectious, a strategy emerged to test widely for the illness and to maximize treatment to suppress the virus to a low-enough level where transmission in the population could be controlled. Strategies then emerged based on these test-and-treat methods to eliminate the epidemic. The discovery of potent drugs to treat HIV infection by the 1990s and use of those agents to eliminate the disease in the population starting in 2013 bolstered trust in biomedical progress and reinforced a confident narrative that epidemic diseases had a discrete start and the potential to be eradicated through scientific means.

Early Years of AIDS as a Fatal Disease

Into the world of relaxed fears about epidemics a new deadly disease arrived suddenly in 1981. Eventually known as AIDS, the frightening disease presented as a group of infections and tumors occurring in otherwise healthy gay men.

Like syphilis, the disease involved multiple organs (brain, eyes, skin, gastrointestinal track, lungs).[1] Symptoms were severe, devastating, and progressive. Furthermore, the disease was almost always fatal. Scientists, physicians, and the unsuspecting public were mystified as to why the unexpected array of debilitating, perilous infections and tumors were suddenly appearing at a time when epidemics had seemed to be a thing of the past.[2] AIDS was a humbling reminder that though experts thought they had vanquished microbial pathogens, humans remained at the mercy of infections. Worse still, modern medicine could not restore them to health. The arrival of AIDS shattered the idea that infectious diseases had been conquered forever.

At the start of the epidemic, AIDS afflicted a group of people whose behavior had been condemned by much of society.[3] During its early years, the disease was thus viewed in a moralistic framework. Victims were perceived as sinners who deserved punishment for violating norms of sexual conduct.[4] Like syphilis, HIV/AIDS was regarded as a fair consequence for those who had made a bad choice. (I use "AIDS" to designate the later stage of infection and "HIV/AIDS" to describe the infection at any point.) Allan Brandt has noted that some people considered the epidemic to be a symbol of deviant sexual behavior and a sign of moral decay. The initial societal response of blame, fear, and exclusion shared similarities with the response to syphilis.[5] Discriminatory proposals were directed against people who had the disease, including quarantines and restrictions of freedom.[6] The initial understanding of HIV/AIDS in the 1980s, through exclusion and blame of unwanted risk groups, was similar to the early understanding of syphilis.

HIV/AIDS afflicted marginalized groups of people whose behavior mainstream society viewed as deviant: gay men (as reflected in the term "gay plague") and intravenous drug users living in urban areas.[7] Victims who were accused of sexual transgression and sinning became diseased, thereby legitimizing the stigmatization of gay men, as Brandt has pointed out.[8] Like syphilis, HIV/AIDS became a symbol that society was ill.

Medical scientists initially struggled to address why a group of life-threatening illnesses (previously known to occur only in people with severely weakened immune systems) would suddenly appear in otherwise healthy homosexual men at the prime of their lives.[9] Scientists postulated an association with a homosexual lifestyle and sought to find a transmissible microbe as a cause.[10] They analyzed semen and lymph nodes taken from people with AIDS, but were unable to find a cause using conventional bacteriological and viral techniques.[11] Nonetheless, scientists remained suspicious of a viral cause. They used specialized techniques to search for newly described retroviruses that had

had been found exclusively in humans with certain types of T-cell leukemias.[12] The first human retrovirus, HTLV-1, had been discovered in 1980 through the use of novel scientific techniques to culture viruses. These involved adding interleukin-2 to cell cultures of T lymphocytes to stimulate the virus to replicate.[13] The second human retrovirus, HTLV-II, was discovered in 1981.[14]

Two groups of virologists working separately used these same techniques to search for and find a retrovirus in lymph glands resected from people with AIDS or AIDS-related complex (ARC). Findings about the virus, initially called HTLV-III and later HIV, were published by Luc Montagnier from the Pasteur Institute in April 1984.[15] Proof of the new human retrovirus was published in four articles during 1984 by Robert Gallo of the U.S. National Cancer Institute. Gallo and colleagues confirmed their finding of HIV in lymph nodes by demonstrating a virally encoded enzyme called reverse transcriptase in the supernatants of the cell cultures, and separately announced they had found the virus that causes AIDS.[16] In July 1984, Jay Levy from University of California, San Francisco, confirmed the findings by isolating a retrovirus in twenty-two of forty-five patients with AIDS and five of ten people with ARC.[17]

Cellular biologists then addressed how a microbe could result in the multifocal spectrum of infections and cancers that came to be known as AIDS. They discovered that the virus attacked and depleted CD4 T lymphocyte cells that circulated in the blood and were pivotal in defending against unusual infections and cancers. With the combined work of virologists and cellular biologists, a novel explanation of the disease was introduced: a retrovirus caused multiorgan infections by attacking CD4 molecules on the surface of T lymphocyte cells, resulting in an array of unusual infections and tumors that consumed a body depleted of T cells.[18] Indeed, this was later shown to be the case when an assay to quantitate CD4 cells was used in clinical practice.[19] Thus, like syphilis, AIDS was a multisystem disease. Unlike syphilis, the pathogenic virus indirectly resulted in multifocal clinical manifestations; the causative microbe depleted CD4 cells, which then predisposed the organism to disease.

Shortly after the discovery of the virus, medical professionals and the public alike extolled the power of science in the realm of AIDS causality and potential control. Regarding viral causation, Anders Vahlne from the Karolinska Research Institute concluded, "The discovery of HIV-1 as the cause of AIDS is one of the major scientific achievements during the last century."[20] Regarding potential applications, Margaret Heckler, then the U.S. secretary of health and human resources, accompanied by Robert Gallo, expressed hope that a vaccine for AIDS could be forthcoming within two years.[21] Gallo acknowledged that historically, identifying a virus was a key step in producing an effective vaccine, as had been the case for influenza, polio, measles, mumps, and rubella.[22] Given these historical models, it is understandable how Gallo would conclude that the same would be true for HIV.

The identification of the virus did not lead to an effective vaccine. It did, however, yield a diagnostic antibody test. As was true for syphilis, the discovery of the microbe proved to be the first step in enabling a serologic test to be developed. Researchers used the diagnostic test, together with the development of quantitative CD4 cell measurements that assessed the strength of the immune system, to plot out the course of the illness over time using blood samples from large numbers of patients with HIV in the absence of therapy.[23] In the sense that the Multicenter AIDS Cohort Study (MACS) was a natural history study to assess prognosis, it was similar to Caesar Boeck's aim with syphilis in 1891. But it was different in design because it was a retrospective study that could be conducted relatively briefly, compared with Boeck's prospective study, which took two decades to carry out.

The cohort study, like Boeck's syphilis natural history study, did map out prognosis. It revealed that people living with HIV could be asymptomatic for eight to ten years before AIDS-associated illnesses occurred.[24] While people still felt well, the quantity of CD4 cells progressively became so depleted (dropping below two hundred cells per cubic millimeter—the point below which technically identifies a person as having "AIDS" as opposed to "HIV") that the cells could no longer provide protection against "opportunistic" infections and tumors.[25] Each opportunistic illness caused serious and debilitating medical symptoms, ranging from breathlessness (pneumocystis), to stroke (toxoplasmosis, lymphoma), memory loss (cryptococcus or progressive multifocal leukoencephalopathy [PML]), diarrhea (cryptosporidiosis), visible skin marks (Kaposi's sarcoma), fevers (cytomegalovirus [CMV], mycobacterium avium complex [MAC]), blindness (CMV), and/or emaciation (MAC).[26] Although effective treatments were available for all of these diseases, death would typically occur in nearly all patients within three years of their onset.[27] Without effective treatment for the virus, the weakened immune system could not be restored, and the disease sufferer would eventually succumb to the illness.

During the asymptomatic period before CD4 T cells declined below the AIDS-related disease level, virologists learned that the virus was actively replicating and being shed in bodily fluids, including semen and vaginal fluids.[28] The medical implication was that a healthy individual who showed no evidence of being diseased could unsuspectingly transmit the virus to their uninfected sexual partners. Medically, this meant that the diagnostic HIV test could determine if an individual was a carrier of a lethal virus for which there was no treatment.

In addition to its medical meaning, a positive test also had social implications. After the HIV serology test was developed in 1985 for the purposes of diagnosis and screening blood for safety, a positive test signified to some the potential danger to infect others with a lethal virus. AIDS was blamed on stigmatized groups whose behavior prejudiced members of society viewed as sinful. Some alarmed citizens called for compulsory testing and the suspension of civil liberties of those who tested positive. In 1986 Lyndon LaRoche, a conservative activist, argued that all who tested positive should be quarantined.[29] Jean-Marie Le Pen, leader of the French conservative party *Le Front National*, advocated the incarceration of AIDS patients in homes that he called "sidatoriums."[30] There was also discussion of discrimination at the workplace, in housing, and in medical care against those who were HIV positive, and of exclusion from routine family gatherings. All these phenomena deprived those who tested positive of the right and liberty to work, to access health care, to have housing, and to enjoy social company.[31] The test had the capacity to further exclude stigmatized people from social interaction. An HIV test could be used for social control—to justify elimination of unwanted behavior from society, as was the case with syphilis and the detention of sex workers during World War I (see chapter 1).

Gay activists struck back against what they successfully argued was a violation of human rights and civil liberties. They argued that the test would be used for discrimination in housing and employment and would deprive patients of their livelihood.[32] This argument was without precedent in public health in the United States. The 1905 ruling in *Jacobson v. Massachusetts* had upheld the authority of states to enforce compulsory vaccination laws, and the U.S. Supreme Court decided that freedom of the individual must sometimes be subordinated to the common welfare, subject to police power of the state.[33] Gay activists argued for anonymous testing and no reporting in order to protect the confidentiality of the individual and protect patients from discrimination.[34] Their message was that their community would behave safely and refrain from engaging in high-risk behaviors to avoid imperiling the survival of the collective.[35] Gay activists encouraged a community norm of concern for the collective, balancing what an individual might want against a concern for the health and survival of the group. The warning of Larry Kramer, founder of the Gay Men's Health Crisis, that gay men should voluntarily change their sexual behavior did not come without a struggle within the gay community. The community was heterogeneous and demonized with internal politics following the sexual revolution of the new gay rights movement.[36] Some factions resisted making concessions by refusing to give up hard-fought freedoms they had won over the previous decade.[37] Nevertheless, as people fell ill, many gay men set a norm of restricting their sexual activity to only include practices that were safer, thereby cooperating with CDC recommendations and taking social responsibility for protecting the health of the community.[38]

With the advocacy of community representatives, a policy of "AIDS exceptionalism" ensued. This policy, unlike that put into place for syphilis, advocated for voluntary anonymous testing and no compulsory testing to avoid violating civil liberties and discrimination in housing and employment. Instead, through peer messaging the representatives promoted responsible behavior using condoms.[39] As a result of these successful arguments, compulsory testing was not adopted.[40] Nonetheless, people with HIV remained scapegoated and were treated with exclusionary practices—victims were avoided socially by those who feared becoming infected via handshakes, dishes, utensils, and toilet seats.[41] Those considered to have committed moral infractions were subject to distancing measures, including exclusion from family gatherings, requests not to touch relatives at mealtimes, and avoidance of restaurants out of fear that gay waiters would spread the virus.[42] The shunning also occurred in workplaces and hospital settings, as some hospital workers would not enter certain patients' rooms, going so far as to leave patients' meals outside their doors.[43]

In the 1980s, historians Elizabeth Fee, Daniel Fox, Virginia Berridge, and others attempted to situate AIDS in the context of the history of other epidemic diseases. At that time, AIDS was almost always fatal and involved mainly gay men who lived in urban locales in developed nations. Historians addressed the disease in a moralistic framework of exclusion and derision of the stigmatized sufferers.[44] They used the idiom of pestilence with its associated fear to make the point that, historically, as much suffering had been caused by blame, isolation, and repression of the feared sufferers as by the microorganisms themselves. Moreover, historian Mirko Grmek pointed out that AIDS had become a metaphor for a culture that spawned major social ills (e.g., illicit drugs, promiscuity) that, like HIV, spread through society.[45]

In addition to fighting for protection against discrimination of HIV-infected persons, AIDS representatives also fought to designate federal funding for AIDS research. They lobbied to increase federal funding for drug development as the virus continued its devastating, unabated spread during the mid-1980s.[46] Representatives claimed that the government was not sufficiently proactive, as patients with AIDS were not part of President Reagan's constituency. Patient representatives were also concerned over a lack of public discussion about the

disease (as had been the case with syphilis), and therefore surmised that optimal efforts to control it, including explicit sexual education, had not been implemented.[47] President Reagan, as is well known, did not use the term "AIDS" in
a public speech until 1985. In addition, his press secretary, Larry Speakes, had
mocked initial questions about the epidemic.[48] Thus, after a period of initial scientific inactivity due to governmental indifference in funding for research,
patient representatives who had faith in the biomedical model lobbied for
increasing governmental funding for antiviral therapies for HIV.[49]

By the mid-1980s, the HIV epidemic instilled new fears when it began to
spread beyond the marginalized "guilty" to groups that people more broadly perceived as "innocent." These included children of HIV-infected mothers and
adults who had received treatments for hemophilia, tainted blood transfusions,
or standard dental care. It began to be understood that an infection could be
acquired without moral deficiency.[50] A similar progression of public understanding had occurred with syphilis in early twentieth century America. Many
tried to distinguish between those who were "innocent" of shortcomings
(e.g., babies with congenital syphilis, wives who contracted the disease from
husbands who visited prostitutes or had extramarital affairs, or those who sup-
posedly caught the disease from a drinking cup, doorknob, or toilet seat) and
those who were infected through a moral infraction (e.g., promiscuous sex).[51]

Not only had the AIDS epidemic reified a distinction between these "innocent victims" and, by implication, "the guilty"; anxieties were exacerbated by
the potential for the epidemic to breach existing boundaries and cause widespread death among the entire population.[52] Although the idiom of pestilence
as just punishment for sinners remained applicable, to some the idea that the
disease would decimate exclusively those who behaved sinfully no longer
seemed to apply. An anguished William Buckley, for example, feared that "there
is no guarantee that the disease will remain confined to . . . homosexuals and
people who inject drugs. . . . If AIDS were to spread through the general population, it would become a catastrophe. . . . Our society is . . . threatened."[53]
According to sociologist Susan Chambre, AIDS activists exploited the heightened concern about the spread of AIDS among the general population.[54] Con-
comitantly, funding for AIDS research increased markedly in the United States
by 1985.[55]

By the early 1990s, AIDS had taken the lives of beloved public figures who
had enriched citizens' lives, which made AIDS victims seem less demonic or
deserving of condemnation and more human. Those who lost their lives had
contributed to diverse professional fields, including acting (Anthony Perkins,
Robert Reed), dance (Rudolf Nureyev), literature (Isaac Asimov), music (Freddy

Mercury), philosophy (Michel Foucault), art (Keith Haring), and sports (Arthur Ashe). The passing of admired public figures helped ease the misguided judgment against all AIDS sufferers.

With federal funding in hand, the search began for a means to restore health by targeting its proximate cause: the HIV virus that depleted CD4 cells.[56] A belief that an antiviral drug could be produced was not unreasonable; by 1979, several had already been developed and licensed to treat viral infections including influenza (Amantadine) and herpes simplex (idoxuridine, acyclovir).[57] By the time the HIV virus was discovered in 1984, the precedence for effective therapeutic antiviral drugs had been set.

Scientists at the National Cancer Institute (NCI) began by choosing a specific drug they believed might have activity against the HIV virus. They decided to first determine whether existing antimetabolites originally developed to prevent cancer cell division might also be effective against the replication of a retrovirus. Investigators at NCI searched their institutions for a library of shelved drugs, and then evaluated them against HIV in vitro. The first drug that demonstrated activity against HIV in vitro was an antimetabolite that had been ineffective against cancer, azidothymidine (AZT).[58] By 1986, AZT had even raised hopes of reversing the clinical course of AIDS by reconstituting the depleted immune system, as researchers demonstrated in an uncontrolled phase I human study.[59] Before AZT could be licensed, however, the U.S. FDA required that a larger placebo-controlled study be conducted.

The FDA mandate unveiled diverging viewpoints about controlled trials. To medical researchers, they were scientific experiments to determine efficacy, but to AIDS activists, they were a means to access otherwise unavailable drugs that held the only prospect of averting an otherwise lethal outcome.[60] The activist group ACT UP (AIDS Coalition to Unleash Power) vigorously opposed the use of placebo as part of a trial for a disease with such a dire prognosis.[61] Medical researchers remained unpersuaded and maintained that without this methodology, physicians would have no reliable information about which drugs would be effective for their patients.[62]

In this divisive atmosphere, the planned twenty-four-week phase II study comparing AZT to placebo in 282 people with advanced HIV disease began in 1986. The trial, however, was terminated at week eighteen with only 10 percent of subjects completing it, when the Data Safety Monitoring Board noted the clear survival benefit of AZT.[63] The board determined that it was no longer ethical to continue the study because equipoise—a true uncertainty about whether a drug is effective or not—was no longer met.[64] Activists intent on avoiding delays fought to expedite in clinical practice the drug's availability for those who needed it, first on a compassionate basis (1986) and then by accelerated FDA licensing (1987).[65]

But AZT used alone as monotherapy did not alter the clinical course of people who were HIV infected. This is because resistance of the virus to AZT developed within six months in people who were taking AZT alone. AIDS activists responded by demanding that the FDA make alternatives available to patients taking AZT.[66] This led to a succession of licensing for a group of drugs, all of which had similar modes of action against HIV: inhibiting the viral nucleoside reverse transcriptase (NRTI) enzymes, known as ddI, ddC, D4T and 3TC, for use as single agents or in combination with another NRTI. However, none of the FDA-approved agents had enhanced potency over AZT or had any substantial impact on the clinical prognosis of HIV.[67] The wait for effective treatments seemed far too long for patients with AIDS, their friends and loved ones, and physicians whose patients were dying from the disease throughout the early 1990s (see Figure 2.1). Gavin McLeod, an infectious disease physician, made a statement resignedly in 1993 that captured the mood of the time about antivirals: "Some progress is being made, but not at a pace equal to the death and devastation inflicted by HIV."[68]

By 1992, the newly formed Treatment Action Group (TAG) began to question the validity of using AZT monotherapy based on limited patient enrollment and short duration of the phase II study.[69] By 1994, a larger placebo-controlled trial (1,749 patients) of longer duration (3.3 years), called Concorde, supported their concerns. The study showed that starting AZT early in the disease did not provide clinical benefit.[70] TAG members affirmed that access to inadequately studied drugs did not always improve survival, speedier approval of potentially promising drugs would not always be better than nothing, and that adequately powered clinical trials were the only reliable means to generate legitimate knowledge about drugs.[71] TAG members eventually worked with scientists based at pharmaceutical companies and in academia to support the development of potent AIDS drugs. TAG favored returning to basic science research to develop more potent agents that had different mechanisms of action than the existing drugs, and conducting larger trials for longer durations to methodically test whether the drugs were truly effective. To do this, they advocated collaborating with pharmaceutical companies and conventional researchers. Although not formally trained as medical investigators, TAG members studied the discipline and worked together with industry. Pharmaceutical companies, in turn, appointed community representatives to their scientific advisory boards.[72] The TAG activists were endorsing the orthodox methodology of basic medical scientists to search

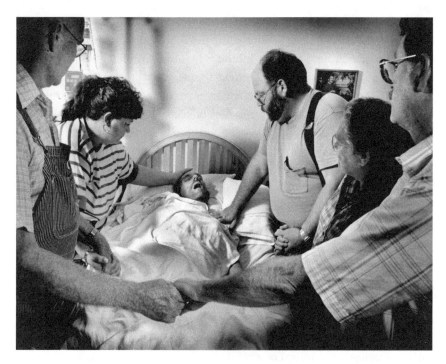

Figure 2.1. Michael Mauch surrounded by family members during the last hours of his life after battling AIDS in the early 1990s, when there were no effective treatments to substantially alter the course of the disease. From *House of Angels: Living with AIDS at the Bailey-Boushay House: 1992–1995*, a documentary photo essay about some of the men and women living with AIDS at a hospice in Seattle, Washington. Used with permission of Saul Bromberger and Sandra Hoover Photography.

for more powerful antiretroviral drugs than existing NRTI agents, and the use of conventional methods (larger placebo-controlled trials) to evaluate their efficacy.

Effective Drugs and HIV as a Chronic Disease

The search for more potent drugs involved engineering chemical compounds that could interfere with targeted areas of the virus's life cycle in CD4 cells other than the reverse transcriptase site. Scientists decided to target virally encoded protease enzymes whose role was to process proteins on the viral surface, thereby preventing infectious viral particles from exiting CD4 cells. Pharmaceutical companies employed medicinal chemists who used three-dimensional computer-generated structures to design molecular compounds called protease inhibitors (PI) that fit into the binding sites of protease enzymes and disabled them.

Unlike previous medicinal chemists, including Ehrlich, who had tested hundreds of compounds by a "trial and error" method of modifying chemical agents, the search for a protease inhibitor involved a different approach, one using computer-driven three-dimensional images of the protease structure.[73] The approach, termed "rational medicinal chemistry," involved chemically engineering a compound to attach to and block the specific binding site of a protease enzyme by mimicking its protein substrate. It differed from traditional antimicrobial developments, where researchers tested chemically modified biological products produced by molds against a "library" of microbes.[74]

The key work in the development of PI agents occurred in 1995.[75] Virologists had noted that resistance to these agents occurred when they were used alone at a certain mutation rate. They theorized that resistance could be forestalled, or prevented entirely, if potent protease inhibitor drugs were combined with two NRTI agents.[76] Investigators found that an ART combination regimen including a three-drug combination (one PI agent combined with two NRTI agents) demonstrated potency in vitro.[77] With TAG members on the board of advisors, phase III studies with large numbers of subjects were conducted for reduced periods of time by using direct serum quantitative viral load as a study outcome rather than clinical outcomes.[78]

These studies found that combination ART was highly potent and reduced viral loads to undetectable levels in most patients when taken properly.[79] Moreover, the undetectable levels were durable as long as individuals continued taking their medicines. By this time, a test to measure the amount of HIV RNA in the blood, a viral polymerase chain reaction (PCR) quantitative assay, became available for use in clinical practice as a surrogate for outcome. Thus, as was the case with syphilis, a blood test, or biomarker, estimating the burden of an organism was included along with clinical parameters as an assessment of outcome.[80] The difference is that quantitative HIV viral load is a genetic marker, not a serological marker like the Wasserman test for syphilis. The word "undetectable" for HIV-infected people became a goal to achieve, as it was linked to control of infection.[81] The studies documenting sustained HIV viral load suppression and CD4 cell boosts with the new PI-containing ART regimens were presented as abstracts during the Eleventh International AIDS Conference, in Vancouver, Canada, to an appreciative audience.[82] By the year's end, two protease inhibitor agents were licensed for use in practice.

Within two years, doctors reported their experience using the drugs in clinical settings and the clinical outcomes of trials. ART restored CD4 cell depletion and reduced mortality, thereby turning AIDS from a death sentence into a manageable disease.[83] Likewise, the fact that practitioners and citizens

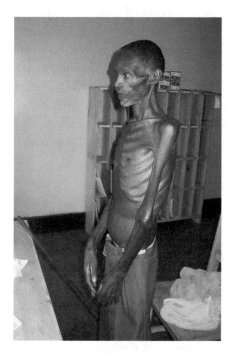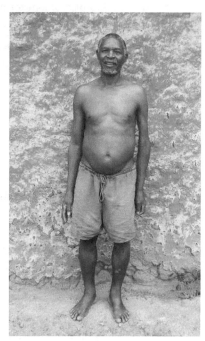

Figure 2.2. Images of one of the first patients enrolled in a community-based HIV- and tuberculosis-treatment program in rural southeastern Rwanda before and after taking HIV medicines and antitubercular medicines. These sequential photographs portray the striking restoration of vitality and health following ART, a response called the "Lazarus Effect." Paul E. Farmer, "Chronic Infectious Disease and the Future of Health Care Delivery," *NEJM* 369, no. 25 (2013). Used with permission of *New England Journal of Medicine.*

no longer viewed AIDS as an invincible killer was reflected in medical texts and popular culture. Medical textbooks no longer included chapters on preparing AIDS patients for death.[84] The last public display of the AIDS Memorial Quilt was held in 1996, marking the end of an era when the ritual of collective grief for deceased victims was visibly enacted on a national stage. In addition, doctors reported dramatic clinical improvements in patients' visible appearance following therapy (specifically, wasting improved). The once prevalent trope of wasting and dying from AIDS now seemed remote. This was an emotionally gratifying moment for all. A person's vitality was restored (a phenomenon called the "Lazarus effect"), as was their lifespan (see Figure 2.2).[85] The virological term "undetectable" became a surrogate for prolonged life, and the disease became defined not by a deadly prognosis, but by viral control and immune restoration.

This was a jubilant moment for people living with HIV, for researchers, for doctors, and for society. It meant that patients were able to "control" their viral load, recover their vitality, and restore their longevity.[86] Follow-up studies confirmed that ART extended the lifespan of individuals who could afford the treatment in developed countries.[87] The introduction of potent ART treatment regimens reinforced confidence in biomedicine for the developed world.[88] The term "undetectable" became a component of a person's identity, underscoring how control of a virus through scientific means restored health and extended the lives of individuals who once had a poor prognosis.[89]

The rational medicinal development of PIs affirmed the value of the application of basic research science to clinical medicine that was practiced by institutions like the National Institutes of Health (NIH). It validated the important contribution that physician scientists played in healing individuals. These successes also substantiated the arguments that Vannevar Bush, head of the U.S. Office of Scientific Research and Development (OSRD) from 1941–1947, had made in the postwar period. Bush advocated for new discoveries in basic science to advance medical treatments.[90] For the development of PI agents to treat HIV, this involved contributions from several scientific fields, namely, molecular biology, cellular biology, medicinal chemistry, and virology.[91] The successful development of these agents also validated the agency of community activists who worked together with scientists to evaluate and deliver new, promising biomedical approaches.

The success of ART reinforced the power of science to harness basic information about disease into effective treatments.[92] The development of PIs was an affirmation of the efficacy and beneficence of the basic biomedical research establishment. Harold Varmus, a Nobel Prize–winning scientist and director of the NCI in the 1990s, when scientists discovered ART, articulated this notion. Varmus's earlier work had been in the recognition of the mechanisms by which retroviruses replicate, and the discovery of how other viruses (e.g., Rous sarcoma virus) led to cancers.[93] Varmus won the Vannevar Bush Award in 2002— an award given by the National Science Board in recognition of an individual whose public service activities in science and technology made an outstanding "contribution toward the welfare of mankind and the Nation."[94] Varmus was the archetype of a scientific insider.

Vannevar Bush had been a catalyst for federal funding of science and medicine in the mid-twentieth century. As head of National Defense Research Committee and the OSRD, in *Science: The Endless Frontier*, his 1945 report to the president of the United States, he advocated for the funding of government science projects during World War II (e.g., the Manhattan Project) and for the funding of science programs in the postwar period.[95] Bush called for an increase in government funding of medical science to "expand the frontiers of knowledge," a requirement for medical advances. Bush's arguments were successful, and the NIH federal budgets, including grants awarded to extramural sites, escalated in the postwar period from less than $4 million in 1947 to over $1 billion in 1966.[96] Bush's vision that the federal funding of science would provide palpable benefits to society resulted in a marked increase in federal grants to support basic science research. Researchers like Varmus carried Bush's scientific spirit to the next generation.

Varmus viewed the discovery of PI drugs as a triumph of scientific medicine along the lines that Bush had envisioned. Varmus summarized this sentiment in a 1998 article he published in *Science* titled "Science and the Control of AIDS." He said the year was worth "celebrating for AIDS research." He noted that the "explanation . . . [for] . . . the dramatic decline in mortality . . . [is] . . . satisfyingly . . . almost entirely based on science: a logical sequence of discoveries has led to highly effective antiviral therapies." He called the discovery of HIV drugs a "triumph . . . [that] . . . exemplifies the potency of molecular medicine—based on full disclosure of viral genes, analysis of viral dynamics and pathogenesis, and development of protein targeted drugs." Varmus said that once we understand the genetic origins and pathophysiological mechanisms of a disease, the "prospects are bright for rational treatments of other complex disorders." He asserted that these understandings could "transform the practice of medicine."[97] Thus Varmus hoped that the prolongation of life through the discovery of HIV drugs would become a model of rational medicinal chemistry that might apply to other fields. *Science* in 1996 deemed the discovery of the AIDS drugs the "Breakthrough of the Year," not only for medical science, but for all of science.[98]

Varmus stated that the "recent success [in developing HIV drugs] has affirmed the vigor of the biomedical research establishment."[99] It also affirmed the capacity of a federally guided, investigator-driven science establishment to collaborate with pharmaceutical companies to undertake drug discovery and development. Varmus credited work done by federally funded independent investigators as "essential" for generating knowledge of the viral life cycle, knowledge on which the rational medicinal therapies were based. This knowledge defined sites of the virus's life cycle for drugs to target. The result was tangible for Varmus: "prolonging the lives of AIDS patients." He attributed this benefit to the advances of basic science—an achievement that resonated with and was fueled by the agency of TAG activists.

With the introduction of potent ART, the way that HIV/AIDS was understood by scientists, doctors, and the public had transformed by 1996. Medical practitioners and citizens no longer viewed AIDS as an invincible killer. The idiom of pestilence with its devastation and fear evolved to a virological framing of disease; the intractable became manageable. A mood of despondency and resignation changed to one of optimism characterized by bold predictions of curing the disease with ART. The confrontational tactics of activists changed to strategies of working in harmony with researchers. Fear of a deadly scourge evolved into complacency.[100]

Yet the problems posed by the pandemic were far from over. As combination regimens were developed, the global demographics of HIV/AIDS had evolved.[101] HIV was never a disease of urban gay men and drug users, as was first believed in 1981. HIV/AIDS had all along been a global disease spread through heterosexual contact between people living in LMRCs. Behavioral recommendations that were promoted in urban gay communities had no impact in LMRCs, where poverty and income inequality—the social determinants of health—did not enable individualized messages promoting safe sex to be effective for people engaging in risky work (see chapter 3).[102]

The excessive costs of ART were exacerbated by the realization that the drugs must be taken uninterruptedly for an entire lifespan. Hopes of curing HIV with ART waned because the virus persists in a subpopulation of latent CD4 T lymphocytes that replicate slowly.[103] Because ART cannot eliminate HIV replication in these reservoirs, attempts to stop ART after suppression of viral load failed.[104] This means that ART must be continued for the duration of an individual's life, posing the risk of side effects (although today's HIV drugs are comparatively less toxic and more convenient to take than the first ones were). The indefinite duration of therapy imposed a cost burden.[105]

The high price of ART (over $30,000 per year for one person), meant that the drugs were unavailable to people who lived in LMICs, where the bulk of HIV/AIDS occurred.[106] Consequently, the life-prolonging benefits of ART were available in wealthy countries, like the United States, which offered drug-assistance plans for low-income people (those with incomes below 500 percent above the poverty line) through federal HIV/AIDS support programs (i.e., the Ryan White Program, authorized in 1990). These benefits did not accrue to LMICs, where treatment was denied because the costs of the drugs far exceeded per capita incomes.[107] This financial reality had an enormous impact in LMICs by the late 1990s: the lives of people who lived in developed countries were prolonged, unlike those in LMICs.[108] In 2001, five years after ART was licensed, the life-saving drugs remained unaffordable for many patients around the world. The quality of generic ART was unproven, and funding for large-scale ART distribution was nonexistent.[109]

The failure to provide ART to LMRCs had devastating impacts on communities, nations, and the world. As historian Randall Packard noted, in LMRCs in African nations, the deaths of young adults left orphaned children to be raised with insufficient adult guidance, and forced AIDS widows into sex work to survive.[110] This situation was compounded by long-term illnesses, resulting in employee absenteeism and a smaller market for goods.[111] By the late 1990s, the average age of death dropped in some countries in Africa by up to ten years.[112] These effects destroyed family structures and communities. Members of the affected population were struck by the disease in the most productive years of their lives, when they were responsible for vital functions in society—harvesting crops, procuring food, teaching students, and providing medical care. As Malawian medical geographer Ezekiel Kalipeni pointed out, the result was a malnourished population in some African communities that culminated in a weakened national defense, which in turn undermined attempts to grow democracies in postcolonial Africa.[113] AIDS and its treatments by the early 2000s had widened health disparities between LMRCs and developed countries.

Soon after the availability of potent ART, a new group of activists became outraged about these inequalities and their consequences to individuals and communities. They objected to the reality that people who could not afford lifesaving drugs continued to die because they did not have access to ART. They argued that the inequitable allocation of expensive ART drugs throughout the world unveiled a problem of humanitarian concern on the basis that health is a human right, and that ART should be available to everyone irrespective of their ability to pay.

These patient advocates, a group of mostly prominent people from divergent backgrounds who fought for impoverished citizens of foreign nations, included, among others, Jonathan Mann (former head of UNAIDS), Peter Piot (director of UNAIDS), Franklin Graham (a Christian Evangelical leader), Paul Farmer (president, Partners in Health), Stephen Lewis (U.N. Special Envoy for AIDS in Africa), Bono (the rock musician), and Greg Behrman (founder of NationSwell). They argued that it was unjust to deny people life-saving drugs because they could not afford them.[114] Their diverse backgrounds allowed their messages to reach a broad, global audience. In the early 2000s, when AIDS was the leading cause of death worldwide for people aged fifteen to fifty-nine, both the U.N. Security Council and the Kaiser Family Foundation called HIV/AIDS a threat to peace and security, arguing that ART in the developing world was medically feasible and morally necessary.[115] The activists made a plea for wealthy nations to donate money for global ART, framing HIV as a major issue of public health and human rights.[116] They focused on the humanitarian aspect of treating HIV in the developing world.[117]

There was resistance from several sources to extending ART globally. The resistance came from some pharmaceutical companies concerned with profits, social conservatives who continued to consider AIDS a moral infraction, fiscal conservatives who were opposed to foreign aid spending, and public health officials who argued that ART was not cost effective and African AIDS programs should continue to focus on purely preventive measures. Some believed that funding global ART would waste money on a program that had not demonstrated an impact, or that donations would be misappropriated by corrupt local governments.[118] Other objections included the lack of infrastructure in Africa and a prejudiced stereotype that Africans were unable to tell time and therefore could not adhere to complex multidrug ART regimens taken throughout the day—concerns that Farmer and his organization, Partners in Health, demonstrated were unfounded.[119]

AIDS activists insisted that no person should be denied life-prolonging drugs. They focused their campaign on discrete goals (distributing ART to an extended number of people), and they addressed a broad political coalition, particularly by including Bono and Graham. This allowed the campaign to reach fans of rock music as well as evangelicals and social conservatives.[120] As historian Victoria Harden has pointed out, once leaders of various political and social groups grasped the devastating impact that AIDS had on communities, society, and the economy, the global response became focused.[121]

As a result of these activities, ART became distributed globally to a growing proportion of people in need of treatment. This was accomplished through a multipronged effort that included increasing funding from donor companies and lowering the price of the drugs. The dramatic increase in AIDS treatments that resulted between 2002 and 2007 represents the largest scale-up in access to medication in public health history; the number of people on ART increased forty-fold during this period, from fifty thousand to over two million people.[122]

One strategy adopted by activists was to confront pharmaceutical companies and promote generic drugs, thereby reducing the price of ART. Once the prices were lower, activists pressured governments to provide more foreign assistance so less-wealthy governments could purchase ART. The activists succeeded in transforming ART from a commodity that the wealthy could afford into a merit good that everyone in need had the right to consume.[123] It also became important to create rational treatment guidelines on practical issues based on evidence about which ART regimens to use, how to monitor therapy, and how to change treatments in case of drug toxicities or resistance.[124] The guidelines were updated every two years to promote standardized use. To encourage donor countries to fund global ART programs, Peter Piot, director of UNAIDS, and Kofi Annan, U.N. Secretary General, sought funding from organizations like Doctors without Borders, Oxfam, and Global AIDS Alliance.[125] In 2002, donors agreed that a new financing vehicle, Global Fund to Fight AIDS, TB, and Malaria should be created, and soon after, U.S. President George W. Bush announced the five-year, $15 billion President's Emergency Plan for AIDS Relief (PEPFAR), which was the world's biggest source of AIDS spending. From a public health viewpoint, the global allocation of HIV drugs represented a landmark achievement.[126]

A multifaceted ART-funding effort was required to reduce prices, promote generic substitution, obtain intellectual property (IP) rights waivers, eliminate duties and tariffs on essential medications, enhance distribution, and encourage local production where feasible. The first countries that reduced the price of ART were India and Brazil, which produced generic formulations with 70 percent reduction in cost. South Africa eventually tried to import less-expensive drugs from India and Brazil, but doing so violated IP rights and required renegotiating an existing World Trade Organization (WTO) international trading agreement to set standards for intellectual property regulation—known as Trade Related Aspects of Intellectual Property Rights (TRIPS)—in 1994. TRIPS posed a problem because the price of drugs yearly continued to exceed the gross domestic product for LMICs.

At the 2000 International AIDS conference in Durban, South Africa, AIDS activists and South Africa's Treatment Action committee formed a protest to insist that U.S. and European pharmaceutical companies make their drugs affordable.[127] The WTO affirmed that an international agreement on TRIPS did not prevent emergency measures empowered by the act, and an exception in TRIPS was made to allow companies to make and sell patented drugs at reduced generic prices internationally, while selling at retail prices domestically.[128] This was decided at the Doha convention in 2001, which indicated that TRIPS should promote access to medicines for all and not prevent states from dealing with public health crises.[129] It allowed donor countries to export drugs to developing countries with a national health problem, as long as the exported drugs were not part of a commercial policy. In 2003, when PEPFAR began, the Bush administration concluded that generic treatments would be a component of an effective strategy to combat HIV.[130] In 2003, the Clinton Foundation announced that it had negotiated with manufacturers to reduce the cost of ART from over $10,000 per year per person to less than $140.[131]

With the negotiation of generic drugs and falling ART prices, the commitment to long-term funding became key since the medicines needed to be taken
for the entire lifespan. Following a two-year effort by AIDS activists, politicians,
multilateral organizations (U.N. and WHO), and outspoken activists, the funding
required to sustain ART distribution was achieved through multiple sources.
These included, among others, the Global Fund to Fight AIDS, TB and Malaria,
which approved initial grants to twenty-six countries allocating $9 billion for
ART globally.[132] The commitment of the Global Fund was followed by the five-
year U.S. PEPFAR, authorized in 2003 and reauthorized in 2008.[133] A challenge
with PEPFAR money, and donations from other countries, was whether it could
sustain funding at $15 billion per year, the amount WHO estimated would need
to be sustained to provide ART globally to the people who needed it.

Some PEPFAR policies, however, have been controversial. For example,
PEPFAR funneled funds only to countries that continued to promote behavioral
change to encourage policies of abstinence and sexual fidelity/monogamy, long
after those tactics were shown to be ineffective for prevention of HIV.[134] In a
study of nearly five hundred thousand individuals in twenty-two countries,
researchers found that PEPFAR funding had no effect on the number of a person's
sexual partners, the age of sexual intercourse, or the incidence of teen pregnancy.
By 2008, U.S. funds continued to flow to abstinence and sexual fidelity programs.[135] In 2016, the U.S. government had invested $1.4 billion in HIV preven-
tion programs that promoted sexual abstinence and marital fidelity, but there
was no evidence that these programs changed sexual behavior or HIV risk. Crit-
ics argued that PEPFAR's funding of an ineffective program came at a cost
because the money could have been better used to fund proven prevention
programs—for example, male circumcision or the interruption of maternal-to-
fetal spread.[136]

Notwithstanding the controversies surrounding PEPFAR, by 2002, the
many ingredients needed to distribute ART to LMICs globally were in place.
Donor countries agreed to provide large amounts of foreign aid and reduce
drug prices through generic programs and the restructuring of IP rights.[137] To
optimize ART allocation globally, WHO set actionable goals. Two such programs targeted meeting a certain number of people who were receiving ART
by a specified date. The first, the "3 by 5" Initiative, launched by UNAIDS and
WHO in 2003, was a global target to provide ART to 3 million people living
with HIV/AIDS in LMICs by the end of 2005. It was a step toward the goal of
making HIV/AIDS prevention and treatment universally accessible for those
in need.[138] The next was the "15 by 15" campaign, which aimed to distribute
drugs to 15 million patients by 2015.[139] These programs succeeded in meeting

their goals, with ART coverage increasing from 800,000 people in 2003 to 17 million people by 2015.[140] The distribution of ART continues to improve, having increased from 500,000 people in 2002 to over 23 million people by 2020 (an estimated 37.9 million people worldwide need the treatment). This has resulted in a 46 percent decline in deaths (from 2 million to 1.2 million per year) between 2002 and 2020.[141] In addition, improvements in affected nations' economies have occurred. As survival rates improved, schools and businesses reopened.[142]

The expanding allocation of ART has been portrayed by the press as a public health victory for individuals, communities, and societies. The *New York Times*, for example, labeled the distribution of ART throughout the world as a "landmark public health achievement . . . [demonstrating] that expensive medicines can be successfully delivered throughout the world and alleviate infection and suffering on a global rather than regional basis."[143]

Public Health Potential and Proposals to Eliminate HIV/AIDS

Programs to eliminate AIDS emerged during periods of confidence in biomedicine.[144] Public health officials reasoned in 2013 that HIV drugs could eliminate the epidemic on a larger scale.[145] Thus, the spectacular therapies not only had implications for restoring health in the individual, but also had potential to eliminate the disease in the population.

The scientific vision for how to eliminate AIDS had evolved. In 1998, after the introduction of ART, scientists wrote that a vaccine was the best way to prevent HIV transmission in the population. Harold Varmus stated, "The still-expanding global dimensions of AIDS are likely to be checked only if science can succeed as admirably with vaccines as it has done with therapies."[146] By 2011, in the absence of an effective HIV vaccine, scientists had begun to consider the dual benefit of ART for prevention.[147]

Their confidence in the capacity of ART led public health officers to design programs to eliminate HIV in the population. These programs extended the benefits of treatment for an individual to the sphere of public health—a premise referred to as "treatment as prevention." The AIDS elimination campaigns were based on the demonstration that ART—by suppressing viral load in blood, semen, and vaginal secretions—renders a patient noninfectious.[148] AIDS investigators argued that a test-and-treat strategy was needed to identify as many infected, untreated persons as possible, to treat them until they no longer were infectious, and to sustain treatment throughout an individual's lifespan.[149] Evidence to support this idea came from two key sources. First, a population study showed that when HIV viral load is undetectable with ART, the transmission of the virus diminishes.[150] The concept that a person whose viral load remained undetectable by complying with ART for years was noninfectious was subsequently referred to as U = U (undetectable = untransmittable).[151] Second, a mathematical modeling prediction that universal HIV testing combined with ART for those who tested positive could nearly abolish AIDS within fifty years substantiated a test-and-treat approach to prevention.[152]

A diagnostic blood test became an indispensable component of elimination plans in order to capture and treat as many people as possible during asymptomatic periods. Accompanying the strategy of using widespread testing for HIV was a reversal of the AIDS exceptionalism idea that had been adopted early in the epidemic when discrimination of stigmatized sufferers was a concern. But now that effective therapies were available for the benefit for the individual and population, the strategy of using widespread testing and reporting replaced prior exceptionalism strategies.[153] The quantitative HIV viral load blood test was used to monitor disease activity in response to ART. As was the case with syphilis, blood tests were used for purposes of surveillance and to ensure that adequate treatment had been achieved.

Citing advances in scientifically proven strategies to treat and prevent HIV/AIDS, U.S. Secretary of State Hillary Clinton called on the world community to join the United States in creating "an AIDS-free generation." The idea of employing "scientific" tools, including treatment to render a person noninfectious, together with modeling predictions laid the groundwork for the gauntlet that Secretary Clinton proposed in 2011.[154] Clinton's plan was more aspirational than an actual campaign as her plan did not lay out specific goals, milestones, or actions. Nonetheless, it presented the feasibility of living in a world free of AIDS based on a test-and-treat strategy.

Clinton presented her proposal in a talk at the National Institutes of Health in Bethesda, Maryland, in 2011. Her speech highlighted three key scientific interventions: using antiretroviral medications in mothers with HIV, which eliminated the risk of vertical transmission; voluntary medical male circumcision, which reduced the risk of female-to-male transmission by more than 60 percent; and offering ART to persons living with HIV, which eliminated the risk of horizontal transmission if the viral load became undetectable. Clinton stated that using these interventions, along with condoms and other prevention tools, offered a historic opportunity to reduce the rate of new HIV infections worldwide. She advocated for individuals to trust in science and to let scientific evidence direct therapy: "We need to let science guide our efforts. . . . In Washington, there are some who wish to live in an evidence-free zone, but it's important that we stand up for science." She did not provide any plans for how to pay for her proposal, and the U.S. government did not make a commitment to increase funding dollars.[155]

The Joint U.N. Program on HIV/AIDS (UNAIDS), unlike the Clinton plan, offered a proposal to eliminate HIV/AIDS within a specific period. As was the case with Parran's proposal to eliminate syphilis, the belief in the power of treatment led to a treatment-as-prevention (TasP) strategy to control the spread of HIV/AIDS. But unlike Parran's campaign or Clinton's plan, the UNAIDS campaign was global. The 90-90-90 plan, issued in 2013, shared the same test-and-treat strategy as Clinton's plan.[156] Unlike Clinton's proposal, the UNAIDS plan laid out explicit milestones for ART coverage and an expedited timeline for ending the epidemic, set by the U.N. Sustainable Development Goal to improve global health over fifteen years.[157] The UNAIDS plan was the first campaign to declare an explicit timeline for ending the HIV epidemic and to provide specific targets for suppressing HIV viral load with treatment.

UNAIDS set an admittedly "ambitious" goal of ending the AIDS epidemic by 2030 (see Figure 2.3). Specifically, the plan stated that by 2020, 90 percent of people living with HIV should be diagnosed; 90 percent of HIV-infected patients diagnosed should be receiving ART; and at least 90 percent of those on ART should achieve viral suppression. The end target was to obtain an undetectable viral load in 73 percent (26.9 million) of the 37 million HIV-infected patients globally by 2020 and to sustain this level of infection for a decade. Based on modeling predictions, the plan stated it would achieve "nothing less than the end of the AIDS epidemic by 2030" if its target milestones were reached in 2020.[158] Unlike Clinton's proposal, the UNAIDS plan set actionable targets, milestones, goals, and timelines, and it addressed funding sources.

In the case of both AIDS and syphilis, the elimination strategies had significant overlap in principle and in design. The scientific basis of the elimination programs for both diseases was a treatment-as-prevention principle, designed to make people noninfectious. Each program stressed the importance of accurate reporting, partner tracing, and notification. Each plan required monitoring of treatment as judged by clinical and laboratory responses. For syphilis, this meant an appropriate decline in the strength of the Wasserman serology, and for AIDS, it involved achieving an undetectable HIV viral load.

In his February 5, 2019, State of the Union address, President Trump proposed a plan to "end the HIV epidemic" (EHE) in the United States by 2030.[159] Trump's goal to eliminate the epidemic within ten years was a familiar timeline that had also been used for syphilis elimination campaigns. Trump credited science for enabling the approach. He said, "In recent years we have made remarkable progress in the fight against HIV and AIDS. Scientific breakthroughs

90-90-90

An ambitious treatment target
to help end the AIDS epidemic

Figure 2.3. Title page of the report outlining the UNAIDS program to eliminate AIDS.
UNAIDS, *90-90-90: An Ambitious Treatment Target to Help End the AIDS Epidemic*
(Geneva, Switzerland: UNAIDS, 2014), www.unaids.org/en/resources/documents/2014
/90-90-90. Used with permission of UNAIDS Commission and Global Advocacy.

have brought a once-distant dream within reach. . . . We will defeat AIDS in America."[160] The Trump plan built on the work of predecessors Bill Clinton (who doubled resources allocated to HIV/AIDS research to $3 billion annually), George W. Bush (who launched PEPFAR and oversaw the country's contribution to the Global Fund to Fight AIDS, TB, and Malaria), and Barack Obama (who developed the first National HIV/AIDS Strategy and pushed for the passage of the Affordable Care Act).

The EHE emphasized biomedical approaches—HIV drugs—used as part of a treatment-as-prevention principle or Preexposure prophylaxis (PrEP) to prevent the spread of HIV.[161] However, the proposal did not discount the need for behavioral approaches (education) and harm-reduction approaches (condoms). The biomedical emphasis of the U.S. EHE program differed from behavioral efforts that were the focus of earlier campaigns (e.g., use of condoms) that had been successful in certain communities, including New York City and Baltimore in the 1980s and 1990s.[162] The difference in these approaches may represent a trend in public health to rely on evidence-based measures to reach benchmarks on time, and because behavioral methods have not been effective across locations.[163] The focus on PrEP as a means of prevention also reflects a reliance on biomedicine to both treat an individual and prevent spread of the illness.

The EHE targeted funding to communities across the United States with the greatest burden—termed "hot spots"—to eliminate HIV. Challenges to the EHE program—including efforts to improve testing and increase PrEP coverage, currently estimated to cover only 100,000 of the 1.1 million PrEP-eligible people in the United States—emphasize the health disparities that exist in these hot spots, primarily located in the southern United States.[164] The EHE campaign enlists "HIV elimination teams" that include patient navigators to help enable people living in hot spots to gain access to treatment facilities (using transportation vouchers, mobile units, etc.) and effective therapies. Alex Azar, the Trump-appointed secretary of Health and Human Services, acknowledged that "we have the tools to end the HIV epidemic . . . within the next 10 years" if the EHE can diagnose as many as possible of the 165,000 Americans who are living with HIV and don't know it, detect growing HIV clusters, and prevent new HIV infections in areas where HIV is spreading most rapidly.[165]

Genomic Therapy: HIV Ushers In Other Areas of Scientific Excellence

AIDS has been at the vanguard of scientific medicine in the realms of rational medicinal chemistry and the use of biomedical tools (e.g., HIV drugs, quantitative CD4 cell counts, and HIV virology) to eliminate the disease in the population.

Gene editing represents another domain where HIV has been at on the forefront of scientific medicine. This technique would allow a "cure" for HIV—an enticing idea that would eliminate the need for lifelong ART. Attempts to cure HIV by using early ART for brief durations failed to sustain a virological response after ART was discontinued because ART cannot eliminate cellular reservoirs of HIV.[166]

The requirement for ART to be continued indefinitely has multiple medical, social, and economic consequences. Medical risks resulting from long-term ART have reduced significantly as refinements in the medicines have eliminated some of the initial side effects associated with them, including a syndrome where both wasting and fat accumulation (called lipodystrophy) occurred.[167] In addition, refinements in formulations now allow for coformulated tablets that are long-lasting, enabling most infected people to achieve and maintain an undetectable HIV viral load by taking one tablet once daily.[168] This contrasts with earlier protocols, in which two to three tablets needed to be taken up to four times daily. But that does not mean that side effects have been eliminated; some ART regimens taken long-term are associated with obesity (a paradoxical situation considering that HIV-infected people once suffered from weight loss and cachexia), diabetes, and cardiac ischemia.[169] In addition, the low-level viral replication that persists below limits of detection can cause chronic inflammation, resulting in vascular disease, renal impairment, bone demineralization and fractures, and cognitive decline.[170] These risks of inflammation typically occur in older people who have taken ART for years—a byproduct of these life-prolonging HIV drugs.[171] Of course, there are also financial consequences to indefinite ART, including challenges of funding the provision of ART to 37.9 million HIV-infected people globally for the duration of their lifetime. These problems contrast with the treatment of syphilis, which was cured with one to three shots of penicillin.

The issues associated with the need for long-term ART underlie the appeal of developing approaches to cure HIV. Several strategies have been employed, including treating with ART combined with a CD4 stimulator (vorinostat). To date, these strategies have been unable to eliminate HIV from reservoir cells.[172]

Another strategy, involving genomic attempts to cure HIV, has achieved success over the past decade. This treatment attempts to eradicate the replication-competent HIV reservoir in CD4 cells by attacking the CCR5 target for genetic therapy. CCR5 is the key coreceptor required for HIV cell entry.[173] The genomic methods used to generate HIV resistance by knocking out CCR5 in the hematopoietic system have included gene editing, gene therapy with zinc, and allogeneic stem-cell transplantation. Gene-editing approaches have used CRISPR (clustered regularly interspaced short palindromic repeats) using an artificial nuclease to create specific genetic edits. Medical researchers have done this in a patient with HIV and acute myelogenous leukemia (AML), where donor cells for a bone marrow transplant (BMT) were subjected to editing with use of CRISPR-Cas9 technology to knock out CCR5 before infusion into the HIV-infected recipient. Immunologist Carl June from the University of Pennsylvania identified the potential to use gene-editing technology to specifically excise integrated HIV DNA from the host genome and thereby eliminate the latent reservoir, avoiding the need for long-term ART use.[174] This strategy holds promise for management of HIV, but its present problem is scalability, as the products have not been studied in large trials, there are no plans to obtain FDA licensing, and gene therapy requires expertise and a high-technology infrastructure to remove CD4 cells, perform gene therapy ex vivo, and then reinsert the cells into the host. Clearly, more convenient delivery systems would be needed to scale gene therapy to manage HIV at a global level.

Nonetheless, among the scientific community, HIV has become recognized as the catalyst for successful ex vivo T-cell engineering for HIV cell-based therapies. June says, "HIV has been at the vanguard of cell and gene therapy for decades, and this trend has continued in genome editing."[175] Genomic approaches remain investigational, have not been licensed for clinical practice, and require high-technology delivery systems.[176] Still, these methods were effective in the small number of patients who have entered clinical trials. They have placed HIV at the forefront of the field of genomics therapy—a widely recognized achievement among scientists, albeit, unlike the development of ART, one that has not been widely covered by the popular press as its high-tech nature excludes global scalability.

Conclusion

There are important parallels between AIDS and syphilis, including how AIDS first appeared unexpectedly as a frightening disease, and how it was initially understood within a moral framework of deviancy. AIDS posed a burden to society by striking people at the prime of their lives. Innovative biomedical therapies provided an efficient avenue to restoring health in the individual patient. Like syphilis, these therapies received widespread attention in the medical and lay press as they lowered deaths and restored vitality—a visual reminder of the emotional impact that treatment of a once-devastating and recalcitrant disease provides to patients, their physicians, families, and loved ones. AIDS, like syphilis, ushered in extraordinary biomedical advances that have been praised by the medical and lay press for their potency and benevolence.

Moreover, as treatment rendered individuals noninfectious, public health officials realized they possessed the tools to eliminate the disease in the population. In the case of both AIDS and syphilis, public health officials were so confident in their potent biomedical tools that they predicted the disease would be eliminated within ten years. The introduction of scientific therapies changed the narrative of each disease from one of recalcitrance to one of control. Biomedicine offered reassurance that AIDS and its consequences for society could be excised.

In chapters 1 and 2, we have explored how two diseases have epitomized the power, efficiency, benevolence, and seemingly limitless potential of biomedicine. In chapter 1, we showed how syphilis bolstered the confident narrative of biomedicine and contributed to the widespread belief in the mid-twentieth century that all epidemics would someday be conquered. In this chapter, we have shown the circumstances under which a clear faith in science has been a throughline from the conviction of patient representatives, who were confident that effective drugs could be developed, to the reassurance that the drugs could restore health in individuals and end the disease in the population. This confident portrayal of science was based on the idea that the might of biomedicine would end syphilis and AIDS and return the world to a state of pre-epidemic normalcy. In chapter 3, we will explore how the actual outcomes of elimination programs have come to delimit biomedicine and challenge the hope that it will provide an end to epidemics.

Chapter 3

Fate of Elimination Campaigns

Public health officials were confident that their scientifically based test-and-treat campaigns would end syphilis and AIDS within a decade following implementation. Each campaign (Parran's in the 1930s, and UNAIDS's in 2013) eschewed moralistic framing, promoted awareness, obtained funding, set goals, and were advertised publicly. However, despite their potential, the campaigns have not succeeded. They fall short because of the complex array of biological, epidemiological, and socioeconomic factors that drive epidemics and interfere with efforts to eliminate them. The exploration of these campaigns sheds light on the promise and limitations of scientific medicine.

Syphilis Elimination Campaigns: 1930s to Today

With funding, effective scientific tools in hand, and the cooperation of the media, Thomas Parran was confident that his campaign would end syphilis. For a brief period, some indicators suggested that his program was working. Clinic facilities for the treatment of VD had grown; public subsidies provided practitioners with diagnostic services and free drugs; and the number of patients receiving the minimum required therapy increased from 15 percent to 60 percent.[1] Nonetheless, these trends were short-lived, and syphilis rates failed to decline from 1936 (318 cases per 100,000) to 1941 (368 cases per 100,000).[2] With the onset of World War II, hundreds of thousands of men were displaced from their homes and mobilized to army camps throughout the country.[3] Parran noted that migration of young adults away from the social controls of their families was conducive to the spread of syphilis because it was associated with an increase in transactional sex. His attempts to optimize case-finding and enter all civilians into treatment proved ineffective under wartime circumstances.

During World War II, the effort to control syphilis was reinvigorated to ensure an adequate number of able-bodied troops. A 1942 increase in federal funding for the project to $8 million annually allowed the addition of rapid treatment centers (RTCs) to develop widespread testing, treatment, and contact tracing to meet wartime needs.[4] As Parascandola has noted, when the U.S. Army adopted penicillin for routine treatment of syphilis in 1944, there was hope that syphilis might be controlled among the troops.[5] With a new tool to fight syphilis, combined with an increase in government funding, rates of the disease began to diminish. When the decline persisted into the 1950s (363 cases/100,000 in 1942 to 109/100,000 cases in 1952), there was speculation that doctors might no longer see cases of syphilis.[6]

As rates continued to fall during postwar times, state and local health departments began to reduce their support of the full-scale public health approach.[7] The federal appropriation of funds for VD control was cut from $9.8 million in 1953 to less than $2 million by 1955.[8] These cuts were accompanied by a rise in rates of syphilis (from 66 cases/100,000 in 1954 to 78 cases/100,000 in 1959), and VD control programs were forced to curtail their approach of testing and treating in RTCs.[9] Noting the continuation of the reversal in the downward trend of syphilis rates in 1962, a disheartened public health expert, Malcolm Merrill, director of the California State Department of Health, remarked, "VD control nearly became another victim of the rhetoric that all communicable disease had been conquered."[10]

Public health officials at the time speculated on why Parran's campaign had failed. Attributing the failure to premature rescinding of federal funding, William Brown, chief of the VD Branch at the CDC (then formally named the Communicable Disease Center), said in 1962, "We learned the law of failure through success—as a disease control program approaches the end point of eradication, it is not the disease but the program that is more likely to be eradicated." Furthermore, he noted that when funding diminished, cases that were subsequently found would "re-seed the population and disease will flourish." He acknowledged the importance of social and behavioral issues, and noted, "We [at the CDC] have not overlook[ed] its [syphilis's] moral, social and economic aspects, and [with] the . . . contributions of the behavioral sciences . . . we are equipped to attack it from every angle." Brown did not elaborate on specific social factors he was referring to or lay out any proposal to address them. Nonetheless, he remained confident that syphilis could be eradicated, stating, "we are on the threshold of eradication. . . . We must work to eliminate the disease completely; we can no longer rest content to reduce syphilis to a low level, and to maintain that level forever." He affirmed his faith in a scientific test-and-treat strategy using penicillin, noting that a "single injection has the power to render the patient rapidly non-infectious."[11]

Uriel Foa, a UNESCO specialist in social research from Bangkok, Thailand, argued in 1962 that eradication would not be possible unless social issues were also addressed. Foa stated, "Behavioral scientists need [to be] invited to join the battle . . . [as] . . . behavioral research [needs] to accompany medical research." He postulated that differential rates of promiscuity among populations, including teenagers and urban adults, who were difficult to reach with traditional messaging, could account for the increase in VD despite potent new therapies. He insisted that approaches must take into account these different patterns of behavior, writing, "Attempts to change the behavioral pattern may be more likely to succeed when they center on the group rather than the individual."[12] Foa, however, did not provide any tangible proposals on how elimination programs should address social issues.

Noting the continued rise in syphilis cases in 1961, Surgeon General Luther Terry vowed to launch a new campaign to eradicate the illness. Terry, a pathologist, had previously served as chairman of the medical board at the National Institutes of Health's Clinical Center. There, he developed an interest in preventive measures that he later applied as surgeon general in his campaign to reduce cigarette smoking.[13] Terry appointed a task force to make recommendations on his campaign to eliminate another public health threat—syphilis. In 1962, he appointed Leona Baumgartner, commissioner of New York City's Public Health Department, as its head. The department's first woman commissioner, Baumgartner, a pediatrician, had experience carrying out municipal programs in disease prevention and childhood nutrition.[14] For her task force proposal, Baumgartner acknowledged that Parran's 1930 campaign would serve as the basis of her recommendations for the new syphilis "eradication" program.[15]

The task force met in New York City on September 13, 1961. Baumgartner reiterated the importance of widespread testing and treating, as well as the reporting of cases to the public health department. She noted that reporting had historically been suboptimal, as private physicians, concerned about confidentiality, were reluctant to reveal the names of their patients to a state office. Baumgartner believed she could improve reporting and contact tracing by reassuring physicians that the information they provided would be kept strictly confidential and that patients' privacy would be protected.[16]

Baumgartner recognized that her program had to go above and beyond Parran's in order to succeed. She believed that Parran's previous attempts at case finding and contact tracing had been hampered by patients' reluctance to be tested and their hesitancy to identify sexual partners because of the persistent stigma associated with the disease.[17] She and Malcolm Merrill maintained that the inability to identify an accurate number of cases and their sexual contacts created a large reservoir of unknown, uncontrolled, and untreated cases.[18] It was this reservoir—the "margin of failure" of 19,000 of the estimated 60,000 new cases of syphilis reported—who did not seek voluntary testing or treatment that drove the continuing epidemic. She identified both the "under-reporting of cases by private physicians to health authorit[ies]" and determining the "margin" of infected, untested people as two key areas that needed improvement.[19] Baumgartner concluded that unless she could identify the margin and improve reporting and contract tracing, then her program would be nothing more than "another crack at an old and familiar enemy."[20] Malcolm Merrill reaffirmed that if the task force could not improve these issues, "then we shall have to live with this disease indefinitely."[21]

Baumgartner elaborated on how she believed she could engage the marginal group. Baumgartner stated that the "margin" consisted of teenagers, male homosexuals, and migrant workers. She believed she could reach these groups by means of a "full, nationwide effort," including by placing educational articles about common syphilis misperceptions in popular journals.[22] In *McCall's* magazine, for example, she sought to debunk what she believed to be widespread overconfidence in the "miraculous powers attributed to penicillin . . . [by] . . . physicians and laymen." She believed that behavioral and social issues, including "the growing moral laxness especially among teenagers due to fundamental changes in society," could be addressed through education.[23]

Baumgartner and her task force elaborated on how they also sought to strengthen case finding, reporting, and tracing. To maximize case finding, she and Warren Davis, chief of program services of the VD Branch at the CDC, sought to extend Parran's efforts by including "cluster contacts," defined as acquaintances of patients, not only their sexual contacts, to maximize the number of cases captured.[24] Davis also maintained that healthcare workers needed to pay more attention to the psychological factors that prevented patients from divulging the names of sexual contacts to health practitioners, who were otherwise unknown to them. Furthermore, Baumgartner, along with Rudolph Kampmeier, professor of medicine at Vanderbilt University, noted that public officials had not been working productively with private doctors and private laboratories to optimize case reporting and tracing.[25] From the 1930s to the 1960s, the reporting capacity of diseases to the national Public Health Service had been strengthened by the Council for State and Territorial Epidemiologists, a new body for deciding national notifiable diseases and updating case definitions.[26] This had not, however, translated into an improved detection of syphilis cases.

Although Baumgartner stressed their importance, she did not provide specific proposals for improving reporting and contact tracing. Baumgartner instead made a plea to doctors and public health officials to improve in these areas. In 1962, she said that due to "the shockingly inadequate reporting of the disease, thousands of individuals who have it are wandering about free to spread it further." She noted that treatment of cases alone without adequate contact tracing and notification would "spread the disease like a forest fire. . . . We have got to find all the people with syphilis. . . . Doctors need to report, we need to interview, test patients and contacts."[27] Baumgartner insisted that this was the only means by which syphilis could be eradicated.

Baumgartner and Terry elaborated on the societal factors they believed were responsible for the growing syphilis problem. Terry identified as factors population mobility (which created more opportunities to form casual sex relationships than were possible in a small community) and the breakdown of older cultural patterns and mores (such as children being less closely supervised in cities than in small towns).[28] Neither Terry nor Baumgartner, however, offered tangible approaches for addressing these issues. Baumgartner also acknowledged that greater insights into human behaviors would be needed to create a successful syphilis elimination program. She said, "We need expanded research into human behavior, into mores, attitudes, motivations. It may help make our present methods obsolete, as we hope they will become . . . [as] we need to know more about prevention."[29] In addition, the two addressed the importance of sustained government funding to subsidize the costs of a syphilis control campaign.[30]

Baumgartner used popular magazines to educate teenagers and heighten public consciousness about the growing problem of syphilis. She postulated that teenagers in the 1960s had not borne witness to the "death and insanity" that had been common outcomes of syphilis before penicillin.[31] William Brown also believed that the increase in syphilis in this group was based in part on the success of penicillin.[32] Baumgartner tried to address the current lack of "inhibition about sexual activity, especially among teenagers" by educating them about the ravages of syphilis, which she believed at one time had been a deterrent to promiscuity.[33] She wrote, "During days of arsenical treatments, people knew about syphilis, feared it and were interested in avoiding it. We have a new generation of people growing up in a . . . new atmosphere of a quick victory of syphilis." She argued for "heighten[ing] the suspicion on the part of the individual that he or she may have the disease—through education, school textbooks, and school hygiene courses. . . . We talk about mass media, and we need to use mass communications."[34]

Baumgartner used the popular press as the vehicle to warn readers about the dangers of syphilis and to counter complacency. Baumgartner's open warnings of the dangers of syphilis had a favorable response, as major magazines, including *Time*, *The Nation*, the *New Republic*, and *Consumer Reports*, called for the medical and public health communities to do something to end the epidemic.[35] Using colorful language in her educational messages to arouse attention, Baumgartner was able to place her syphilis eradication campaign high on the national agenda.[36] She wrote, for example, "We need to put magic in our materials so they will appeal to our audience, so they will enlist willing, enthusiastic support for this drive." She said, "Injecting penicillin is simple. Finding the patients who need it is another problem. We will succeed only as we accept syphilis control as an exercise in human behavior extending far beyond the traditional limits of medicine." Baumgartner identified overreliance on quick, efficient biomedical cures without addressing broader social issues as an impediment to achieving eradication. She wrote that the "elimination of this sorry plague will only come from . . . breaking the atmosphere of blissful confidence" in biomedical cures. Baumgartner then made a playful appeal to young people, stating, "Together, it is possible that we can bring to a practical end the twisted history of this unattractive and twisted organism."[37]

Baumgartner continued her use of colorful language to remind her medical and lay audience about the dangers of complacency. She referred to the syphilis rates, which had declined during the postwar period, from 1947 to 1955, but then began to climb as funding dropped after 1955. She wrote, "The torrent of information that had poured from radio, newspapers, televisions, and magazines slowed to a trickle. Editors moved on to other things. Meanwhile, syphilis moved on to other people. If the problem was solved, the syphilis organism did not know it."[38] Here, Baumgartner identified the problem of complacency as a threat to eradication campaigns, including a lack of attention from the media and from the government to sustain funding.

While Baumgartner sought to increase public awareness of the dangers of syphilis, Terry sought to obtain federal subsidies for his anti-VD program. Terry, like Parran, maintained that he was justified in seeking federal funding for a national public health problem. With the advocacy of the surgeon general, the Community Health Services and Facilities Act, enacted by the Eighty-Seventh Congress, was signed into law by President John F. Kennedy on October 5, 1961. It funded grants to the states for the expansion of medical services facilities like nursing homes and medical programs for general public health and outpatient services. It also extended and strengthened the 1946 Hill-Burton Act, which enabled the federal government to provide funding to the states for the creation of new treatment clinics.[39] Based on the task force's recommendations, these federal funds were to be used for comprehensive national anti-VD efforts, including medical services (facilities to find, diagnose, and treat individuals with syphilis), epidemiological services (officers trained to interview patients, trace their contacts, and bring patients into treatment), and educational activities.[40] The federal subsidies to control syphilis had increased from $3 million per year in 1955 to $9.5 million in 1964.[41] Baumgartner asserted that without such a multifaceted, well-funded program, the epidemic would fester, as control efforts would be limited to "mere firefighting" that would not "eliminate permanently the conflagration."[42]

Baumgartner provided an accelerated timeline for "the eradication of syphilis." She said that if the comprehensive program recommended by the task force "can be secured and developed to the required level by 1963 . . . the epidemic spread of syphilis in this country can be stopped within ten years."[43] On the basis of the task force's report, President Kennedy in February 1962 recommended, and Congress endorsed, what he termed "the initiation of a major 10-year program of Federal grants and direct action aimed at the total eradication in this country of this age-old scourge of mankind."[44] The goal of eradicating syphilis was reaffirmed by President Lyndon B. Johnson after he assumed office.[45] William Brown, chief of the Division of Venereal Disease, said in a presentation at a VD conference at the University of Oklahoma that even though some people may be skeptical, "two Americans will land on the moon [and] . . . the target date for the eradication of syphilis from this country is two years after the expected moon landing." The implication from Brown's analogy was that scenarios that may have once seemed implausible, like landing humans on the moon—or eradicating syphilis—could be achieved if people had the technology and the will. Brown was confident that humans had the technological means—diagnosing and treating syphilis—to "eradicate it [syphilis] right on schedule."[46]

At the start of the campaign, Baumgartner continued to recognize that her public health campaign would require more than effective biomedical tools. She wrote, "Scientifically, the tools are available to eliminate the problem. . . . [One may think] that takes care of the problem. . . . Yet that is not the case. . . . The problem has not been solved. . . . We have been here before, we are back again for another crack at an old and familiar enemy." Baumgartner recognized that "our tools for diagnosis and treatment are good," but the problem lay in "human behavior . . . of . . . not only those who contract syphilis and pass it on to others but also Health workers who have not brought to all who need them the excellent weapons the laboratories have provided."[47] She again recognized the need to remind physicians to cooperate with reporting.

Thus, Baumgartner's program attempted to address the perceived gaps in Parran's program, both moral and social. In addition to educating the largest audience possible, Baumgartner also promoted open discussion and stressed the burden of the disease on the individual and the country. She pointed out the social problems that could thwart elimination strategies in evasive populations, such as teenagers.[48] Despite these complications, the goal of her plan was to eradicate syphilis in ten years (see Figure 3.1).

Nonetheless, Baumgartner and Terry's plan failed. The rates of syphilis fell from 69 cases/100,000 when the campaign started in 1962 to fewer than 31 cases/100,000 in 1966 but then relapsed to the baseline by 1972, with 68 cases/100,000.[49] Terry's campaign failed to secure sustained funding as syphilis was overtaken by other priorities.[50] In fact in 1966, the task force had expressed concern that the level of federal funding that was made available per year was insufficient to fully implement the activities they recommended.[51] But the lack of sustained funding was not the sole reason for the campaign's failure.[52] Despite Baumgartner's attempts to define syphilis as a medical disease, it was difficult to completely escape the moral framework that had prevented some from being tested or the reluctance to reveal contacts. These factors compromised both Baumgartner's and Parran's attempts to maximize case finding.[53] Additionally, we do not know how effective education had been in moderating sexual behavior; Baumgartner did not outline the measures offered to teenagers in the 1960s.

Reformers, from the social hygienists in the 1920s to Baumgartner in the 1960s, had faith that education could be a primary means of altering sexual behavior and that individuals would cooperate. But the efficacy of this intervention for STDs has yet to be verified, especially in the absence of standardized strategies, such as providing explicit instructions on safe sex, or having trusted leaders deliver the messaging. Furthermore, though Baumgartner identified the social issues that led to a vulnerable environment, as mentioned, she outlined no specific ideas for how to resolve them. Despite their own warnings, Baumgartner and Terry did not offer anything substantively different from earlier eradication programs, and their campaigns suffered an identical fate.

Syphilologists at the time speculated on why the program had failed. Vernal Cave, director of the New York City Health Department, implicated insufficient funds and workers, incomplete reporting, and incomplete case finding as reasons for the failure of the program. Cave lamented, "Sadly, [when] we proceeded in the direction of syphilis eradication, we also began to

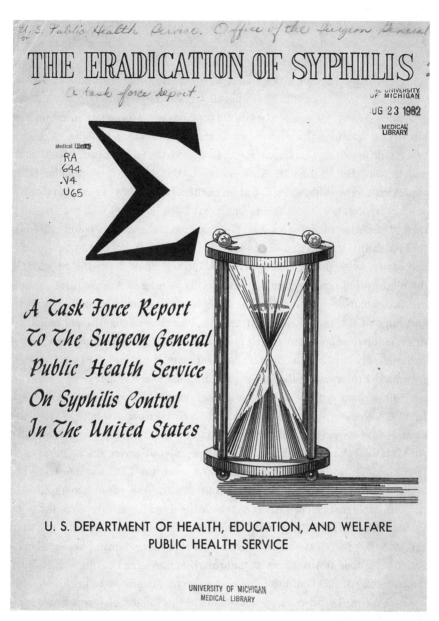

THE ERADICATION OF SYPHILIS

A task force report.

A Task Force Report
To The Surgeon General
Public Health Service
On Syphilis Control
In The United States

U. S. DEPARTMENT OF HEALTH, EDUCATION, AND WELFARE
PUBLIC HEALTH SERVICE

Figure 3.1. Title page of the report produced in 1962 by the task force headed by Leona Baumgartner. The hourglass imagery reinforces the campaign's position that it was only a matter of time before syphilis would be eradicated. Used with permission of U.S. Government Publishing Office.

eradicate our control program. . . . History was repeating itself and the axiom that 'history teaches us that history teaches nothing' stood up.'" He continued, "We have come to the realization that no communicable disease can be brought under control by treatment alone."[54] William J. Brown stated that "penicillin is not the 'dragon killer' we thought it was in the 1950s, when we referred to the illness as a 'dying disease.'"[55] Thus, by the late 1960s, there was a growing realization that biomedical solutions alone would not be sufficient to control syphilis.

Public health experts Hunter Handsfield, from the University of Washington, and Edward Hook, from the University of Alabama, writing decades later, expanded on these ideas. Prior public health officers, they wrote, had trouble reaching groups they identified as "marginal," that is, groups who shared a mistrust of government and medicine. They assumed interviewers could influence these marginal populations and elicit the information needed to control the spread of disease. But, according to Handsfield and Hook, they failed to consider the relevant political, cultural, and economic features of the groups. Gay men and promiscuous women could lose their jobs if they were identified as such, and migrant workers faced deportation as branches of government collected information to support their firing or deportation.[56] Consequently, these groups had difficulty trusting that public health officials would maintain confidentiality with the information that had critical implications for their lives.

Subsequent syphilis elimination programs in the United States followed. In 1999, when syphilis was at its nadir (2.1 cases per 100,000 people), the Centers for Disease Control and Prevention (as the CDC by then was formally titled) issued the National Plan to Eliminate Syphilis from the United States (see Figure 3.2).[57] Despite the overall low rates, the CDC was motivated to act, as syphilis remained a severe public health problem in geographically concentrated areas where African Americans lived in poverty. Syphilis rates in these areas were thirty-eight times higher for African Americans than for whites.[58] The CDC sought to eliminate this long-standing health disparity, stating that it would be a "landmark achievement . . . to significantly decrease one of this Nation's most glaring racial disparities in health."[59] This campaign, unlike prior ones, addressed the influence of race on the incidence of syphilis.

Otherwise, the 1999 plan was similar in design to previous ones. It used widespread testing and treatment to provide early, specific diagnosis and treatment of symptomatic and asymptomatic individuals prevent further transmission of syphilis to their partners.[60] The plan used the word "elimination" in place of "eradication," which earlier programs had used. It defined elimination as cessation of "sustained transmission," characterized by a reduction of syphilis

The National Plan to Eliminate Syphilis from the United States

Figure 3.2. A title page from the report outlining the CDC's 1999 syphilis elimination campaign. CDC, *The National Plan to Eliminate Syphilis from the United States* (Atlanta: U.S. Department of Health and Human Services, October 1999), www.cdc.gov /stopsyphilis/plan.pdf. Used with permission of the CDC.

to 1,000 or fewer cases in the United States, or a rate of 0.4 per 100,000 people.[61] Though the CDC document did not articulate why they changed terminology, it is possible they concluded that, in the wake of the prior programs, eradication was an unattainable goal.

The 1999 CDC campaign was based on a 1997 Institute of Medicine (IOM) document titled *The Hidden Epidemic*, which outlined a path to ending syphilis and other STIs in the United States. The IOM report sought to provide health services for racial minorities (African American, Hispanic), the homeless, incarcerated people, sex workers, and transgender groups in addition to the "margin" groups Baumgartner had targeted earlier (adolescents, men who have sex with men [MSM], and migrant workers). The IOM report, and the 1999 CDC campaign to follow, stressed the need to mobilize community groups to improve surveillance and treatment in targeted populations.[62] Thus, the IOM report and the CDC campaign targeted high-risk areas, acknowledged racial disparities, and involved community stakeholders to deliver services (testing, treatment, reporting) in a culturally sensitive fashion. The 1997 IOM document acknowledged the problems of privacy, confidentiality, and underreporting but, like prior programs, did not provide specific strategies to address them.

The CDC plan elaborated on social problems that fueled syphilis in the 1990s. It mentioned poverty, sexism, homophobia, illegal drug use (including use of crack cocaine), the sex industry, distrust of government, and the legacy of Tuskegee. It also expanded on the difficult-to-reach, disenfranchised populations they referred to as the "core"—including the homeless, people living in weak community infrastructures, and those who lacked education.[63] The plan identified the economic consequences of syphilis, including the loss of productivity and wages due to absenteeism.[64] While noting these social issues, the plan offered no specific proposals on how to correct them.

The 1999 syphilis program sought to change the method of surveillance. The CDC no longer recommended intensified screening of the whole population, premarital testing, or routine testing of hospital patients. The CDC acknowledged that the yield in these populations was too low and occasional false positive cases would occur—as happens when a nonspecific test is used as a screening test in sites where the disease is not highly prevalent. The CDC advocated widespread testing for high-risk populations such as commercial sex workers, antenatal women, risk-taking MSM, and those entering detention. Like earlier campaigns, it stressed educating the public by having open discussions about STD prevention and STD-related services. To succeed, the CDC acknowledged that eliminating syphilis required ongoing resource investment. Early budget estimates were set at $80 million annually, of which the federal portion was estimated to be approximately $39 million.

Following its launch in 1999, the CDC campaign achieved some successes in targeted populations. The numbers of cases among women and African Americans initially decreased every year, and congenital syphilis, which peaked in 1991, had declined by more than 90 percent in 2003. Between 1999 and 2003, there was a 95 percent reduction in primary and secondary syphilis in women, and a 92 percent reduction in congenital syphilis. The Black-to-white ratio went from 28.6:1 to 5.4:1, demonstrating an encouraging trend in the initial disparities within four years of the program's launch.[65]

The early successes were short lived. Elimination goals were not achieved by the 2005 target date, possibly due to increases in syphilis among MSM. Indeed, more than 60 percent of primary and secondary cases were occurring in the MSM population. In addition, the decline in syphilis rates between 1990 and 1995 had been attributed to AIDS mortality among this population, and the relapse could have been due to enhanced HIV survival with antiretroviral therapy.[66] The campaign's acknowledgement of social considerations in interfering with elimination efforts was not translated into effective policy. Furthermore, funding never reached the targeted amount.[67]

A revised CDC effort, the Syphilis Elimination Effort (SEE), was launched in August 2005, when the CDC convened a Syphilis Effort Consultation meeting (see Figure 3.3).[68] The CDC had a funding agreement with fifty-nine state, local, and territorial STD programs to conduct SEE activities for eight years, until 2013.[69] A revised (higher) elimination goal was set: 2.2 cases per 100,000 population (overall) by 2010. It specified different targets based on gender and race; the target for men was 4.2 per 100,000, and for women 0.38 per 100,000. The Black-to-white target ratio for 2010 was 3:1.[70] The plan sought to attain these goals by enhancing public health services, boosting outreach programs, and implementing culturally competent services and interventions that the 1999 plan had already identified.[71]

Again, the 2005 SEE effort failed to reduce rates of syphilis to the new targets by 2010. By 2009, more than 50 percent of all syphilis cases reported to CDC were among Black Americans, and overall syphilis rates were 4.5 per 100,000 people.[72] The disease remained geographically concentrated, thereby failing to rectify the health disparities that the CDC sought to reverse.

Despite the twentieth-century eradication campaigns and the twenty-first-century elimination campaigns, syphilis is raging both in the United States and globally. From 2013 to 2016, the rate of syphilis increased among both men and women in the United States, and in every age group, race, ethnicity, and

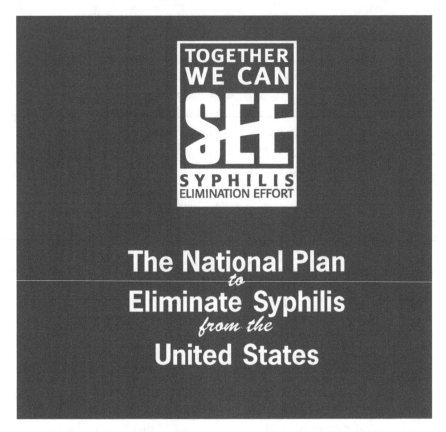

Figure 3.3. A title page from the CDC's revised 2005 plan. CDC, *The Syphilis Elimination Program Assessment and Findings Monograph: Lessons Learned* (Atlanta: U.S. Department of Health and Human Services, 2005). Used with permission of the CDC.

region.[73] In 2016, rates of primary and secondary syphilis remained higher among men (15.6 cases per 100,000 males) than women (1.9 cases per 100,000 females), and were highest in the West and South (see Figure 3.4).

In addition, syphilis remains concentrated among particular populations: MSM, urban, African Americans, and Hispanics. In fact, in 2017, among 27,814 cases of primary and secondary syphilis in the United States, 16,155 (58.1 percent) cases occurred among MSM; Black Americans had 23.1 cases per 100,000 persons; Native Hawaiians/Other Pacific Islanders had 12.9 cases per 100,000 persons; Hispanics Americans had 10.9 cases per 100,000 persons; American Indians/Alaska Natives had 8.0 cases per 100,000 persons; white Americans had 4.9 cases per 100,000 persons; and Asian Americans had 3.9 cases per 100,000 persons.[74] In every group, the incidence and rates of

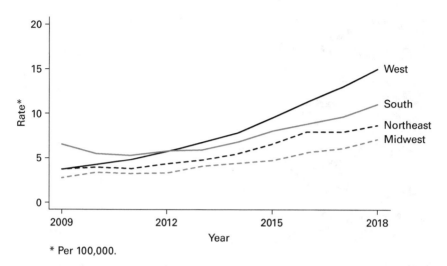

* Per 100,000.

Figure 3.4. Increases in cases of primary and secondary syphilis, recorded by region, 2009–2018. CDC, *Sexually Transmitted Disease Surveillance 2018* (Atlanta: U.S. Department of Health and Human Services, 2019), figure 36, www.cdc.gov/std/stats18 /STDSurveillance2018-full-report.pdf. Used with permission of the CDC.

syphilis are substantially greater than the 1999 CDC target for elimination by 2005 (defined as 1,000 or fewer cases, or a rate of 0.4 per 100,000 population overall). Syphilis has remained a major hazard for society despite the implementation of programs designed to eliminate it.

With syphilis remaining a major threat, a new 2021 STI control plan by the U.S. Department of Health and Human Services (HHS)—titled the *STI National Strategic Plan for the United States, 2021–2025*—has out laid goals to prevent new STIs by improving screening and treatment.[75] The HHS plan addresses syphilis and other STIs and identifies the rise in STIs as the impetus for the plan.[76] The Office of Infectious Disease and HIV/AIDS Policy (OIDP), which is part of HHS, convened an STI Federal Steering Committee composed of twenty federal agencies and offices to develop the plan.[77] The committee has laid out the STI plan's goals, strategies, and action steps, including implementing a program that uses new technologies in STI diagnostics, therapeutics, vaccines, research, and surveillance.[78] It also lists as a goal addressing the individual, community, and structural factors and inequities that contribute to the spread of STIs, such as stigma and social determinants of health (see Figure 3.5).[79] Thus, there is an all-inclusive test-and-treat program that addresses biological as well as social factors that determine risky behavior. Nonetheless, the funding source for the proposal has not been resolved, and it is too premature to know what the fate of the 2021–2025 HHS National Strategic Plan will be.

A. Vision

The United States will be a place where sexually transmitted infections are prevented and where every person has high-quality STI prevention, care, and treatment while living free from stigma and discrimination.

This vision includes all people, regardless of age, sex, gender identity, sexual orientation, race, ethnicity, religion, disability, geographic location, or socioeconomic circumstance.

B. Goals

In pursuit of this vision, the STI Plan establishes five goals:

1. Prevent new STIs

2. Improve the health of people by reducing adverse outcomes of STIs

3. Accelerate progress in STI research, technology, and innovation

4. Reduce STI-related health disparities and health inequities

5. Achieve integrated, coordinated efforts that address the STI epidemic

Figure 3.5. A summary of the aims of U.S. Health and Human Services, *Sexually Transmitted Infections: National Strategic Plan for the United States 2021–2025* (Washington, DC, 2021), 30, https://www.hhs.gov/sites/default/files/STI-National -Strategic-Plan-2021-2025.pdf. Used with permission of HHS.

AIDS Elimination Programs: 2013 to Today

Campaigns to eliminate AIDS are based on a design similar to the ones for the syphilis programs. The key features of today's UNAIDS plan—its premise (treatment as prevention) and design (test and treat)—resemble those of the syphilis plans. The UNAIDS plan, like the syphilis plans, emphasizes the importance of carrying out widespread testing, getting all people into treatment to render them noninfectious, and obtaining central subsidies for implementing the plan. But there are several differences, including in scale (the UNAIDS campaign is global, whereas the syphilis plans are national) and therapy duration (treatment for HIV/AIDS is for a lifespan, whereas for syphilis it is one shot in most cases). According to the UNAIDS plan, "The world will need to combine political will . . . and sufficient financial resources to sustain lifelong HIV treatment for tens of millions worldwide."[80] The 90-90-90 plan does not provide specific methods on how to maximize case detection or attain the sustained funding needed to carry out the program for its duration. Public health experts are uncertain about whether the UNAIDS goals can be met by 2030.[81]

Presently, the UNAIDS campaign is meeting its targets in some locales but is falling short in multiple locations in the United States and globally. Overall, of the three targets (90 percent tested by 2020, 90 percent of those tested treated, and 90 percent of those treated undetectable by 2020), none have been reached, according to the data for the interim 2020 target date. In terms of the percentages, approximately 83 percent of people with HIV globally knew their HIV status in 2020.[82] The remaining 17 percent still need access to HIV testing services. In addition, of those who know their status, 86 percent are being treated with ART. Furthermore, 88 percent of those receiving ART have an undetectable HIV viral load.[83] Thus, only 64 percent of the global HIV-infected population presently have viral suppression (83 percent tested × 86 percent of those treated × 88 percent of treated who are undetectable)—which is below the 73 percent UNAIDS viral suppression target (90 percent × 90 percent × 90 percent) globally for 2020.[84] Thus, ART uptake overall in 2020 is lower than UNAIDS targets. Moreover, there are several geographic locales (e.g., India, China, Pakistan) where ART uptake is much lower than elsewhere. Across the world, the targets are presently being met inconsistently.[85] Rates remain particularly high among high-risk, vulnerable populations, which include racial (e.g., African Americans) and ethnic (Hispanic) minorities in the United States.

Thus, many HIV-infected people presently living in LMICs who are eligible for therapy still do not receive it. Consequently, the death rate from HIV/AIDS, although reduced by more than 55 percent since the peak of 1.2 million in 2010 and 1.7 million in 2004, before ART was distributed widely, remains substantial, at 770,000 per year worldwide. In addition, the disease continues to spread. The number of newly infected per year, although reduced 38 percent from its peak at 2.6 million before ART distribution, has remained stable at 1.5 million per year.[86] On a more positive note, 92 percent of pregnant women with HIV received ART, compared with 49 percent in 2010. This prevents the vertical transmission of HIV to babies during pregnancy and childbirth and also protects maternal health.[87] Despite the considerable progress made, the 2020 UNAIDS milestones have not been met by their target date, and the burden of the disease remains unevenly distributed in the world. HIV/AIDS still takes a substantial toll on individuals, families, communities, and nations.[88] Today, the disease remains one of the world's most serious public health challenges.[89]

In 2019, Present Trump laid out a specific plan to End the HIV Epidemic (EHE) in the United States based on biomedical advances (see Figure 3.6).[90] The goal of the EHE program was to reduce new cases by 75 percent in the first five years and by 90 percent in the following ten years, averting more than 250,000 HIV infections in that period.[91] The goal also included enrolling every American infected with virus (1.1 million people) in treatment and reducing new HIV infections by 75 percent by 2024.[92] Trump committed $291 million to this project in his 2020 budget proposal.[93] It is too early to tell if the EHE program is on target for success, as the five-year milestone date is not until 2024.[94]

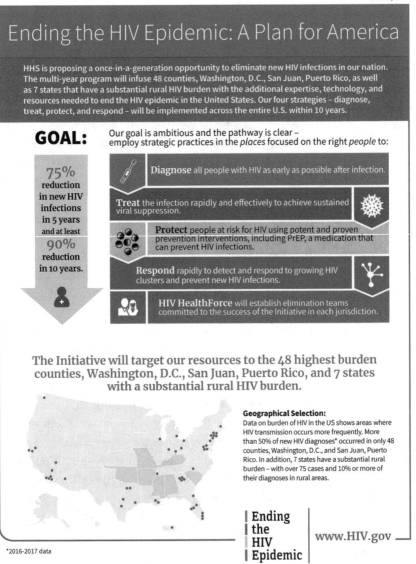

Figure 3.6. A summary of President Donald Trump's "Ending the HIV Epidemic: A Plan for America," Alex Azar, secretary, HHS, February 6, 2019, 1, https://www.hhs.gov/sites /default/files/ending-the-hiv-epidemic-fact-sheet.pdf. Used with permission of HHS.

AIDS and Syphilis Campaigns Fall Short Despite
Their Potent Biomedical Tools

Elimination plans have not reached their goals despite having the scientific potential to do so. There are multiple dimensions to the reasons why these programs have fallen short of their goals, both scientific and social.

Biological and epidemiological properties of HIV and syphilis impede elimination programs. A prolonged asymptomatic period of contagion and the diseases' spread in private settings make it difficult to capture individuals who need to be identified, treated, and contact traced. This challenges accurate surveillance, the sine qua non for control programs. In asymptomatic people, a high-HIV viral load in genital secretions or the presence of spirochetes in a chancre can spread infection.[95] AIDS and syphilis differ from the only human epidemic that has been eliminated globally to date, smallpox, which is contagious only during overt signs of disease (e.g., visible rash).[96] In addition, the most effective biomedical tool for prevention, a vaccine, has been elusive due to an inability to map key elements of immunity of HIV and syphilis.[97] The spread of STDs in nonpublic settings challenges accurate contact tracing because people may be reluctant to divulge private information to public health officials they do not trust. The transmission of smallpox can be more easily tracked as it frequently affects household contacts.[98]

Logistical factors, including lack of appropriate facilities, infrastructure, and manpower, also interfere with elimination campaigns. Creating the proper infrastructure for testing, treating, and retention in care is necessary as diseases now increasingly occur in rural areas worldwide.[99] This includes having an adequate supply of medical personnel who have expertise in HIV, not just in urban areas, where experts tend to be available, but also in rural areas, both globally and in the United States.[100] In the United States, for example, there are shortages of qualified HIV-treating physicians to cover geographically dispersed rural areas where there have been outbreaks associated with intravenous drug use.[101] Also, a lack of adequate facilities staffed with expert physicians knowledgeable about ART and about how to handle toxicities, treatment failure, and drug resistance is a mounting problem.[102] Potential strategies to address the growing number of HIV patients who reside in rural areas globally include telemedicine and mobile health units.

Concomitant epidemics (syndemics) interfere with elimination programs and fuel their spread. Drug dependence created by the opioid epidemic, for example, threatens compliance with medical regimens and increases risk of transmission due to sharing of needles or failure to use condoms when a person is disinhibited when high.[103] The need to provide competent drug addiction management, including provision of long-acting opioid treatment, is key to achieving adherence to HIV medication regimens.[104] Management of mental health issues, in addition, are also necessary to assure linkage to care and adherence to HIV medicines.[105] Surges of new epidemics, such as COVID, indirectly interfere with HIV/AIDS programs by creating clinic closures that disrupt their availability for non-COVID conditions like syphilis and AIDS. Consequently, COVID surges can disrupt linkage to HIV care, threaten medication adherence, and impede outcomes of elimination plans.[106] The COVID pandemic may also impact LMICs globally because lockdowns and border closures can interrupt production of medicines and distribution of generic HIV drugs, potentially increasing their cost.[107]

The moral framing of syphilis and AIDS continues to interfere with public health efforts to eliminate them. Historians have emphasized how the judgment of venereal diseases by social hygienists persisted beyond the introduction of science and interfered with early twentieth-century public health efforts to handle STDs.[108] The moral undertone of discussions about syphilis, although not as evident in public health efforts today, has persisted. People with STDs continue to feel ashamed and guilty. Stigma deters many from being tested and receiving treatment, as some prefer to keep their diagnosis secret.[109] In fact, in 2018 the CDC reported that eight of ten people with HIV continued to report feeling internalized stigma.[110] This shame impacts patients, preventing them from revealing their status to their employers, coworkers, and family members.[111]

The issue of internalized stigma may be mitigated for some who reach "undetectable" HIV status while on ART and who are therefore uninfectable (U = U).[112] Nonetheless, the challenge to discover cases and care for all patients diagnosed with syphilis, AIDS, or other STIs is best mitigated by empowering those who feel stigmatized so they will not be reluctant to get tested. An easing of negative feelings may also encourage the patient to reveal the identity of their contacts, who can then also be tested. Empowered STI patients will not resist obtaining the health care they need to remain healthy, thereby preventing the spread of disease to others.[113] Strategies to mitigate stigma, including counseling by respected peers, are being implemented for AIDS, syphilis, and other STIs, but their effectiveness remains unestablished.[114]

Some elected officials have been reluctant to use effective programs (e.g., PrEP, treatment of drug dependence, needle exchange programs, licensing and medically examining sex workers), out of fear of encouraging behaviors they consider morally distasteful.[115] The idea that moral reformers consider the real cause of disease to be depravity and not a microbe was reflected in the abstinence-only HIV-prevention programs promoted by President George W. Bush as part of his PEPFAR program, long after they were shown to be ineffective.[116] These priorities also continue to be reflected across other health initiatives, such as by those who decline the HPV vaccine, which effectively reduces cervical cancers, out of fear of encouraging proscribed behavior in preteens.[117] Likewise, those who forecast that elimination of HIV will be possible if a vaccine becomes available must acknowledge that some may hesitate to use an HIV vaccine out of fear of encouraging sexual promiscuity.

The moral framing of STDs continues to threaten the process of finding and reporting cases and tracking contacts, which public health officials have relied on to control syphilis.[118] Parran, for example, believed he could capture cases and their contacts with a "Wasserman Dragnet." Baumgartner sought to eliminate the "margin of failure," and the current UNAIDS plan seeks to diagnose 90 percent of cases. But can any campaign realistically overcome the hurdles involved in capturing the majority of infected people? In addition to problematic moral framing, biologic factors (asymptomatic periods of contagiousness) and epidemiologic issues (tracking contacts in private settings) present difficulties. These factors, as well as the socioeconomic issues outlined next, characterize both syphilis and AIDS and weaken the assumption that epidemics of STDs can be ended at all.

Syphilis and AIDS show that biomedically based public health programs must address socioeconomic factors that drive epidemics and create risky environments that confound disease elimination campaigns. Katinka de Wet, a sociologist at the University of the Free State in South Africa, and public health experts Richard Crosby, professor of public health at the University of Kentucky, and Ralph Diclemente, professor in the Department of Social and Behavioral Sciences at the College of Global Health, New York University, argue that elimination campaigns have not adequately taken social sciences into consideration.[119] Medical investigators from Luther Terry's 1962 task force and from the IOM in 1997 also acknowledged the need for elimination programs to address social issues.[120] The medical anthropologist Paul Farmer noted a tendency for public health approaches to seek predominantly biological solutions about what are in fact "biosocial phenomena."[121] Scholars from diverse backgrounds have insisted on the continued need for public health programs to address social issues in conjunction with biomedical issues.

Authors have elaborated on the socioeconomic factors that influence disease outcomes, which are the social determinants of health. African Americans, for example, experience lower economic status, fewer job opportunities, and greater risk behaviors, including transactional sex and intravenous drug use.

Lower economic status is also associated with less access to preventive information and health care.[122] Residents of lower-income neighborhoods exhibit social risk factors, including higher rates of drug use and high-risk sexual norms that create high-risk populations and vulnerable environments.[123] The persistence of disease in these populations and environments—inner-city, predominantly African American neighborhoods in the southeastern United States, adolescents, people using illicit drugs, incarcerated individuals, people who have migrated due to work or refugee status, transgender populations, among others—has thwarted the biomedical efforts to eliminate diseases.[124]

Social determinants both create a vulnerable environment for the spread of HIV and syphilis and interfere with attempts to control these diseases. These include gender-power imbalance, leaving female sex workers unable to negotiate use of condoms with their clients and creating conditions where women are victims of violence. Determinants also include poverty and lack of educational opportunities, which create environments where people assume risky behaviors to survive or to seek escape from their dismal circumstances.[125] Poverty, especially in regions where there are income inequalities, leads women to enter the sex industry, or others to inject drugs.[126] Poverty can also lead to displaced populations (e.g., migrant workers), who might assume risky behavior and sexual disinhibition when removed from the constraints of their usual social circles.[127] It can also lead to crime and incarceration, another environment that is prone to the spread of STDs and disruption of care, both during incarceration and following release.[128] Likewise, armed conflict and natural disasters create displaced populations that are removed from normal communal restraints and therefore susceptible to unprotected promiscuity. Introduction of newer technologies has created social conditions that lead to novel environmental vulnerabilities. Computer-app dating services that do not require identification information, for example, have increased the number of contacts with anonymous partners who cannot be traced.[129] Numerous social factors create these risky environments for infection and interfere with elimination programs.

Racism interferes with patients' trust in doctors and therefore threatens adherence to medical advice, retention in care, and cooperation with medication.[130] Mistrust has been particularly evident in African Americans living in the southern United States following Tuskegee (chapter 4).[131] These marginalized populations, both within a country and across nations, account for what Baumgartner in 1962 called the difficult-to-reach "margins"—or disenfranchised populations, to use today's terminology.[132] These populations account in part for the inconsistency in eliminating epidemics and the geographic "hot spots" of STDs that persist in the United States and globally.

The syphilis elimination plans—the UNAIDS 90-90-90 plan and the EHE plan—acknowledge the importance of social issues, but they have not provided tangible strategies to resolve these problems. The UNAIDS plan states, "Urgent efforts are similarly needed to scale up . . . prevention strategies . . . to eliminate stigma, discrimination and social exclusion."[133] But like the syphilis programs of the 1940s, 1960s, and 1990s, the UNAIDS plan fails to outline an approach to "eliminate" them. Furthermore, neither the AIDS nor the syphilis programs have addressed how they would sustain funding to reach their accelerated goals within one generation (as set forth by Parran in 1936 and Clinton in 2011) or one decade (as set forth by Terry in 1962, UNAIDS in 2013, and EHE in 2019).

The global scale of the UNAIDS campaign, as well as the appearance of new, unexpected social and behavioral problems, creates new complexities in elimination campaigns. The need to provide costly ART for a lifetime compounds the existing challenges of sustained funding, retention in care, medicine adherence, and loss of follow-up that are especially pertinent in LMICs, which are battling overburdened health systems and shortages of staff and medicines. Furthermore, unexpected HIV outbreaks (including via needle-sharing and in multigenerational, rural populations addicted to prescription narcotic drugs) underscore the difficulties of HIV surveillance.[134] These difficulties are compounded by the growing number of people under the influence of drugs (e.g., methamphetamine) and the growing popularity of soliciting anonymous sexual partners through the internet.[135] The significance of socioeconomic factors for public health campaigns has prompted public health expert Hunter Handsfield to state, "Biomedical strategies are inherently insufficient to control any STD."[136] Over the years, public health officials have increasingly offered structural interventions to address social determinants that influence risky behavior at the environmental level, as outlined in chapter 6.[137]

Budgetary and political factors are also obstacles to achieving elimination campaign goals. It can be difficult to sustain adequate funding for campaigns, particularly during times of vacillating economic stability.[138] For several syphilis campaigns, funding has been reduced as infection rates began to decline, and funding was no longer thought to be necessary as other, more pressing political priorities arose. Similarly for HIV, because UNAIDS does not provide subsidies, it is unclear whether the projected incremental costs of approximately $26 billion per year can be achieved. At the end of 2019, for example, only $18.6 billion was available—an inadequate 70 percent of what is needed to achieve UNAIDS goals.[139] It remains to be seen whether the political will of local and international communities that is needed to support the plan can be sustained for decades. Funding programs of donor countries are at risk of dropping in priority, particularly during periods of transition between administrations, thereby jeopardizing PEPFAR, the Ryan White program, and EHE.[140] Furthermore, LMICs cannot contribute the necessary remaining amount, as even discounted prices of drugs remain above per capita incomes. Nonetheless, to keep the global AIDS response on course, UNAIDS is calling for yearly HIV investments in LMICs to rise to a peak of $29 billion by 2025—a goal that may be unattainable.[141] For these reasons, some experts are uncertain whether society can end the HIV epidemic within the UNAIDS-specified time frame.[142]

Syphilis and AIDS underscore the problem of how to customize a general campaign to local regions in a culturally sensitive manner. This is particularly relevant given variations in the risks that "drive" epidemics in different locales nationally and globally, ranging from intravenous drug use in some regions (e.g., inner-city areas in the United States and Eastern Europe; rural United States) to unsafe activities between MSM (e.g., Down Low populations in southeastern America) and heterosexual transmission in women (in, e.g., sub-Saharan Africa). Prevention-and-control combination programs, according to WHO, must have the flexibility to allow for tailoring to the particular risk behavior that drives HIV in a specific locale.[143] When a program is sensitive to a culture, the messaging resonates with stakeholders living in that community.[144] Challenges arise in how to recruit and fund peer leaders and facilitators so that public health messages (e.g., get tested, enroll in care, etc.) will influence the behavior of members of the community.[145] Peer education remains an effective tool with long-term impact for behavior change among high-risk HIV groups worldwide (e.g., sex workers, inner-city populations).[146] Scaling this model to global, diverse communities (e.g., Eastern European drug users) is a significant challenge, as is enlisting peer leaders to communicate the messaging.

Campaigns against AIDS and syphilis have made bold predictions by identifying ambitious goals of successful elimination programs within specified timelines. It could be argued that there are several advantages to this approach: to galvanize workers toward achieving a specific, time-sensitive goal; to inspire collaboration to accomplish difficult tasks; to make elimination a priority that is supported by tax funding. Phrases like "ending AIDS" and "AIDS-free generation" are emotional, and they reinforce deeply rooted Enlightenment ideals of human control over unpredictable natural events. But promoting programs with bold predictions can have real downsides when programs fail to meet their goals. Feelings of burnout or resignation may develop among workers if target milestones are not achieved by the designated dates. Another risk is the fostering of mistrust in public health officials and the medical system for promising results that do not materialize.

Individual responsibility cannot entirely be discounted as a factor for people who do not adopt harm-reduction behaviors because they believe they are perceived to impinge on personal liberties. Historically, blame has been placed on all individuals with STIs for contracting the disease; the disease itself implied an underlying character defect and a degree of irresponsibility. To some extent, identifying social determinants of illness takes responsibility away from the individual and locates the vulnerability in environmental factors. But even with provisions (insurance coverage, culture-appropriate case-managers to help navigate medical needs), some people cannot maintain their medical care—and, by proxy help to eliminate the epidemic. Some are unwilling to adhere to their medicines—often due to medication fatigue or mistrust in science, or the use the use of illicit drugs that can derail a pill-taking routine. The consequence of not complying with ART is the risk of spreading the virus. Rectifying risky environments, mitigating social determinants of HIV, and making provisions for engaging people in care in culturally respectful ways will result in a greater number of people who meet their treatment targets (an undetectable viral load). For the remaining patients, newer insights into lack of adherence with medical advice is needed.

Legal issues can interfere with efforts to eliminate epidemics. Laws in several states—those, for example, that prevent addiction treatment, needle exchange, or syringe purchasing—are examples of counterproductive laws. Adherence to treatment is impossible if adequate management of drug dependence is not provided.[147] Similarly, laws that make homosexuality illegal interfere with strategies to improve testing and retention in care in those locations, as they discourage gay individuals from being tested.[148] Laws that penalize same-sex intercourse contribute to a perpetuation of stigma and discrimination. In many African nations, laws criminalizing homosexuality may be fueling the epidemic, as they dissuade key populations from seeking treatment and healthcare providers from offering it. Laws against needle exchange programs and same-sex intercourse are directed toward eliminating the unwanted behavior—drug use and same-sex intercourse—and interfere with efforts to control the epidemics. Changing these laws is an important structural intervention to rectify vulnerability of the legal environment.

Conclusion

Biomedical tools are powerful and necessary, but as this chapter shows, they are insufficient to end epidemics. Public health programs must be comprehensive and seek to rectify socioeconomic factors that lead to risky behavior and interfere with elimination campaigns. All campaigns, from the syphilis campaigns in the 1930s to the HIV and syphilis campaigns of today, have acknowledged the importance of changing the social environment that leads to risky behavior, including stigma, discrimination, poverty, and discrimination against women. But none have provided a practicable road map to rectify these socioeconomic factors, which drive epidemics and challenge elimination campaigns.

Consequently, the stories of AIDS and syphilis shed light on the boundaries of biomedicine. They testify to the ingenuity of our biomedical therapies and reinforce their power to heal individuals. But they unveil the limitations of biomedicine in the realm of public health. AIDS and syphilis continue to pose threats to individuals, families, and communities—particularly in LMICs and poor inner-city regions in developed countries—despite scientifically feasible campaigns to eliminate them. The narrative of biomedicine has evolved from a 1950s confidence in the potency of anti-infectives and vaccines to eliminate epidemics, to a more measured picture today. The narrative began with the promise of living in an epidemic-free world (chapters 1 and 2) but now rests in the reality that people must live with epidemics and their control programs (chapter 3). The view of biomedicine as triumphant and having limitless powers has yielded to a more modified view of biomedicine as having limited powers—as necessary but insufficient to eliminate disease in the population.

Likewise, an examination of elimination campaigns alters the narratives of AIDS and syphilis themselves. It has become evident that the goal of elimination is elusive. Biomedicine has not provided the neat, bookended closure desired. Rather than terminating the syphilis and AIDS epidemics, biomedicine becomes a part of their ongoing narrative. The promise of biomedicine to end the devastation to individuals and burden to society eventually becomes tempered by the reality that the epidemics persist unevenly in the population. Individuals learn to live with this enduring reality, and with the biomedically based efforts to eliminate them. Syphilis and AIDS, and their associated medical and social undertakings, have become part of our human experience. The following chapter will show how the histories of AIDS and syphilis can be used not only to shed light on the limitations of biomedicine, but also to illustrate notorious situations that have undermined elimination programs.

Chapter 4

Legacies of Mistrust

Syphilis and AIDS

Events throughout the AIDS and syphilis epidemics have fueled mistrust in science, doctors, public health officials, and the government. Ethical lapses during human experimentation and research and in patient care have led to public outcry that medical investigators are callous. Notable coercive public health interventions have deprived individuals of their livelihoods, leading some to question whether public health officials have the best interests of patients in mind. Government inactivity has led to suspicions that some elected officials involved in public health policies do not care about the lives of disease sufferers. Finally, government prioritization of the economy over public health has produced suspicion about the motives of government. These episodes, like the spectacular advances (chapters 1, 2) and limitations (chapter 3) of elimination programs are a part of the complex legacy of syphilis, AIDS, and biomedicine. The episodes reinforce the long historical roots of suspicion of biomedicine, medical scientists, and public health that have been reflected in cultural representations of scientific medicine.

Ethical Lapses Involving Syphilis and AIDS

Ethical violations in human experimentation involving syphilis and AIDS have gained the attention of the popular press. These notorious episodes have resulted in a public impression that patients' well-being is not the foremost concern of doctors and other officials, who can exploit people for ulterior motives—for example, to acquire new knowledge (as in the case of researcher Udo Wile), to validate racial prejudices (as occurred in Tuskegee, Alabama), or to advance a particular ideology (as exemplified by South African president Thabo Mbeki). Together, these episodes reinforce a notion that patients are often misled by doctors and officials and treated as a means to an end, rather than being treated purely for the benefit of the patient. The conducting of trials of unclear benefit that exploit vulnerable populations is part of the legacy of syphilis and AIDS.

From 1913 to 1917, Udo Wile, a professor of dermatology and syphilology at the University of Michigan, performed, without consent, experimental brain puncture in patients with paresis from syphilis. His research premise had potential therapeutic implications: if living spirochetes were in the brain, direct installation of Salvarsan into the brain might be beneficial. Salvarsan given in the usual routes, through IV (intravenously) or IM (intramuscularly), had not been effective in treating syphilitic paresis. But Wile did not directly state this potential therapeutic utility. Furthermore, the study utilized an experimental trephining operation in a vulnerable and impaired population.[1] The study, therefore, had no clearly stated purpose and was potentially hazardous. Wile's procedure involved drilling a hole, then inserting a long needle through the skin and bone, "push[ing] firmly and deeply into the cortex . . . [of the brain, then removing] . . . by suction, a . . . cylinder of brain substance . . . into the syringe."[2] Wile performed brain punctures on six patients institutionalized at Pontiac State Hospital in Michigan without informing them or their representatives about the procedure or its risks.[3] Wile did find living spirochetes in brain cortex tissue of these six patients based on rabbit inoculation studies.[4] But he did not address the therapeutic significance of his findings.[5]

Wile's human experiment was denounced in lay periodicals and the medical press shortly after his publication. He was accused of exposing patients to a potentially harmful procedure for no direct therapeutic purpose or clear benefit to the subjects, and of not informing subjects of his intention.[6] Wile's experiments were viewed even in their day as a breach in medical ethics.[7] But debate over the use of incapacitated subjects without consent continued as some doctors argued that patients with paresis would die anyway, as standard therapies were ineffective.[8] Nonetheless, as historian Susan Lederer has pointed out, Walter Cannon, president of the American Medical Association (AMA) Council on Defense of Medical Research, viewed Wile's experiment as unethical because of its improper use of human subjects in experiments.[9] AMA president William Williams Keen agreed that Wile's case demanded condemnation.[10] Newspapers emphasized the unethical nature of Wile's work.[11] But the sentiment was not uniform.[12] This revealed a public divide between the defense of potentially helpful research and the need for protection from unscrupulous doctors. Furthermore, Wile technically was not in violation of the AMA's

1847 Code of Ethics, which made no mention at the time of rights and responsibilities surrounding human research.[13] Notwithstanding these considerations, Wile's use of invasive methods aroused an outcry among physicians and the lay public.

The medical profession has recently criticized the pathologist Aldred Warthin (chapter 1) for his controversial early twentieth-century views about eugenics. Warthin's concern for the maternal transmission of syphilis formed the basis of his views toward eugenics. At the 1928 Race Betterment Conference in Battle Creek, Michigan, Warthin proposed that religion and the concept of forgiveness of sin paradoxically harmed humans by enabling the transmission of syphilis.[14] To compensate for what he viewed as religion's tacit sanctioning of reproduction for all humans, he encouraged students contemplating marriage to examine their ancestral backgrounds to avoid the transmittal of syphilis between mother and infant. Warthin believed that the only means to improve the collective hereditary "germ plasm," or cellular material that is passed on from generation to generation, came through the voluntary application of eugenics.[15] He did not define the unfit germ plasm according to race or ethnicity, but attributed it to a group including what he referred to as "the insane, feeble-minded, the drunkards, dope-fiends and prostitutes, suicides, and the criminal."[16] He argued that the church, by advocating reproduction regardless of the quality of germ plasma, contributed to the decline of the race. He asked his medical students to pick mates based on their germ plasm qualities instead of romantic attraction. Although Warthin's views have not received national attention, in 2019 the Department of Pathology at the University of Michigan publicly announced its decision to remove two endowed collegiate professorships in Warthin's name because of his eugenic views.[17]

Thomas Parran, U.S. surgeon general from 1932 to 1948 (chapter 1), was himself involved in controversy. During his sixteen-year service as surgeon general, the USPHS carried out the Tuskegee and Guatemala syphilis studies, which exploited vulnerable populations and deprived sufferers of effective therapy. Although the extent of Parran's involvement in approving, funding, and providing oversight for these human experimentation studies is unestablished, the fact remains that his role as the surgeon general was to oversee the USPHS. It is puzzling to reconcile his documented advocacy for widespread testing and treatment as an essential component of his U.S. eradication campaign with the fact that he oversaw a study in Tuskegee that systematically withheld treatment from African American men. Due to his involvement in these studies, the University of Pittsburgh decided to remove Parran's name from a campus building in the School of Public Health in 2018, and the American Sexually Transmitted

Diseases Association removed his name from its Lifetime Achievement Award in 2013.[18]

The most publicized example of ethical misconduct regarding human experimentation of syphilis is the USPHS study carried out in Tuskegee, Alabama, from 1932 to 1972. Susan Reverby and others have written extensively about this experiment, in which effective treatment was denied on a racial basis to underprivileged, poor sharecroppers over the course of four decades.[19] The Tuskegee experiment began as a test-and-treat eradication trial, but rather than shuttering it in 1932, when the trial was defunded during the Great Depression, USPHS officials repurposed it as a study of untreated syphilis.[20] The revised intention was to prove a racist hypothesis that Black men were more likely to develop cardiovascular damage than neurologic damage because their brains were less developed than those of white people. The study withheld therapy to four hundred black men, then correlated clinical findings with postmortem examinations. The USPHS officers were able to recruit volunteers into the study by promising treatment to men who had no other access to medical care. Subjects were deprived of the best available treatments at the beginning of the experiment: Salvarsan, and penicillin when it later became available.[21] From 1936 to 1970, six peer-reviewed articles were published in medical journals, one every four to six years, documenting that those with untreated syphilis died at higher rates than those without the disease (see Figure 4.1).[22] USPHS officials did not end the study until 1972, when an employee of USPHS leaked the story to the Associated Press and an ensuing *Washington Star* article exposed the study as a racist, unethical abuse of state power by public health officials.[23]

Objections to the Tuskegee study were interrogated by venereologists. Rudolph Kampmeier, for example, claimed that many of the subjects who had enrolled had had pre-existing late syphilis for at least twenty-five years, and that most with long-standing neurological and cardiac syphilis would not have improved with penicillin.[24] Did Kampmeier's objection have any empirical basis? At the time, there were no controlled trials to address whether penicillin would or would not benefit people with late neurologic manifestations of syphilis.[25] Nonetheless, researchers withheld therapy that had the potential to improve the lives of subjects with advanced syphilis.

In addition to causing unnecessary suffering for individuals, the Tuskegee study and its legacy exacerbated a breakdown of trust among Black people, physicians, and government officials due to ethical violations in human experimentation that had happened before, including, among others, unethical gynecological procedures performed on African American enslaved people by the nineteenth-century U.S. surgeon J. Marion Sims.[26] The Tuskegee-fueled

MORTALITY COMPARED

The relative mortality of syphilitic patients compared to nonsyphilitic controls is shown somewhat differently in Figs. 2A, 2B, and 3. As all previous workers in this study have found, the most striking single feature distinguishing the syphilitic group from the nonsyphilitic is that the death rate is higher among the syphilitic men. Exactly how and why more of the syphilitic group has died is not clearly discernible, but the penalty which the syphilitic patients have paid in terms of life expectancy is well documented.[5]

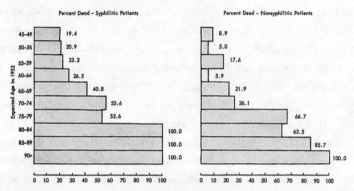

Fig. 3.—Mortality of syphilitic and nonsyphilitic patients, compared by percentage of each age group who have died during study period.

In Fig. 3, the mortality percentages of the deceased, by age group, are compared. Here again is seen the higher mortality of the syphilitic patients in each age group, with the exception of the 75- to 79-year-old category, where the death rate for nonsyphilitic is higher than that for syphilitic men. Such a difference serves to point out how the diseases of the aged enter the picture and seem to level the differences in the mortality experience of the men as they enter their later decades.

Figure 4.1. Page from a 1955 medical publication describing the Tuskegee experiments. It indicates increased death rates due to syphilis. Despite this finding, treatment was withheld from the study subjects who had syphilis, and the study was continued for another seventeen years after the publication of this report. From L. S. Shuman, Sydney Olansky, Eunice Rivers, C.A. Smith, and Dorothy Rambo, "Untreated Syphilis in the Male Negro: Background and Current Status of Patients in the Tuskegee Study," *Journal of Chronic Diseases* 2, no. 5 (November 1955): 543–558. Used with permission of Elsevier Inc.

mistrust has compromised health care utilization by Black men and other minorities today, as outlined in this book in the context of HIV and COVID (chapters 2, 5).[27]

The USPHS conducted a separate syphilis study from 1946 to 1948 in Guatemalan prisons to assess whether taking penicillin immediately after sex would prevent syphilis and other VDs. This goal was defensible because it was unknown whether penicillin was useful in this context. The study was flawed, however, because it exploited underprivileged communities by deliberately exposing prisoners to syphilis.[28] The purposeful transmission of potentially life-threatening STDs in Guatemala had been approved by USPHS officer John Cutler and funded by the NIH. In the study, prostitutes with active syphilis were paid to have sex with prisoners in Guatemala City's central penitentiary. Some subjects were infected by having sex with uninfected prostitutes who had been directly inoculated with infectious material on their cervices. The study enrolled fifteen hundred subjects but ended prematurely because it proved difficult to transfer disease. It was never published. The CDC and NIH later deemed the study unethical because researchers deliberately exposed subjects to serious health threats, did not obtain consent of study subjects, and used vulnerable populations. President Obama's 2011 presidential commission concluded that the experiments had violated ethical standards of 1946, even though there was little regulation of medical experimentation at the time.

As these examples show, ethical breaches in human experimentation have taken place in the context of syphilis in studies where medical investigators were willing to sacrifice their subjects' well-being to gain medical knowledge. Objections to these incidents have been well publicized in the lay press. In addition, just as a public apology was issued to the survivors of Tuskegee by President Clinton in 1997, an apology was extended to Guatemala by President Obama.[29] The revelations about Tuskegee and Guatemala deepened entrenched suspicions about scientists and doctors, and have contributed to reluctance on the part of minority populations to participate in medical studies or adhere to medical care.

Several incidents that occurred during the AIDS epidemic have also fueled mistrust in medicine. The stereotyping of Africans as primitive and incapable of following complex ART regimens was an obvious example of structural racism perpetuating medical inequalities. In addition, insufficient trust was evident in 1986, for example, when activists objected to medical investigators using placebos during randomized trials (chapter 2). Investigators did not violate the ethical standards of the day, but some citizens became suspicious that doctors and governmental officials were not doing everything possible to save the lives of patients.[30] Although the investigators had not misled subjects, they were accused of being callous for not caring about the well-being of their subjects.[31] Investigators, on the other hand, maintained that they could not know with certainty whether a drug could be effective unless it was part of a trial using an untreated control group (see chapter 5).[32] A more notorious controversy emerged in the late 1990s in a study conducted in nine countries in Africa, when a control group of HIV-infected pregnant women was given placebos rather than effective ART regimens, which by then were available to prevent vertical transmission. This raised legitimate ethical objections about a contradiction between how subjects were being treated in sponsor countries and in LMICs, and underscored inequalities between clinical practice standards in sponsoring countries and African countries.[33]

A recent ethical lapse involving gene editing in a non-HIV-infected person has fueled long-standing mistrust in medicine and physicians. In 2018, He Jiankui, a Chinese physician, claimed that he had genetically edited the embryos of twins before they were implanted in their mother's womb. He infused gene-edited (CCR5 deleted) cells into an embryo that was not HIV infected for the presumed purpose of protecting the fetuses against HIV infection. The two girls were not HIV infected, but the genetic edit would, according to the researcher, protect the girls from acquiring their father's HIV infection. His experiment was unethical because the safety of the procedure was unknown, and there are established, safer ways to prevent HIV infections. He had resorted to unethical practices to achieve what he claimed was a greater good. His experiment drew criticism from scientists around the world.[34] As a result, He's work is another highly visible example of an ethical lapse in human experimentation.

In the 2000s, an episode in South Africa raised concerns about mistrust in government in the context of public health. President Thabo Mbeki denied that a virus caused AIDS.[35] Mbeki based his ideas on the work of Peter Duesberg, a one-time prominent cancer researcher from the University of California, Berkeley, who switched the focus of his research to AIDS. In 2000, Mbeki appointed Duesberg to a panel of AIDS advisers along with other researchers who denied a viral cause of AIDS.[36] The resultant governmental policies prevented the rollout of ART in South Africa at a time when 20 percent of the population tested HIV positive. Mbeki refused to purchase ART on the grounds that buying the drugs would fuel the profit of developed nations that had exploited Africa since colonization.[37] Mbeki lost the chance to prevent high rates of AIDS-related mortality and to reduce South Africa's high rates of HIV prevalence. Studies estimate that the withholding of ART during Mbeki's administration led to as many as 330,000 preventable deaths. HIV denialism and Mbeki's failure to implement government-sponsored ART occurred during a time when the benefits of ART were well known.[38]

Duesberg has never withdrawn his belief in HIV denialism. He has maintained that HIV is an incidental "passenger virus" and that AIDS is caused by environmental toxins.[39] Duesberg has also been accused of fraudulent research.[40] He is under investigation at Berkeley for having made false claims in a paper.[41]

Duesberg's HIV denialism and alleged misconduct may have tarnished an ide-
alized image of the medical scientist as beneficent that reached its apogee in
mid-twentieth-century America.

Misguided, Coercive, and Indifferent Public Health Efforts

There have also been misguided public health attempts to control syphilis and
AIDS. These attempts sought to regulate behavior according to societal norms
rather than focusing on scientific public health approaches. With syphilis, in
the early 1900s, the social hygiene movement targeted removing social evils,
and some physicians were reluctant to use Salvarsan for fear of converting what
some viewed as a moral infraction into a medically treatable disease.[42] For AIDS
in the early 2000s, PEPFAR-associated restrictions required that prevention
funds be devoted to abstinence and fidelity, long after these methods had been
shown to be ineffective.[43] There are many current-day examples of these attempts. For example, some elected government officials have been hesitant to
adopt needle exchange programs because of a concern that they encourage drug
habits, though studies show otherwise.[44] Likewise, some religious groups in the
late nineteenth century in the United States resisted the adoption of regular
licensing, inspection, and regulation of brothels in fear that such measures perpetuate rather than eliminate prostitution.[45] Others have been slow to institute
PrEP out of concern that it would encourage sexual promiscuity. Outcomes have
suffered when public health programs have regarded diseases like AIDS or syphilis as a means of controlling sexuality.

Syphilis and AIDS have also been associated with historical instances of
unnecessarily coercive public health practices at the expense of civil liberties.
The government has at times gone too far in the name of hygiene to abridge the
rights of those perceived as potentially threatening the greater good. To control
rates of syphilis, there were mandatory detentions of sex workers and closures
of brothels during World War I and postwar (see chapter 1).[46] In this case,
public health officials rescinded people's livelihood for years to protect the
public good. For AIDS, there was talk of compulsory testing and quarantining
those who tested positive—an abridgement of a person's individual rights (see
chapter 2).[47] These coercive measures were never adopted for AIDS, in part
because of challenges from patient representatives.[48] For both syphilis and
AIDS, these well-publicized compulsory measures came at a cost to individuals, whose personal freedoms were rescinded or threatened with abridgement.

There have been notable periods of government inactivity in the realm of
public health. For syphilis, there have been repeated episodes of premature
rescinding of funding for elimination programs.[49] The inability to commit the

sustained funding needed to eradicate the disease has in part been responsible for the failure of elimination programs.[50] Furthermore, when AIDS was uniformly fatal in the 1980s, President Reagan did not provide federal funding for clinical care or research programs (see chapter 2).[51] Due to the exposure of governmental inactivity by patient representatives, federal funding for AIDS research expanded substantially by 1985, and approval and licensing processes for drugs were streamlined.[52] When a splinter group of AIDS activists, Treatment Action Group, worked in harmony with pharmaceutical companies to encourage basic research as the best path forward, potent HIV drugs were developed.[53]

Episodes Involving Syphilis and AIDS Bolster a Critique of Biomedicine

To recap, the misapplication of scientific medicine in the context of syphilis and AIDS research and treatment has eroded trust in biomedicine, physicians, and government officials. Marginalized populations have felt they were misled by doctors who behaved unethically by exploiting patients for the sake of advancing knowledge or reinforcing prejudices. These well-publicized lapses in the handling of both syphilis and AIDS have also intensified a legacy of suspicion and mistrust of science, medicine, and public health and have interfered with efforts to control them. Mistrust in physicians, in turn, undermines the beneficent, powerful narrative of biomedicine that had reached its apogee in the mid-twentieth century.

Suspicion and critique of scientific medicine and doctors, in fact, have long historical roots independent of syphilis and AIDS. This critique has been evident in both historical events and cultural representations of scientific medicine since the 1800s. In the nineteenth century, when physicians at the Paris School of Medicine were correlating premortem observations of large numbers of patients with postmortem findings, a concern developed that doctors were becoming more interested in the advancement of science rather than in patients' overall well-being.[54] It was during this period that European and American fictional works addressing the callousness of doctors and the misuse of science in medicine became popular. In her famous 1816 novel, *Frankenstein*, for example, English author Mary Shelley depicts protagonist Victor Frankenstein's motivation to become a medical investigator following his mother's death. Victor's investigations are so successful that he can create life. But when his male creation requests that Victor create a female companion, he refuses to comply out of fear of originating a self-propagating breed of human-made creatures.[55] The creature then retaliates against Victor's family. Shelley portrays medical science as powerful, but suggests that doctors can be callous and cause harm when they misuse science.

American author Nathanial Hawthorne later wrote *Rappaccini's Daughter*, an 1844 novel about an Italian medical researcher, Giacomo Rappaccini, who studies the effects of poisonous plants on humans.[56] Rappaccini grows the plants in a garden and tests them in humans. He chooses to give the plants to his daughter. She survives by developing resistance to their effects, but in the process she poisons others, including her neighbor Giovanni. Hawthorne, like Shelley, depicts the productive and destructive powers of scientific discovery, and the whims of medical investigators as central to those powers.

The nineteenth-century critique of medical science in literary works continued with the work of antivaccinationist British playwright George Bernard Shaw prior to the introduction of regulatory agencies in the early twentieth century. Vaccine opposition had been present in the United States since inoculation of pustular material from people with smallpox was introduced into the skin of an uninfected person in the early eighteenth century, and in England since the introduction of vaccination for smallpox in the late eighteenth century. Since the early nineteenth century, opponents of smallpox vaccination feared that the dangers of vaccination outweighed any possible benefit. Antivaccination leagues developed in the early 1800s in reaction to Edward Jenner's vaccination, with their objection stemming from sanitary concerns over scoring the flesh on a child's arm with a quill.[57] In addition, opposition in England throughout the nineteenth century was based on religious objections (because the substance derived from an animal), scientific objections (due to a belief that vaccines wouldn't work because disease came from miasma, not contagion), and political grounds (based on the view that vaccines violated personal liberty). Objections to smallpox vaccination persisted in America, as noted by historian Judith Walzer Leavitt, among German immigrants in Milwaukee at the turn of the twentieth century.[58] At the time, American pharmaceutical companies had been vigorously promoting vaccines targeting a wide range of microbes without systematic testing. This occurred prior to the development of FDA regulations for safety and efficacy.[59] To people like Shaw, this indiscriminate practice gave the impression that physicians were acting primarily for their own profit.

Shaw showcases these themes in his 1906 play *Doctor's Dilemma*, in which Shaw depicts a physician investigator, Alonso Ridgeon, who develops a life-saving cure for tuberculosis.[60] But he does not have enough of the product to treat all his patients. When deciding who gets curative treatment, Ridgeon's judgment is clouded by his attraction to the wife of one of his patients, and he decides on that basis to withhold the drug from his patient. Shaw implies that medical scientists do not always make decisions objectively, nor can they escape their self-interests.

The critique of biomedicine and its practitioners extended beyond these literary works to include challenges from a range of academicians. In his 1959 critique of biomedicine, *Mirage of Health*, René Dubos, who was head of microbiology at the Rockefeller Institute, contests any notion that biomedicine could render epidemic diseases obsolete. As civilizations unfold, he reasons, unforeseen consequences of human activities will alter the environment such that they will inevitably unleash new infectious epidemics.[61] Epidemiologist Thomas McKeown pointed out in the 1970s that the decline of several epidemic diseases had preceded the advent of vaccines and chemotherapy.[62] The control of these diseases could not have been credited to biomedical advances, he reasoned, but rather to better sanitation and nutrition. Philosopher Michel Foucault interrogated the objectivity of scientific knowledge itself. He considered the categorization of diseases by medical experts during the Paris School as an exercise in using their special knowledge to exert social control over behavior deemed undesirable.[63] Foucault asserted that medical scientists are not more noble or objective than others; they are prey to bias and unfairness like anybody else.

To compound this multifaceted literary and academic critique of biomedicine, society has also become disillusioned with medical scientists in the wake of recent historical events. Episodes of misconduct tarnished the moral image of medical scientists perpetuated in Sinclair Lewis' popular 1925 novel *Arrowsmith* and Paul de Kruif's 1926 book *Microbe Hunters*.[64] For example, the image of the selfless investigator may seem hard to reconcile with scientists who have engaged in public disputes over credit for scientific discoveries (including the dispute between Robert Gallo and Luc Montagnier about who deserved credit for the discovery of the HIV virus).[65] In addition, the portrayal of medical scientists as truth-searchers may not seem appropriate in today's times given accusations of fraudulent research.[66] The idea that researchers are ethically and morally superior to members of other professions has been tarnished by recurring ethical breaches in medical experimentation, such as those committed by J. Marion Sims, Udo Wile, and the Tuskegee and Guatemala researchers, and by the involvement of USPHS investigators and Surgeon General Thomas Parran.[67] These notorious events have been compounded by the major horrors of Nazi medical experimentation, including forced sterilization and euthanasia of the enfeebled, demented, and handicapped.[68]

Suspicion of biomedicine in both fiction and actual historical circumstances has also been fomented by instances of medical products that have caused direct harm to patients and society. These occurred even throughout the twentieth century, after the FDA began to require safety inspections. There were harmful vaccines due to inadequate inspection, including the live-virus Park-Kolmer vaccine in 1934 (resulting in polio and paralysis in twelve children), and the Cutter polio vaccine of 1955 (which was linked to seventy vaccine-associated cases).[69] In 1998, the British physician Andrew Wakefield claimed that autism was related to the vaccine for measles, mumps, and rubella (MMR), which he maintained had not been properly tested before being used.[70] The paper received wide publicity, and MMR vaccination rates began to drop because parents were concerned about the risk of autism after vaccination.[71] The idea still has a following, though the paper has since been retracted and larger epidemiological studies have shown no correlation between MMR vaccination and autism.[72]

In 1974, critiques of modern scientific medicine were reinforced by philosopher Ivan Illich's challenge to the discipline. Illich argued that society had become too dependent on biomedicine.[73] This trend, he argued, had become harmful to the health of the individual and society, especially since the achievements of scientific medicine have had shortcomings, such as iatrogenic diseases (including the rise in multidrug-resistant organisms), the increasing number of people living with chronic incapacitating diseases, and the inhumane care received by dying patients with chronic, terminal diseases.

The critique of modern medicine and its dependence on biomedicine is also reflected in contemporary cultural representations, including television. Television programs today do not depict scientific doctors per se, as they were portrayed in *Arrowsmith* or *Microbe Hunters* in the early twentieth century. They depict clinicians who practice in the era of biomedicine. The sometimes unflattering portrayal of physicians reflects negative and distrustful feelings toward doctors and the dark side of medicine, while also reflecting the appeal of such narratives.[74] The ways in which physicians are portrayed has changed drastically during the last fifty years. Today's television doctors are fallible and concerned mainly with their personal lives rather than the welfare of their patients. This portrayal contrasts with earlier medical dramas, in which physicians such as Drs. Marcus Welby, James Kildare, and Ben Casey were depicted as saintly heroes who could do no wrong and were slavishly devoted to their patients.[75]

Conclusion

There is a long-standing sentiment held by some and reflected in cultural representations of scientific medicine that the ideal of biomedicine has not fulfilled its promises.[76] As this chapter has shown, multiple well-publicized episodes involving syphilis and AIDS have fueled that sentiment. No matter how impressive the technical achievements of scientific medicine may be, the confident belief in the benevolence and nobility of medical scientists is not embraced by all, particularly in marginalized populations. Today, a significant faction of society shares an antiscience and vaccine-hesitant orientation, and they mistrust the neutrality and expertise of medical scientists.[77] This enduring historical skepticism of the medical enterprise, bolstered by the misapplications of biomedicine in AIDS and syphilis and by the cultural representations of medicine today, is also evident in COVID, the subject of the next chapter.

Chapter 5

COVID

Familiar Patterns Emerge

Syphilis, AIDS, and COVID share parallel narratives. Each has been characterized by the promise of novel biomedical products to eliminate a devastating epidemic. But the histories of AIDS and syphilis provide perspective on how socioeconomic factors that drive these epidemics interfere with our efforts to eliminate them. Due to notorious historical events associated with their management, AIDS and syphilis exemplify the mistrust in medicine and the concern for protecting personal liberties that underlie many people's actions today. As a result, we have experienced COVID and its elimination efforts unevenly, influenced by racial and economic disparities. AIDS and syphilis provide perspective on what it means to live with COVID and the epidemic narrative in the biomedical era. We will begin by exploring COVID chronologically.

Initial Pandemic Period: January 2020–December 2020

The disease now known as COVID suddenly appeared in Wuhan, China, in December 2019. Widespread community global transmission ensued due to international travel during the Chinese Lunar New Year holiday.[1] The causative pathogen, a respiratory virus to which the global population had no immunity and for which there was no vaccine, was identified in record time: three weeks after the first case.[2] Two weeks later, the genome of the novel coronavirus had been sequenced and shared among scientists around the world at an unprecedented pace.[3] The rapid identification of the virus and its genetic makeup offered hope for an early, effective vaccine.[4] The disease was unpredictable, ranging from asymptomatic to causing severe respiratory symptoms. The death rate (1 percent) was high enough to cause global alarm, but low enough to enable continued transmission.[5] The world's nations, having previously braced themselves for the possibility of infections originating abroad and spreading to their countries (e.g., Zika, Ebola), developed a heightened alarm in February 2020, when CDC scientists predicted a massive spread of the novel coronavirus among the global population.[6]

Initially, leaders of both wealthy (e.g., Trump in the United States, Boris Johnson in the U.K.) and middle-income (Jair Bolsonaro in Brazil) nations downplayed predictions of a widespread pandemic.[7] Some leaders were trying to maintain an optimistic appearance during an election year (Trump), or were concerned that widespread lockdowns would be bad for business.[8] With escalating numbers (800,000 confirmed cases globally) by March 2020, however, nations around the world implemented behavioral restrictions (e.g., lockdowns, masking, and stay-at home orders).[9] But these measures came too late, allowing the pandemic to reach every nation as cases skyrocketed during the first surge, in March through May 2020.[10] The restrictions left millions without jobs and drove billions into isolation due to closings of schools, theaters, bars, restaurants, sporting events, public gatherings, churches, temples, mosques, museums, and libraries.[11]

In the United States, the pandemic disproportionately affected people of low income and racial minorities employed in frontline jobs (e.g., custodians, bus drivers) that did not allow them to work remotely from home.[12] These groups tended to reside in crowded homes or apartments, sometimes poorly ventilated, that did not provide adequate space to enable isolation or quarantine.[13] Hospitals attempted to cope with soaring numbers of patients that exceeded capacity by converting nearby structures into makeshift medical units. Moreover, healthcare facilities cancelled routine procedures and office examinations to accommodate the surge of patients with COVID, as supplies of protective gear dwindled.[14] Meanwhile, there was a shortage of standard supplies (personal protective equipment [PPE], ventilators, medicines), and difficult decisions were made about how to allocate limited resources.

Fear was rampant from the start, as doctors and nurses anguished over decisions about rationed resources and made judgments about treatments at a time when there was little certainty about therapies.[15] The pandemic forced everyone to struggle with the idea that their patients, families, or they themselves were vulnerable. As death rates rose, people became alarmed as they saw images of empty streets during lockdowns and corpses stacked in makeshift freezers. The trajectory of the pandemic was uncertain at a time when there was no vaccine and no effective treatment.

Initial lockdown measures were successful in reducing transmission by the end of May 2020. But many countries were eager to return to pre-COVID lifestyles. U.S. government leadership lifted restrictions prematurely before rates had sufficiently declined.[16] In addition, some groups refused to wear masks or distance socially, framing the public health restrictions as a violation of individual liberties. In the United States and other nations, a second wave of infections occurred in October 2020 that was most severe in states or regions that had eased restrictions early.[17] At this point, some responded to the returning virus with renewed dismissiveness about public health restrictions, whereas others would not let their guard down.[18] The public's confidence in science and its prescriptions was not uniform.

There was a mixed public response to scientific recommendations regarding other aspects of COVID. Most people were confident that science would yield an effective vaccine.[19] Other citizens and government officials, including President Trump, dismissed scientists' ability to judge the severity of the pandemic or forecast its potential for extensive global transmission.[20] Others became impatient with the methodical pace of science to assess the utility of drugs (e.g., ivermectin and hydroxychloroquine) and advocated their use in practice without adequate study.[21] This reflected an intolerance of the deliberate pace of science. Others, however, maintained faith that biomedicine would yield effective drugs and prophylactics in time through traditional clinical trials.[22]

The U.S. government funneled large sums of money to pharmaceutical companies in an unparalleled effort to promote expeditious discovery, testing, and mass production of effective vaccines (a program named Operation Warp Speed).[23] Trump's goal was to have an effective vaccine by presidential election day, in November 2020.[24] In the meantime, without effective vaccines or drugs, people began to wonder what the eventual consequences of the pandemic would be for families, societies, individuals' lives, and the economy. During this unprecedented moment, some began to refer to the 1918 influenza pandemic as a historical analogue to provide perspective and commiseration.

Connections between COVID and the 1918 influenza were obvious. Influenza, like COVID, had frightening symptoms, a significant mortality, resulted in rapid spread in crowded situations that involved international population migration, and was caused by a respiratory virus (identified in 1931).[25] The initial downplaying of science was also a shared feature. U.S. President Woodrow Wilson initially trivialized the illness's significance, as he did not want to project a weak image of the United States during World War I. Consequently, the homecoming of troops after armistice on November 11, 1918, was followed by widespread community transmission. Because the surge exceeded the capacity of hospitals to care for the ill, field units were built, and armories were used to house patients. In addition, ancillary staff (nurses, attendants) were assembled, and funeral homes were soon overwhelmed with the dead. Wearing masks, implementing restrictions to ban large gatherings, and closing movie theaters and schools all reduced transmission. Furthermore, locales that implemented early restrictive population measures of longer durations avoided rebounds compared with cities that delayed restrictions.[26] These public health recommendations were contested by organized antimask leagues. Certainly, multiple features of 1918 influenza share parallels with those of COVID today.

There are additional reasons that 1918 influenza is an apt analogue for COVID. In 1918, the public was surprised that a new epidemic had occurred and that a vaccine employing what was thought to be the responsible pathogen, the Pfeiffer bacillus, was ineffective.[27] At the epidemic's onset, the public had a growing confidence that science could control epidemics, based on the availability of treatments (antisera and chemotherapy) and prophylaxes (vaccines) against certain infections.[28] This is illustrated by the comment of William Braisted, then surgeon general of the U.S. Navy, prior to World War I: "Infectious diseases that formerly carried off their thousands, such as yellow fever, typhus, cholera, and typhoid, have all yielded to our modern knowledge of their cause and new consequent logical measures taken for the prevention."[29] At the start of the epidemic, Rufus Cole, a pulmonologist from Rockefeller Institute stationed at Fort Devens, expressed dismay that the Johns Hopkins pathologist William Welch, who symbolized the promise of scientific medicine, was unable to find a cause or cure for the unknown disease.[30] He said, "It shocked me to find out that the situation . . . was too much even for Doctor Welch."[31] The poet and pediatrician William Carlos Williams said, "We hadn't a thing that was effective in checking that potent poison that was sweeping the world."[32] Victor Vaughan, dean of medicine at the University of Michigan Medical School, stated, "Doctors know no more about this flu than 14th century doctors had known about the Black Death."[33] Thus, 1918 influenza reminded physicians that humans remained vulnerable to epidemics they could not control.

COVID's frightening symptoms and rapid spread throughout the population could also be compared to those of the 1348 Black Death. Each had an impact on the economy, triggering inflation due to the diminished supply of goods. Like COVID, Black Death also influenced societal customs; for example, the sudden increase in the number of dead precluded individual burial. The Italian Renaissance writer Giovanni Boccaccio talked about bodies being stowed "tier upon tier . . . showing no . . . respect to dead people." Black Death, like COVID, provoked reminders from writers and doctors not to abandon their social obligations to one another. Boccaccio considered those who ran away from the sick "inhuman."[34] The French surgeon Guy de Chuliac summoned physicians to honor their duty to provide care for their patients, even though they could "accomplish nothing," as they could not alter the course of their patients' infection. De Chuliac wrote, "I . . . did not dare to leave lest I lose my good name," even though he became infected with plague himself.[35] Likewise, during the early COVID period, healthcare workers continued working while risking endangering themselves at a time when there were PPE shortages, no vaccines or drugs were available, and the virus was more virulent than today's strains.

COVID can also be compared with the 2003 outbreak of severe acute respiratory syndrome (SARS) in China, which also involved the sudden occurrence of a novel coronavirus that had potential to spread globally. Unlike with COVID, during the SARS outbreak, early implementation of dramatic public health measures (e.g., travel restrictions on international flights, quarantine of the exposed, mask wearing) ended in a self-limited, geographically contained epidemic without widespread community transmission or pandemic spread.[36] SARS in 2003 serves as an example that containment is possible if public health programs acknowledge the serious potential of an epidemic and implement restrictive measures early in its course.

Despite COVID's alarming nature when it first appeared in 2020, several nations minimized its severity and delayed early implementations of restrictions.[37] The United States missed opportunities for surveillance, contact tracing, and the activation of the Defense Production Act, which would have mandated businesses to produce necessary items, including PPE and ventilators.[38] Government officials from the United States, Brazil, and U.K. also failed to adopt centralized guidelines for widespread testing and schooling.[39] Indeed, countries that lacked a centralized approach and ignored the advice of experts had the fastest rates of virus spread.[40] Despite dismissing scientific recommendations, Trump displayed a confidence in biomedicine by allocating $12 billion toward Operation Warp Speed.[41] His narrative of a harmless, vaccine-preventable virus would not perturb the image of strength and wealth of the United States during an election year.

Trump's ideas resonated with some citizens, who prioritized their rights to defy scientific recommendations and gather in large crowds without wearing face masks. The Sturgis, South Dakota, Motorcycle Rally in August 2020 was one example. Those among the 250,000 unmasked participants who acquired coronavirus at the rally dispersed the virus after they returned to their hometowns.[42] The rates of spread continued to climb after the holiday season at the end of 2020, as families who lived in multiple houses congregated and a more transmissible variant of COVID emerged.[43] The United States had higher rates than anywhere else in the world as of February 2021, after Trump had left office.

As COVID shows, the cost to minimize the severity of a pandemic is the missed chance for containment. The dilatory response of the United States and other nations caused unnecessary human suffering and societal consequences.[44] Nonetheless, throughout 2020 Trump continued to underestimate the severity of the pandemic.[45] He maintained that work restrictions, stay-at-home orders, and advice by public health experts to restrict crowds or wear face masks were unnecessary.[46] Government inactivity persisted throughout 2020. Given the asymptomatic spread of the virus, stopping its spread would have required widespread and rapid testing, timely isolation of the infected, and quarantine of the exposed.[47] Even by February 2020, when the pandemic had spread to 150 countries globally, involved over fifty million people worldwide, and resulted in over 290,000 deaths, government officials, including in the United States, Brazil, and U.K., continued to downplay its significance, thus missing opportunities to contain its spread.[48]

President Trump continuously blamed the United States' economic rival China for introducing the virus to the nation.[49] Blaming the marginalized had insidious effects, reinforcing preexisting prejudices that labeled these groups as dangerous and unworthy of integrating into society. It also introduced the idea that the virus Trump called "Chinese" was not harmful to white citizens because of an implicit assumption that it preferred to infect those of Chinese origin. This may have provided a false sense of reassurance for anxious mainstream groups that they were not vulnerable to the disease. It may also have served to absolve the government of any sense of accountability—implying the government should not be responsible for fixing a pandemic that was not their fault. Blaming the marginalized outsider is a recurrent historical pattern—as the responses to syphilis and AIDS underscore—that societies often display when new epidemics arise.

During the wave from March to May 2020 wave, citizens adhered resignedly to restrictive measures, including virtual learning, which disrupted classrooms and deprived students of in-person social interaction.[50] By May, the pandemic plateaued, but public health officials warned not to reopen the economy too soon, in spite of President Trump's insistence that "we have met the moment and we have prevailed."[51] In June, Trump encouraged several states to lift the lockdown before CDC target infection rates were met, stating the virus would "fade away" on its own.[52] By June, states that had prematurely reopened their economies experienced increased rates of infection compared with states that continued economic restrictions—a finding that underscored the lack of centralized guidelines regarding when to revoke work restrictions and stay-at-home orders.[53]

Trump's relationship with science, however, remained unpredictable. While dismissing scientific recommendations, he continuously supported vaccine development.[54] The president, believing that CDC predictions of widespread disease threatened the economy, made an executive decision to soften CDC messaging by creating the White House's own coronavirus task force, led by Vice President Mike Pence.[55] Trump also disputed CDC director Robert Redfield's claim that wearing masks was essential, saying in September 2020 that Redfield had "made a mistake. . . . A vaccine is much more effective than masks."[56] Trump, who refused to wear a mask, developed COVID himself two weeks later.[57] At the time, a communications official in the Trump cabinet, Michael Caputo, accused government scientists at the CDC of sedition.[58] While the White House was editing the CDC's recommendations, Trump appointed Scott Atlas, a neuroradiologist at Stanford Medical School who saw no need for shutting down society, as an advisor on the coronavirus task force.[59] Atlas proposed an unproven strategy to achieve herd immunity without a vaccine.[60]

By the end of 2020, false narratives mounted online. They included conspiracy theories such as the notion that the Chinese government had manufactured the virus as a biological weapon.[61] By December, following the release of the vaccine, unsubstantiated narratives promoted by the website ZeroHedge created uncertainty among some citizens about the vaccine's safety.[62] Others remained uneasy because of the lingering logistical concern that it would take months to mass produce and distribute a vaccine to the 380 million people in the United States and eight billion people in the world who needed it.[63]

Biomedical Breakthrough: Vaccines, December 2020 to March 2023

Highly effective vaccines were produced in record time, taking just one year of development. U.S. studies proving the vaccine's efficacy were released in November 2020. Tedros Ghebreyesus, director-general of the WHO, predicted that "the end of the COVID pandemic is in sight" if the vaccine were to be given to enough people globally.[64] When two pharmaceutical companies responded by scaling up manufacturing of the mRNA vaccines, Ghebreyesus's forecast seemed plausible.[65]

Scientists portrayed mRNA vaccines as a biomedical triumph. The one for COVID was the most rapidly produced vaccine ever and among the most effective. The vaccine bypassed traditional methods, which use live attenuated virus, inactivated vaccine, or subunit vaccine and customarily require years to develop.[66] Its perceived advantage over traditional vaccines is that it does not require a virus to produce protective antibodies. By avoiding the lengthy development process, scientists constructed an mRNA vaccine within a month of the genome's report.

Though mRNA vaccines had been a promising technology before COVID, scientists first had to overcome biological hurdles before mRNA products were ready for human use.[67] Researchers in the 1970s found that when mRNA from one species was introduced into a more complex type of cell, it was inactivated by the host cell's enzymes (ribonucleases).[68] The destruction of mRNA before it could translate a foreign protein became an impediment to research. Investigators found that adding gene sequences at the beginning and end of the mRNA protected it from enzyme destruction. A second hurdle emerged because external RNA triggers an immunological response that can inactivate it prior to translation. By 2005, researchers modified the mRNA so that it produced its protein before it was destroyed.[69] Another hurdle was how to engineer delivery of vaccine into the cell as mRNA is too large to traverse cell membranes. To overcome this obstacle, scientists used lipid nanoparticles (LNP), which required storage at low temperatures to remain unstable. Though the vaccine's 2020 arrival in the spotlight seemed sudden, the technology for an effective COVID mRNA vaccine had been in development for decades.[70]

With the pandemic threat of COVID and the rapid sequencing of the coronavirus genome, the stage was set for the development of an mRNA COVID vaccine.[71] Crucial to the rapid and successful development of COVID vaccines was the cooperation between government (the NIH), private pharmaceutical companies, and academic research groups, and funding by government.[72] The large numbers of subjects willing to enroll in clinical efficacy trials during the pandemic enabled well-powered trials to be conducted in an unprecedentedly short period.

The press heralded COVID mRNA vaccines as scientific marvels.[73] As had happened with syphilis and AIDS, groundbreaking biomedical developments using novel scientific mechanisms offered the promise of controlling the disease in the population. Anthony Fauci, director of infectious diseases at the National Institute of Allergy and Infectious Diseases, called the development of two effective COVID mRNA vaccines a "spectacular scientific breakthrough . . . a historic moment . . . a triumph of . . . biomedical research that was . . . done in record time."[74] Dan Longo, a cardiologist at the Brigham and Women's Hospital, Boston, stated that the COVID vaccine "is a triumph. . . . [It] holds the promise of saving uncounted lives and giving us a pathway out of what has been a global disaster."[75] These views of the vaccine's benefit show the confidence that physicians had in the capacity of their new biomedical tool to control COVID.

Despite the enthusiasm, some remained skeptical about vaccine safety given the accelerated schedule of the studies. Among Democrats, some were suspicious that Trump had pressured the FDA to bypass the usual safety measures so that the announcement of a safe, effective vaccine could be made by election day.[76] New York governor Andrew Cuomo proposed appointing an independent council of experts to review the vaccines' efficacy data before they were used in his state.[77] Notwithstanding his skepticism, the vaccines were approved by the U.S. FDA for an Emergency Use Authorization (EUA) clause in December 2020. They were mass produced for eligible individuals in the United States and intended to be distributed through an effort that included private volunteers and pharmacies, and National Guard sites.[78] Groups at highest risk for acquiring the virus (e.g., essential workers) or developing severe disease (e.g., the elderly, those with weakened immune systems) were targeted to receive the vaccine first.

By January 2021 public health officials had become hopeful about the ability to vaccinate a sufficient percentage of the population, initially estimated to be 70 percent, to achieve the herd immunity needed to end the pandemic.[79] It is notable that there was no formal campaign to end COVID by a specified date, as there had been with syphilis and AIDS. When the initial vaccine rolled out, the United States used motivational language that evoked emotions of nationalism and patriotism. President Joe Biden (elected in November 2020) had a stated goal of achieving "Independence from the virus" by July 4, 2021, indicated his confidence in the vaccine campaign.[80]

Despite the aggressive rollout of an effective vaccine in December 2020, COVID has persisted. Too few people have received the vaccine, and public health measures (e.g., social distancing, mask wearing, testing, isolation, quarantine) have been sporadic.[81] Both globally and in the United States, vaccination rates have consistently been lower than initial estimates to end the pandemic. Meanwhile, the threshold to achieve herd immunity has increased from 70 percent to 90 precent due to the circulation of highly transmissible variants. In the United States, the flagship of the world's biomedical establishment, only 60 percent of the population had been fully vaccinated by January 2022, a figure that did not place the United States among the top fifty nations worldwide in terms of vaccination rates. In addition, global vaccination goals (targeting 70 percent of the world's population by mid-2022) have not been met. LMICs with vaccination rates around 20 percent have been the origin of variant strains that spread globally along international travel routes.

Likewise, vaccination rates have been highly variable according to regions within wealthy nations.[82]

The Kaiser Family Foundation (KFF) survey of December 2020, which tracked public attitudes and experiences with COVID vaccines, showed that hesitancy was highest among young people (in the thirty to thirty-nine age bracket), rural residents, Republicans and Black adults. Among those who were hesitant to get vaccinated, the main reasons were lack of trust in the government to ensure the vaccines' safety and effectiveness (55 percent), concerns that the vaccine was too new (53 percent), and additional concerns about the role of politics in the development process (51 percent).[83] A November 2021 KFF study showed that the 15 percent of the population who chose not to be vaccinated remained consistent in their decision, and that the threat of new variants did not influence their decision.[84]

The ongoing replication of the virus among susceptible unvaccinated people has enabled additional mutant strains to develop. Some variants have shown a selective advantage in terms of enhanced transmission, as evidenced by those that have become dominant, such as the Delta variants and Omicron subvariants. The unmet goal of achieving full vaccination means that herd immunity will not be reached, and the virus will not be eliminated from the population.[85] The long-term fate of the pandemic may be subject to viral evolution, potentially resulting in seasonal infections akin to nonepidemic influenza, especially now that there are vaccines and oral drugs available that can reduce hospitalizations and mortality.

Within the first month of the vaccine's release in January 2021, the initial allocation in the United States was too low and demand exceeded supply.[86] The U.S. government had not paid enough attention to operational issues in distribution to various sites.[87] By December 2021, demand no longer exceeded supply; forty million people eligible for vaccination in the United States had refused to get one. Meanwhile, the pandemic continued in successive waves, primarily affecting the unvaccinated, and being concentrated particularly but not exclusively in conservative states with lower inoculation rates and more relaxed attitudes toward group gatherings.[88] That too few people have been fully vaccinated in developed nations has been a problem that has also extended to LMICs.

The allocation of COVID vaccines, as was true for HIV medicines, created a humanitarian problem globally. Vaccine distribution drove health disparities further, as vaccines were delivered to wealthy nations that purchased them first. Too few doses have been allocated to LMICs. Biomedical interventions, AIDS and COVID show, can exacerbate pre-existing inequalities.[89] The engagement of activists has resulted in the willingness of leaders in some countries to waive intellectual property (IP) rights and facilitate technology transfer (TT) in order to allow people in LMICs access to vaccines and medicines.[90] The need for this became evident with the emergence of Omicron subvariants by January 2022. Vaccines, along with boosters, provided the greatest protection, albeit incomplete, against these variant strains.

Vaccines have also exacerbated pre-existing inequalities within wealthy nations. The lowest vaccine rates in the United States are in the poorest neighborhoods.[91] To address socioeconomic inequity, the CDC in December 2020 first recommended prioritizing vaccines to go to "frontline essential workers," including grocery and transit workers.[92] Inequalities have been heightened by shortages in vaccine products and inadequate infrastructure to deliver them, particularly in low-income communities where rates of disease spread and risk of death are highest.[93] Vaccine inequalities have also been influenced by ideological factors, including a mistrust of science and government that persists today.

As the number of people who received the vaccine plateaued in the summer of 2021, another COVID surge began. Independence from the virus by July 4, 2021, as Biden had hoped, did not materialize. The maximum number of people who accepted vaccination by choice had been reached, and the numbers of unvaccinated people, for reasons of inadequate production, uneven allocation, or incompatible ideologies, were too high to reach the targeted goal. The portion of the population who would not take the vaccine, both in the United States and globally, was high enough to threaten the prediction that a vaccine would curtail the pandemic.[94]

Reluctance to receive recommended vaccines, however, preceded COVID.[95] Factors contributing to this reluctance in high-income countries have traditionally included lack of confidence in public health officials, complacency that the disease is not as bad as public health officials predict, the disruption of daily schedule involved in getting the shot, belief that side effects from vaccine are worse than disease, and a concern for self-interest over collective responsibility.[96] In LMICs, a mistrust in science also undergirds the concerns for safety and a lack of acceptance of the risk calculations made by public health officials.[97]

By December 2021, after a third peak in August had subsided, the situation remained unchanged with a fourth surge of COVID due to the Omicron variant. By January 2022, this became the dominant strain in the United States and globally. At that time in the United States, many were fatigued and mistrustful of scientific recommendations, a situation compounded by initially confusing messages and fluctuations regarding whom should receive booster shots in August 2021 and whether vaccinated individuals needed to wear face masks.[98]

The shifting messages persisted in December 2021, when U.S. health officials backed booster vaccinations as evidence mounted that the booster would provide greater protection against the severity of the Omicron variant.[99]

The fourth wave lingered into January 2022. Unlike in prior surges, a larger proportion of the population had been vaccinated: 25 percent in LMICs and 65 percent in developed countries.[100] The realization that the pandemic could not be eliminated given incomplete vaccination rates led many countries, apart from China, to avoid the restrictive strategies used during the first wave, in March 2020. The revised public health approach was to acknowledge the widespread nature of the virus, which had become milder, while recommending modifying day-to-day affairs (e.g., masking, distancing, showing vaccine passports, taking rapid tests, staying home if respiratory symptoms arose, adopting "testing-to-stay" in school policies). This approach favored allowing people to live productive lives by following public health recommendations. As an editorial in *Nature* in January 2022 stated, "For those who had hoped that 2021 would be the year that put the pandemic in the past tense, the Omicron variant is a harsh reminder that it is still very much present. Rather than laying plans to return to the 'normal' life we knew before the pandemic, 2022 is the year the world must come to terms with the fact that SARS-CoV-2 is here to stay."[101]

There remained, however, persistent anxieties about how to live safely and conduct a rewarding life—particularly for people at high risk for disease progression. By 2022, citizens across the world became exhausted by what they viewed as intractable cycles in which the virus continued its surges and spread, risking severe disease in vulnerable groups. The vaccinated began to regard the unvaccinated as unnecessarily perpetuating these cycles.[102] Some lived complacently without following sensible restrictions, and others were unsure how much and when they could ease their vigilance. Many vaccinated people became uncertain about whether it was safe to attend large gatherings that might include unvaccinated people, or whether and when to get tested. These persistent dilemmas became part of living with the pandemic and turned seemingly trivial choices about whether to attend family gatherings into important public health decisions. Some vaccinated people remained frustrated that the pandemic could not be eradicated due to a lack of cooperation from the unvaccinated, an issue that the WHO had cited as a top-ten global threat before COVID appeared in 2019.[103]

Many unvaccinated people in the United States harbor a deep mistrust in medical experts and government officials. Some of the mistrust is likely attributable to the numerous missteps of public health and government officials in handling COVID from its start—including downplaying its significance, missing an early opportunity to develop a reliable rapid test, delaying advice to wear masks, recommending untested therapies (including convalescent plasma), questioning the decision to grant an EUA for the vaccine (in December 2020), and providing unclear guidance on who needed a mask (July 2021).[104] The mistrust was compounded by inconsistent advice regarding who needed a booster shot during 2021.[105] Surely this shifting of advice further undermined trust in scientists and governmental officials among citizens—even those inclined to "follow the science" and its recommendations.

But this mistrust predates COVID, and some of it is intertwined with the history of syphilis and AIDS (chapter 4). It has compromised the ability to reach the vaccine coverage required to end the epidemic.[106] Some individuals continue to have lingering doubts about the safety of a vaccine that was so rapidly produced, and are concerned that the vaccine was rushed to project a triumphant image in time for Trump's attempt at re-election.[107] Even after rigorous scientific trials were conducted and medical scientists attested to its safety, by January 2022, up to 60 percent had not received boosters despite the rising percentage of cases that were due to Omicron subvariants.[108]

The mistrust of science has provided a permissive environment for the spread of misinformation globally. Online falsehoods about insufficient testing escalated in December 2020, soon after the first Pfizer vaccines were administered.[109] The misinformation persisted, providing narratives that some of the unvaccinated population, already mistrustful of science, found credible. Suspicion of science is also present in LMICs, including in Africa. In African countries, the mistrust stems from medical investigators from developed countries conducting experiments on people from LMICs without proper consent or compensation, as well as on the development of treatments and technologies without consideration for historically disadvantaged communities. During the colonial period, insensitive research studies conducted on Africans resulted in biomedical errors and accidents, creating legacies of skepticism.[110]

There have been attempts to coax unvaccinated individuals to voluntarily get shots. Programs have tried incentives (e.g., payment, lottery tickets, a day off work, or a ticket to a sports event).[111] Mandates increased vaccine uptake, but not enough to curtail the course of the pandemic. Biden initially avoided mandates to prevent a backlash, then employed them when voluntarism failed. Mandates in the United States have been imposed at the workplace (e.g., hospitals, various corporations), the state level (requiring vaccination in, e.g., school workers, hospital workers, municipal workers), and the federal level (government employees). By November 2021, COVID surges in Europe were so extreme that the Austrian government mandated all citizens to receive a vaccine—a decision that engendered backlash from conservative groups. Nevertheless, Biden's mandates within the United States, which included federal employees and businesses with more than one hundred people that are subject to OSHA enforcement, increased vaccine rates.[112] By January 2022, however, the U.S. Supreme Court had repealed some of Biden's mandates for OSHA-enforced companies with greater than a hundred employees.[113]

Although mandates have increased vaccination rates, the percentage of fully vaccinated people (68 percent of the population in the United States) has remained well below the number needed to end the pandemic (90 percent) and prevent emergence of variants originating from LMICs (e.g., Delta, which emerged in India in March 2021, and Omicron, which emerged in South Africa in November 2021).[114] The remainder of unvaccinated people in wealthy nations like the United States are mostly individuals who are ideologically opposed to having the government tell them what to do, or are mistrustful of scientists or government officials.[115] Carrot-and-stick approaches, combined with expanding the age range of those eligible for vaccination, increased the percentage of vaccinees, but not at a rate high enough to prevent the emergence of new variants that perpetuate spread.[116] The percentage of unvaccinated people who have accepted vaccination because they needed encouragement, wanted an incentive, or were mandated or persuaded by friends, workers, relatives, or trusted messengers, has plateaued.[117]

The initial discussion about achieving herd immunity ceased once it became clear that existing vaccine strategies would not reach the target. The percentage of the population that was vaccinated has been consistently below that needed to achieve herd immunity.[118] Vaccines were less effective against the Delta and Omicron variants.[119] Breakthrough infections occurred, despite vaccination, months after immune levels waned with the Omicron variant.[120] Due to the reduced vaccine efficacy over time, additional boosters have been needed to provide sufficient immunity against emerging variants.[121] Nonetheless, the percentage of boosted adults has remained low globally. For these reasons, the initial hope of achieving herd immunity is no longer considered tenable by scientists.

The unlikelihood of reaching herd immunity underscored a need for continued social-distancing measures in high-risk groups. Although no longer recommended for the general population, the need for continued behavioral change, including masking in large indoor areas, may remain necessary in certain locales (e.g., within hospitals) for several more years and for those in high-risk groups.[122] If surges recur, as some predict, it may mean resuming wearing masks for the general population in areas such as airports, obtaining rapid antigen tests prior to family gatherings and attending only if proven negative, abstaining from attending large gatherings (concerts, sports events), and conducting business, when possible, remotely by Zoom. Since the fall of 2022, many people have resumed most of life's activities and rhythms, recognizing that the virus is unlikely to disappear. This sentiment has grown, especially since we now have vaccines and therapies that turn COVID into a manageable virus, akin to seasonal influenza.[123] A global strategy of scaling-up COVID vaccines and drugs, together with making rapid antigen testing more available and affordable, will be needed to diminish disparities in health.

By the fall of 2022, COVID had come to represent the sort of risk that most vaccinated people unthinkingly accept in other parts of life. Nonetheless, policy issues remained, including determining which precautions should continue, when they should be reinstated, and how long others should remain in place (e.g., offices remaining partially empty; hospitals and schools requiring everyone to wear a mask). It also remains uncertain how long individuals need to worry about another COVID surge, and how long they will need to organize their lives around COVID. Masks, for example, have inhibited communication, remote office work has hampered collaboration, and social isolation has caused mental health problems.[124] COVID fatigue can make these issues fade into the background of people's lives until a new, unpredicted surge occurs. Indeed, the United States endured a fourth surge in January 2022, and by fall of 2022 we had experienced the emergence of a new rise in cases caused by Omicron subspecies mutations with the potential of widespread transmission. The course of the pandemic remained unpredictably erratic, as mRNA vaccines do not provide complete protection against subvariant strains, including BA.5, which became dominant in July 2022.

Thus, despite the availability of an effective vaccine, some remain unsettled by the uncertainty of the pandemic's trajectory. Experts have debated whether a new surge could be caused by a variant that combines the rapid spread of today's XBB.1.5 subvariant with the high virulence of the Delta strain.[125] Furthermore, given logistical problems with vaccine delivery, disregard for following protective precautions, and vaccine hesitancy, it is uncertain whether the spread of COVID can be controlled globally, and what failure to control will cost patients, society, and the economy. Anxieties that people had in the first part of the pandemic, although no longer as conspicuous, continue three years in (when this book was completed).

With persistent barriers to achieving optimal vaccine coverage, those who are at high risk of severe disease (e.g., the immunocompromised, the elderly, those with diabetes, obesity, or chronic lung conditions) have braced themselves since the start of the pandemic with a readiness to adopt permanent behavioral adjustments like wearing masks and avoiding large crowds in airports and shopping centers.[126] To what extent life for all people will resemble pre-COVID times remains speculative. Indeed, the unpredictability of living with the virus has been a defining aspect of the current situation.[127]

The influence of politicization on effective COVID responses has been an issue from the pandemic's start.[128] The intrusion of ideological partisanship into basic scientific and policy questions has affected the U.S. public health response.[129] Political polarization has hampered an effective pandemic response by preventing people from joining together in solidarity to achieve a common goal of public health. In addition, one's views on the effectiveness of drugs like hydroxychloroquine has reinforced political allegiances, rather than raising the question for impartial clinical study.[130] Evidence for mask wearing and vaccine mandates became colored by the suspicion that adherence to these recommendations was a yardstick of one's political devotion.[131] Petitioning people who live in democratic countries to "follow the science" is unlikely to persuade those who are antigovernment, vaccine hesitant, or suspicious of scientists' recommendations. Science does not have the neutrality or authority to convince the mistrustful to adopt its recommendations.

The relationship between politics and public health, however, is not straightforward. Authoritarian countries like China that use vaccines with low efficacies (Sinovac) and that have upheld "Zero COVID" cases as targets reimposed unpopular restrictive lockdown measures into December 2022. The government response led citizens angered by the oppressive nature of government surveillance to protest the stringent restrictions.[132] The continued lockdown also had global economic repercussions, perpetuating inflation due to supply chain disruption.[133] The Chinese government's response to COVID shows that there is no straightforward solution for how governments should handle epidemics. Governments in the United States, Brazil, and U.K. have been excoriated for downplaying the epidemic and missing an opportunity for early containment. China, in contrast, has shown that failure to reverse lengthy restrictions can be counterproductive and cause unnecessary damage to the economy and livelihoods.

When the founder SARS-CoV-2 strain appeared in January 2020, the economic effects of COVID included shortages of frontline workers such as policeman and repairman, and also supply chain shortages, making goods more scarce and more expensive.[134] These economic effects persist today. Furthermore, there is uncertainty as to what will happen to the disease abroad, as several nations that handled the pandemic well at first had outbreaks later, including Cambodia, Indonesia, and Russia. Safety is not guaranteed for people in groups that are at high risk of developing severe infection. Despite widespread complacency about the pandemic today, and its overshadowing by other pressing world events, people cannot feel secure that we have adequately addressed COVID. Uncertainties remain about how long its economic consequences will last, the potential need to reinstate restrictions due to a surge from a highly transmissible and virulent virus, or how to persuade unvaccinated or partially vaccinated individuals to get vaccinated or boosted.

As of November 2022, some people were anxious that the general public's complacency about the pandemic signaled an ominous future. With loosening of restrictions, and travel and socializing returned to normal, threat of another rise in COVID loomed at the end of 2022.[135] Public health experts were concerned about Omicron subvariants like BQ.1.1, which can evade existing immunity from recent infection or from vaccines, including the reformulated Pfizer and Moderna boosters designed for BA.5 variants that had previously dominated. Moreover, the newer variants can evade monoclonal antibodies like Evusheld, which had previously protected immunocompromised people at the highest risk for disease progression. Despite these concerns, a fifth surge had not yet materialized by March 2023.

Some have estimated that adults and children who remain unvaccinated in the United States will never be persuaded to accept vaccination.[136] Some suggest that the United States has reached a ceiling of persuadable people, one that is lower than the threshold needed for broad immunity from Delta or Omicron variants. Indeed, the number of adults receiving a first-time vaccine has plateaued, and only 20 percent of children ages five through eleven have received vaccines.[137] As of May 2022, 67 percent of U.S. citizens had been fully vaccinated. Unproven strategies to reach the population of unvaccinated people include approaching them in a compassionate manner rather than stigmatizing them as irrational opponents, and mobilizing groups of relatives of unvaccinated people who succumbed to COVID to sponsor vaccine drives aimed at increasing vaccination rates.

Patient representatives have played a role in advocating for the care of sufferers of COVID and for research into long-term sequela.[138] An advocacy group called COVID Survivors for Change has lobbied for mental health treatment, disability benefits, and paid sick leave for people with chronic sequela of COVID. Furthermore, some COVID survivors have called for the United

States to avoid returning too quickly to normalcy, and view Biden as paying too little attention to issues confronted by long-COVID patients and high-risk, COVID-susceptible individuals.[139] Their advocacy is reminiscent of that of AIDS representatives, who accused the government of indifference in the early part of the epidemic.

As of March 2023, when this monograph was completed, most people behaved in a complacent fashion that put pandemic considerations on the back burner. They considered COVID to have become a tolerable threat, similar to a common cold, that required no specific precautions. But others who were at greatest risk for progressing to severe disease continued to take daily precautions and hope for the day when the virus wouldn't restrict their lives any longer.[140] The increase in vaccination rates that will be necessary to achieve this goal will require cooperation and solidarity. But it remains difficult to foster the bonds between fellow citizens required to successfully manage the pandemic in today's atmosphere of divisiveness and polarization.[141]

As of March 2023, a cautionary weariness had also developed, particularly among those at highest risk for disease progression. At the end of each wave, citizens became lulled into thinking that the dangers were behind them, only to realize that they may need to re-adopt restrictions in the future. This uncertainty prompted a persistent anxiety about whether a boost in vaccination rates caused by mandates would raise coverage high enough to eventually eliminate severe disease.[142] If not, would the disease be endemic on a permanent basis, or might a new variant emerge that is more contagious than Omicron subvariant BA.5 and as virulent as Delta? How common and severe might these breakthrough infections be, particularly for people at high risk? Will existing vaccines still be effective against new variants, or will new-generation COVID vaccines be required? Will yearly boosters that contain protection against newly emerging variants be necessary? Underlying a mood of complacency is some degree of anxiety about these uncertainties, particularly for those at high risk.[143] Forecasting the course of the virus has been a humbling endeavor even for experts. Living with the virus entails some frustration that it remains a concern three years into the pandemic.

U.S. government and public health efforts have shown signs of readiness to live with the pandemic. Rapid antigen testing has been scaled up to minimize the impact of social isolation, schooling, and devastating effects on the economy. Biden used the Defense Production Act to increase the production of rapid testing kits.[144] By January 2022, the use of these tests enabled social gatherings and sporting events to occur, provided that attendees tested negative on the day of the gathering. Testing also allowed children to stay at school rather than quarantine from home if exposed to someone with COVID.[145] These approaches indicate a pragmatic effort to adapt to the persistent pandemic while minimizing the effect on social, psychological, and economic well-being. Today the focus in most countries is to enable citizens to live a life as fulfilling as possible, rather than ending the epidemic.

The oral drug Paxlovid prevents disease progression for people who are at elevated risk.[146] It also protects the work force (by reducing the number of days away from work), the economy (by preventing reductions in the work force), and prevents hospital overflows (by reducing hospitalizations). The availability of oral treatments, coupled with rapid testing, changed the nature of the pandemic into something more akin to a temporary virus, much like the common cold, even for unvaccinated people.[147] Despite a relaxed concern about COVID, however, hospitalizations, ventilation, and deaths still occur. There were on average 1,320 deaths per day globally from December 2022 through March 2023, composed mainly of unvaccinated and high-risk patients.[148] Thus, the perception of COVID as a trivial common cold is not true for all people, and may prove false if more virulent variants emerge. For these reasons, Paxlovid plays a key role in preventing severe disease in high-risk people and in LMICs where vaccination rates are low and the infrastructure to deliver intravenous treatments (monoclonal antibodies) may be unavailable.

The humanitarian motivation for donor countries to supply these drugs and vaccines throughout the world is obvious as more than half of deaths have occurred in LMICs where vaccination rates have been suboptimal. However, self-interest is also involved, as continued viral spread across the globe could lead to the virus spreading to developed countries again.[149] But partnerships between governments and private entities to accomplish vaccine distribution have been precarious. The United States had a partnership with Emergent BioSolutions, for example, which led to the disposal of millions of doses of the J&J vaccine due to contamination. Nevertheless, Biden vowed to increase production of mRNA vaccines that the United States could ship throughout the world.[150] Activists had been pushing Biden to pressure Pfizer and Moderna to share their patents and technology with manufacturers overseas to enable production of vaccines and drugs in LMICs.[151]

COVID adds a new dimension to a narrative of confidence that peaked in the mid-twentieth century. Epidemics like AIDS, syphilis, and COVID often carry the promise of ending within an expedited time frame due to innovative biomedical products. But underlying social, economic, and biological issues challenge this notion. We continue to live with these epidemics, and efforts to eliminate them persist.

Inability to Control an Epidemic Despite the Availability of Potent Biomedical Tools

With COVID, like syphilis and AIDS, we have the scientific means to eliminate the epidemic. Anthony Fauci, in fact, said about COVID, "When you have 75 . . . million people eligible for vaccination who don't get vaccinated, you will have continual smoldering spread of the infection. . . . It's frustrating because we have the wherewithal within our power . . . to suppress it."[152] AIDS and syphilis provide perspective on why our scientific tools have not reached their potential for COVID.

Issues that have involved AIDS and syphilis, including mistrust of science and its methods, scientific denialism, and disinformation, provide perspective on the difficulty of controlling COVID today. Medical ethicist Henry Beecher had identified scientific misconduct in human experimentation as a problem prior to the episodes that emerged with AIDS and syphilis.[153] A review of the latter can provide insight into the medical mistrust that underlies the hesitancy of some people to receive COVID vaccination.

Vaccine adherents have viewed the unvaccinated as irresponsible for allowing preventable spread of COVID, increasing the burden on hospitals, and increasing the rates of death.[154] The vaccinated incriminate the unvaccinated for not following the logic of science. Their refusal has, as President Biden said, "cost us all" by increasing the risk that the virus finds nonimmune hosts to continue its spread and develop mutations.[155] As discussed, however, the present approach of imploring the unvaccinated to "follow the science" has not succeeded.[156]

One untested approach to improving vaccination rates would be to foster communications between the two sides. It remains speculative whether the unvaccinated would be receptive to such approaches or whether the vaccinated would be willing to embrace them. Current public health approaches have included mandates and incentives to encourage vaccination among the unvaccinated.[157] Mandates have increased vaccination rates where they can be enforced (e.g., among federal workers, employees of federal contractors), but they cannot reach individuals who do not fit into these categories.[158] Likewise, incentives (e.g., time off work, lottery tickets) only appeal to some people.[159] It remains uncertain whether those who are resistant to mandates or incentives can be persuaded.[160] Why presently unvaccinated people refuse shots has not been systematically examined. A foundational belief of the unvaccinated may be a loss of trust in science.[161] An impasse ensues when the unvaccinated

become increasingly inured to pleas to follow a science they may compre-
hend but do not trust. Furthermore, the vaccinated have become angered by the
preventable harm caused by the unvaccinated. Hospitals overwhelmed with
COVID patients can compromise the care of patients who have non-COVID illnesses. The chance of gaining cooperation diminishes as the unvaccinated
become increasingly entrenched in their positions and the vaccinated grow
embittered.

A mistrust in science among the unvaccinated has bred the dissemination
of disinformation promoted by right-wing media (e.g., Fox News, Sinclair Broad-
cast Group). The belief in alternate theories and remedies has flourished while
the confidence in orthodox science and its methods has fractured. The bureau-
cratic missteps that have occurred since the start of COVID have certainly eroded
confidence in science and governmental officials.[162] By illustrating the ethical
violations of some scientists, the histories of AIDS and syphilis show that mistrust stems from deeper historical roots. An acknowledgement of this record by
public health officials could establish a common ground and enable communication between otherwise opposing groups. The historical record could cite episodes of unsafe polio vaccines in the 1930s and 1950s to reinforce that today's
COVID vaccines fulfill rigorous safety criteria.[163] It could acknowledge that
serious side effects (e.g., myocarditis) are less common with vaccination than
with naturally occurring disease.[164] Also, there is no evidence to support concerns about coronavirus vaccines containing a microchip or being derived from
fetal tissue.[165] This approach could acknowledge that vaccines are not risk free,
but they are less risky than getting the disease. An examination of the historical
record could hypothetically facilitate communication by enabling the unvaccinated to feel understood and willing to engage in a discussion.

The denial of scientific expertise has been evident throughout COVID as
people have defied scientists' advice that vaccines are necessary and that the
disease was a severe public health problem requiring restrictive measures. This
denial has had detrimental consequences for society. But the COVID pandemic
is not the first time scientific denialism has caused harm to individuals and society. History is in fact replete with circumstances where the dismissal of scientific findings has led to perilous societal consequences.

Significant denialism occurred during the AIDS epidemic (chapter 4). At
the turn of the twenty-first century, South African president Mbeki insisted that
poverty, rather than a virus, caused AIDS.[166] Mbeki based his views on the opin-
ions of Peter Duesberg, whose theory was rooted on arguments used by opponents of germ theory from the late nineteenth century. Duesberg acknowledged
that HIV was present adventitiously in tissue but claimed that it was not

pathogenic. He noted that HIV had not fulfilled Koch's postulates. Using an animal model, Koch established these criteria to provide proof that a bacterium isolated in culture from a diseased tissue was the causative pathogen and not simply an accidental finding (chapter 1).[167] Duesberg did not acknowledge that doctors in the late twentieth century had routinely accepted microbes as the cause of disease in humans, even without an animal model to fulfill Koch's criteria (e.g., cytomegalovirus, or CMV).

Duesberg's argument, although flawed, gained credibility by receiving the support of another respected scientist, Kary Mullis, who won the 1993 Nobel Prize in Chemistry for coinventing the polymerase chain reaction (PCR) technique. Duesberg served on a Presidential Advisory Panel on HIV organized by Mbeki in July 2000, where he sanctioned avoiding the use of drugs to treat HIV. Based on the advice of Duesberg, Mbeki elected not to implement a national treatment program for AIDS and banned the use of ART in healthcare settings from 2000 to 2003. When cases of HIV continued to climb, the South African cabinet overruled Mbeki and approved a plan to make the drugs available. The delay in treatment, however, resulted in several hundred thousand preventable deaths. Mbeki's denial of a retrovirus as the cause of HIV has had enduring repercussions for South Africa, where HIV rates remain the highest among neighboring nations.[168]

Another episode of scientific denialism involving HIV/AIDS had damaging global consequences. After the CDC determined in 1985 that there was no risk of HIV transmission via casual contact, some remained unconvinced and chose to continue their exclusionary practices (chapter 2). AIDS sufferers were avoided by individuals who feared becoming infected by casual contact even though medical evidence indicated otherwise.[169] The social exclusion of sufferers compounded their physical suffering.[170]

Cultural representations illustrating the dangers of medical scientific denialism preceded AIDS. A century beforehand, the playwright Henrik Ibsen addressed the consequences of denying medical and scientific advice. In his 1882 play *An Enemy of the People*, Ibsen conjured a tale about a medical doctor who revealed the harmful effects of tainted products that a prosperous tannery had discarded into the drinking water supply of a tourist town.[171] The town's mayor denied the diagnosis of the physician—whom he rebuked as the people's "enemy"—on the basis that his conclusions threatened the growing economic stability of the town's citizens. The mayor made the decision at the expense of the health of his town's residents, who became poisoned by consuming the tainted water. Ibsen's fictional illustration in the late nineteenth century of the perils of scientific denialism foreshadowed actual epidemics.

Bubonic plague, for example, appeared in the booming port city of San Francisco in 1900. A group of scientists commissioned by Surgeon General Walter Wyman to investigate the outbreak used scientific techniques to diagnose plague.[172] Elected public officials, however, worried that word of plague would be bad for the city's profitable tourism business. They denied the commissioners' findings. Consequently, no definitive action to control the disease was taken until 1903, when neighboring states threatened an embargo against goods traded from California unless the state took steps to manage plague. By the time California officials implemented effective antiplague strategies, the disease had spread via rats to prairie dogs in surrounding rural areas. Because of such delays in implementing containment measures, plague endures as an illness, albeit in small numbers, in the southwestern United States.

Another example of the dangers of scientific denialism is the outbreak of measles in the United States between 2010 and 2019. Several citizens disregarded scientific advice that measles remained a concern in the United States. Unlike those who lived in the 1960s, before the measles vaccine became available, most families had not personally witnessed the ramifications of the disease.[173] Headed by celebrities like Robert Kennedy Jr., an antivaccination movement maintained that vaccines were less safe than medical doctors indicated, particularly due to an association with autism (a claim that had been discredited). Kennedy and others argued that taking the measles vaccine was essentially a losing proposition because there was more to lose (permanent autism) than avoiding a disease (self-limited measles). Misinformation websites concluded that orthodox medicine had misled the population, and that vaccines were unsafe, unnecessary, and ineffective.[174] These arguments found resonance in various regions of the country, including parts of California and New York, where inadequate vaccine levels permitted measles outbreaks to occur following exposures during airport travel. Similar outbreaks of measles have occurred throughout the 2010s in other U.S. communities.[175]

The medical impact of chronic traumatic encephalopathy (CTE) also illustrates the hazards of scientific denialism. By 2005, a group of scientists concluded that CTE was the cause of a progressive neurodegenerative disease among some veteran football players in the National Football League.[176] NFL executives, however, denied the findings.[177] They claimed the evidence was insufficient to establish any association between repeated head trauma and CTE. The NFL did not invest in technology designed to diminish the damaging effects of head contacts, enforce protocols to remove players with concussions from continued play, or create deterrents for helmet-to-helmet hits by penalizing them until years later, in 2016. At that time, a senior NFL executive officially acknowledged a connection between repeated head trauma and CTE.[178] Although the diagnosis of CTE remains contested by some neurologists, delaying the adoption of protective measures resulted in neurological damage done to players who had experienced repeated serious head contact.

As illustrated, then, scientific denialism has perpetuated irreversible harm to the population. To illustrate how science can be cast in doubt by those who find that it conflicts with their interests, Naomi Oereskes, a science historian, has documented examples where science deniers have influenced the debate over tobacco, second-hand smoke, acid rain, chlorfluorocarbons, ozone depletion, and climate change.[179] This book adds to Oereskes work by illustrating how medical epidemics—plague, measles, CTE, and AIDS—can also serve as cautionary tales about the hazards of ignoring the recommendations of scientists. Historically, science, although powerful, has never had the power to override other ways of deciding what constitutes the health of a population—either physical health or economic well-being. The results of science are adopted when they align with the broader concerns of the community, including considerations not to jeopardize the economic strength of a company or community.

As is true of science denialism, scientific misinformation is not new to COVID. It also was evident during the HIV epidemic. BBC journalist Edward Hooper postulated in his 1999 book *The River* that the poliovirus vaccine campaign was responsible for HIV/AIDS.[180] Hooper claimed that kidney cells harvested from monkeys to grow polio contained simian immunodeficiency virus (SIV) and were therefore responsible for spreading HIV.[181] Hooper's widely publicized assertions were refuted by straightforward evidence that none of the cells used to grow polio contained HIV or SIV.[182] Unlike the spread of today's COVID misinformation, this episode of HIV misinformation could not have been disseminated widely on social media, which did not exist at the time.[183] The production of scientific misinformation is not unique to COVID, but the rapid dissemination of unverified knowledge claims to a broad audience through social media is unprecedented.

Challenges to the necessity of performing scientific trials to verify drug efficacy have preceded dangerous epidemics like COVID. At the onset of COVID, there was an experimental basis for supporting the use of drugs that were licensed to treat other diseases (e.g., hydroxychloroquine, ivermectin). But there were no clinical trials showing their effectiveness against COVID. In the context of a pandemic crisis, some argued for the use of these drugs in routine clinical practice, rather than as part of a clinical trial, which would include a placebo to gauge effectiveness.[184] The ethics of withholding a potentially useful drug during a lethal epidemic was debated during the early phase of COVID.

This debate has also occurred during prior epidemics.[185] Investigators have raised concerns about denying potentially effective agents to people who have a serious disease that lacks effective treatment, particularly during epidemics.[186] Historically, medical scientists have maintained that the only way to obtain reliable data is to conduct trials that include an untreated control group.[187] At the heart of the dispute lies the principle of equipoise: an uncertainty of whether a treatment is effective.[188] Since researchers cannot be certain whether treatment is advisable before clinical trials are performed, there is no distinct line defining equipoise or its absence when a study is begun.[189] Even in nonepidemic settings, doctors can be conflicted about whether to administer a drug or to ask a patient to enter into a controlled trial.[190] Their dilemma is compounded in epidemic settings, when there is a heightened risk of withholding potentially beneficial therapy by randomizing to a control group patients who may have a poor prognosis and the potential to spread an untreatable infection.[191] During COVID, doctors were confronted with the dilemma of whether to prescribe licensed drugs for off-label indications, or to study these agents as part of a clinical trial.

This controversy, which has long historical roots, arose soon after comparative clinical trials emerged. In the late nineteenth century, investigators began to embrace controlled trials. They allowed physicians to overcome biases they believed hampered their ability to evaluate therapeutics impartially.[192] The demand for more rigorous research standards intensified during the early twentieth century in response to new medical opportunities following the availability of chemical products such as Ehrlich's Salvarsan in 1910. The use of controlled trials accelerated during the influenza pandemic in 1918 to test the efficacy of the Pfeiffer bacillus.[193] By the 1920s, controlled trials were being used more often to test the effectiveness of the expanding volume of antisera, vaccines, and chemical compounds.[194] In several epidemic settings preceding COVID, a sense of urgency has been associated with the risk of withholding therapy for study-enrolled subjects.

This pressing need became evident in the early AIDS era. In 1986, as outlined in chapter 2, AZT raised hopes of reversing the disease's lethal course.[195] The FDA mandate for a placebo-controlled study underscored conflicting viewpoints about these trials. To medical researchers, they were essential experiments to determine efficacy, but to AIDS activists, they obstructed access to effective drugs.[196] In this divisive atmosphere, the planned twenty-four-week phase II study comparing AZT to placebo was terminated early when a survival benefit of AZT was noted.[197] Activists fought to expedite the drug's availability first through a compassionate basis (1986) and then by accelerated FDA licensing (1987).[198] By 1992, TAG patient representatives questioned the efficacy of

AZT based on limited patient enrollment and the short duration of the prior study. TAG's concerns were substantiated in 1994 by a larger placebo-controlled trial of longer duration showing that AZT did not provide clinical benefit.[199] TAG members affirmed that providing speedier access to promising but unstudied drugs is not always better than nothing, and that adequately powered clinical trials are the only reliable means to evaluate therapeutics.[200]

The same dilemma about the appropriateness of conducting placebo-controlled trials also emerged during the 2014 West African Ebola crisis. These ethical concerns, coupled with the logistical challenges of conducting trials during emergency situations, impacted the research that took place during the outbreak. Clinical trials evaluating promising therapies at their early stage of development (e.g., favipiravir) were consequently carried out in open-labeled studies using historical controls.[201] Some medical researchers, however, maintained that Ebola treatment trials using historical controls were invalid, arguing that the improvement in supportive care of patients during the epidemic (e.g., Ebola Treatment Unit availability) could have led to improved outcomes.[202] They concluded that without a clinical trial using concurrent controls, results are uncertain, and no reliable therapies were able to be ascertained.[203]

Polio was another epidemic where this controversy played out. By the 1930s, fear of a lifelong paralysis that randomly struck children had become widespread.[204] Some physicians, having witnessed the consequences of polio firsthand, were reluctant to withhold potentially helpful but otherwise unavailable interventions from young children assigned to a control group, including a trial using convalescent serum.[205] Reticence to heed earlier advice continued into the 1950s, including from virologist Jonas Salk. Others, like epidemiologist Thomas Francis, advocated for a placebo-controlled design to assess promising polio interventions.[206] In 1955, after conducting the largest placebo-controlled trial in medical history, Francis announced the efficacy of the formalin-killed Salk vaccine in a public forum.[207]

The debate over the necessity of clinical trials during a pandemic like COVID unmasked a predicament that risks eroding trust in a healthcare system willing to withhold potentially effective treatment during a crises. History shows that doctors continue to need rigorous placebo-controlled trials to reliably assess potentially effective therapies, such as hydroxychloroquine for COVID. The challenge is to do so in a way that both respects patient rights and satisfies scientific rigor. A potential solution is to involve community stakeholders in recognizing the importance of using available scientific methodologies (e.g., the stepped wedge trial) that minimize the length of time untreated controls groups go without intervention while maintaining statistical power to assess efficacy or harm.[208] Similarly, efforts could to made address scientific mistrust by highlighting the historical benefit of using interventions guided by randomized controlled trials, which have allowed doctors to assess the efficacy of vaccines against polio and drugs to treat AIDS, while avoiding the dangers of promoting untested drugs like hydroxychloroquine. To minimize distrust, physicians must be transparent in acknowledging to their patients the difficulty of withholding potentially effective drugs when consequences of doing so are high.

These stories reveal a fundamental aspect of science that makes science trustworthy. Naomi Oereskes has argued that scientific results are trusted because science, by its very nature, is a collective enterprise, and its findings are always verified through vetting and peer reviews.[209] This view is an extension of Ludwig Fleck's earlier idea of thought collectives: what makes something a fact is that experts agree on it.[210] Oereskes argues that scientific communities rely on collective institutions and peer consensus to accept or reject research results, which makes science as a whole reliable. Oereskes affirms the reliability of scientific claims if they emerge from a healthy scientific ecosystem. The dilemma over the use of randomized controlled trials during AIDS and COVID provides insights into Oereskes' arguments by showing how patience with the time-consuming methods of scientists breaks down during times of urgent epidemic threats.

COVID, AIDS, and syphilis also provide examples of situations where trust in science breaks down due to perceptions that scientific advice threatens civil liberties. Some citizens refuse COVID vaccination and ignore social-distancing recommendations because they believe these measures impinge on their personal freedoms. There have been instances during AIDS and syphilis when the government has gone too far in abridging the freedom and livelihood of individuals in the name of public health (chapters 1 and 2). These episodes illustrate how coercive public health measures, unlike the recommendations made today to help contain COVID in nonauthoritarian societies, can revoke the personal liberties of citizens. In the case of syphilis, the U.S. government arrested female prostitutes and detained them in reformatories for years (from World War I to 1953) to protect soldiers from the disease.[211] American women who had proven or suspected venereal diseases, or who were considered "promiscuous," were forcibly placed in detention centers and quarantined without due process, thereby depriving them of their livelihood and violating their civil liberties.

Likewise, when an HIV test was developed in 1985 for diagnosis and screening blood, some alarmed citizens called for compulsory testing and the indefinite quarantining of those with positive tests (chapter 2).[212] Gay activists protested what they argued was a blood test that would be used for discrimination in housing and employment and therefore a violation of civil liberties.[213] Instead, they proposed practices like members of the gay community assuming responsibility to notify their partners, and committing to measures that reduced harm (e.g., using condoms, closing bathhouses).[214] Many voluntarily restricted their behavior (e.g., by having sex only with protection), setting norms of safe sex without compromising pleasurable activity to protect public health.[215]

These AIDS activists highlighted a distinction between denying personal liberties (e.g., detaining sex workers, quarantining people who test HIV positive) and modifying behavior by adopting harm-reduction measures. They showed how coercively revoking civil liberties differs from the voluntary limiting of behavior for public health purposes. The behavioral modifications of gay activists in the 1980s—like the COVID recommendations made today for social distancing, mask wearing, and avoiding crowds—are inconveniences that do not revoke personal freedoms or threaten an individual's livelihood. Gay men were willing to accept these inconveniences to protect public health. The activists' actions in the early 1980s showed that it was possible for members of a community to willingly alter their behavior to maintain public health without sacrificing personal liberties—a precedent that remains important for COVID today.

Public Health Measures Expose Socioeconomic Inequalities and Turn Them into Health Disparities

The histories of AIDS and syphilis also provide a basis for understanding how medical interventions have fueled underlying health disparities during COVID. The life-saving HIV treatments of the 1990s exacerbated pre-existing socioeconomic inequalities because they were available to people living in wealthy nations but not those who resided in LMICs.[216] Activists rectified this inequality by advocating for funding from donor countries, elimination of IP laws and technology transfer arrangements, production of generic drugs, and improvements in health infrastructure in LMICs (chapter 2).[217] Nonetheless, a disproportionate number of AIDS and syphilis cases globally and in the United States still involve underprivileged populations due to poverty, lack of healthcare infrastructure and access to medicines, ongoing systemic racism, and mistrust of public health officials.[218] Consequently, treatment campaigns have exacerbated the persistence of these diseases among racial minorities, highlighting the need to address the socioeconomic factors that interfere with the ability of public health measures.

To achieve disease control, COVID elimination campaigns, like those of syphilis and AIDS, must also address socioeconomic issues. This is necessary to ensure compliance with social-distancing measures and an acceptable rate of vaccine delivery.[219] According to health policy expert Marcella Nunez-Smith, COVID public health strategies must address housing stability, food security, educational equity, and pathways to economic opportunities.[220] In addition, Stanford University pediatrician Rhea Boyd maintains that control strategies must include structural approaches targeting housing reform, universal worker protection, and an increase in minimum wage to reverse long-standing racial inequalities.[221] Strategies also need to include a message from a peer groups to advocate for vaccination and address mistrust in science and the government. Clyde Yancy, a cardiologist at Northwestern University, has argued for COVID programs to target economic development in vulnerable communities.[222] Policy experts and physicians have pointed out that campaigns to control COVID must include structural programs to address vulnerable environments, a notion reinforced by the histories of syphilis and AIDS.

Also like syphilis and AIDS campaigns, COVID elimination campaigns need to include structural interventions that mitigate unsafe behaviors. These include, among others, lessening the stigma that prevents people from wearing face masks, providing housing that allows poor people who do essential work to safely isolate while at home, ensuring universal protections for workers while on the job, and advocating for an increase in minimum wage, which could begin to reverse racial health inequities (chapter 6).[223] In addition, governmental strategies must address the challenge of distributing a limited supply of vaccines to people who need them most, such as frontline workers unable to work remotely, and to disadvantaged populations living in vulnerable environments, such as residents of inner cities, the homeless living in shelters, inmates in overcrowded jails and prisons, migrating workers in LMICs, or those residing on remote Native American Indian reservations.[224] Until strategies that address these socioeconomic issues are implemented, efforts to handle COVID, as has been the case with syphilis and AIDS, will accentuate underlying racial and social inequalities.[225]

As was the case with the global distribution of life-saving anti-HIV drugs, the COVID vaccination effort has unveiled a similar humanitarian problem: vaccines are primarily distributed to wealthy countries, leaving resource-poor countries underserved. The same is true for distributing oral drugs like Paxlovid, which can prevent hospitalizations and deaths from COVID.

With COVID today, socioeconomic and racial inequalities create environmental conditions that hamper containment strategies. Long-standing structural inequalities are behind the disparities.[226] Impoverished Americans, particularly Black and Hispanic people, often live in crowded homes, tenements, or boardinghouses. Under these circumstances, they cannot isolate from others when sick.[227] In addition, buildings in low-income areas are often left out of plans to improve indoor air quality, forcing the children and adults who live, work, and attend school in them to breathe substandard air indoors.

At times, authorities have advocated for staying at home as the best way to avoid COVID. African Americans and Latinos disproportionately belong to a segment of the labor force that lacks the capacity to work from home, a factor that places this community at higher risk for contracting the virus—both at work and at home.[228] African Americans are also at greater risk of severe disease once infected because they are less likely to be insured, more likely to have existing health conditions that predispose them to severe disease (e.g., diabetes), and less likely to have primary care physicians.[229] Furthermore, they often live in segregated neighborhoods that lack job opportunities, stable housing, and grocery stores with healthy food. The social determinants of health that explained the heightened vulnerability of persons of color to COVID include unequal access to education, employment, housing, and justice. In addition, therapies and preventive measures may not be equally available to racial and ethnic minorities due to reduced access to medical care and the lack of universal healthcare coverage. Health policy experts like David Blumenthal argue that these issues must be addressed in a centralized fashion to enable adequate vaccine distribution and coverage.[230]

Thus, COVID, like AIDS and syphilis, has impacted persons of color and of lower socioeconomic status at much higher rates. Biomedical techniques designed to eliminate the disease may exacerbate these disparities. For COVID, then, increased infections among Black people result from inadequate access to healthy foods and habitable housing—as well as the innate biases of physicians.[231] They also result from joblessness; a mistrust in science, physicians, and government officials; limited access to care (e.g., due to a lack of transportation); and limited capacity to distribute treatments to underserved neighborhoods.[232]

The persistent economic and logistical barriers that impede adequate vaccine distribution to LMICs, poor inner-city areas, and remote rural areas pose humanitarian problems, threatening to deepen global inequities and divide countries with access to vaccines from those without.[233] Uneven distribution of biomedical products—whether life-saving HIV drugs or effective coronavirus vaccines—exacerbates underlying social inequalities and creates health disparities. The ability of wealthier nations to buy vaccines while poor nations cannot has led to what Tedros Ghebreyesus, head of the WHO, has termed a "catastrophic moral failure."[234] As has been the case with AIDS, organizations (e.g., GAVI Alliance and COVAX) have proposed strategies that view vaccines as a merit good, emphasizing the need to improve vaccine distribution to poor nations and to enhance global vaccine coverage. But even with the help of these organizations, there have not been enough vaccines to achieve adequate global coverage.[235]

The humanitarian problems posed by the unequal global distribution of COVID vaccines have historical precedent. During the AIDS pandemic in the 1990s, life-saving drugs available in wealthy nations took years to reach Africans who needed them. While mortality rates from the disease dropped in the United States during that period, they remained static in Africa. The eventual global distribution of ART, facilitated by the lobbying of activists, required the cooperation of drug companies with governments of LMICs to ensure adequate distribution during the emergency. A similar approach is needed to allocate COVID vaccines globally to those in need. This underscores an ongoing humanitarian crisis, as vaccine rates have remained low in LMICs while people in wealthy countries receive COVID vaccines.

As has been the case with syphilis and AIDS, biomedical advances involving COVID—vaccines and treatments—have turned pre-existing socioeconomic inequalities into healthcare disparities.[236] Developed nations where large portions of the population have been vaccinated experience lower rates of overall disease, severe outcomes, and deaths compared with LMICs, where there are problems in affording and distributing drugs to populations who need them.[237] This may be compounded by inequities in the availability of oral treatments such as Paxlovid that have the potential to reduce COVID deaths. Vaccines and therapies for COVID can, like interventions for HIV, widen pre-existing economic inequalities and turn them into health disparities. IP waivers, generic production of drugs, and contributions from donor countries, as has been done for HIV/AIDS, can mitigate these disparities.

For COVID, as was true for syphilis and AIDS, there have not always been straightforward solutions for developing strategies to rectify disparities that result in persistent disease in vulnerable communities.[238] For example, there were limited supplies of vaccines during their early rollout in 2020, which exposed a dilemma of whether to vaccinate all essential workers or whether to include minorities (who were poor and had borne the greatest risk for infection), the elderly, and people with serious medical conditions (who were dying of the virus at the highest rates).[239] Notwithstanding these dilemmas, as the COVID pandemic has matured, it persists unevenly both globally (affecting mostly LMICs) and within wealthy countries (concentrated among people who are at high risk of developing serious disease).

Additional social factors, such as stigma, can also interfere with COVID control programs. Stigma is a less overt factor in COVID than with syphilis and AIDS, but it plays a role in threatening adherence to public health recommendations. For COVID, people of Chinese origin who live in the United States report feeling stigmatized by the rhetoric of the "Chinese virus."[240] Furthermore, some individuals, including Trump, attached stigma to those who wore face masks, whom he derided as weak, unmanly conformists who disturbed the sensibility of those who prioritized personal liberties above all else.[241] Stigma surrounding COVID persists, polarizes, and undermines public health attempts to control the disease.

Stigmatization and polarization have also surrounded COVID vaccination. The chance of rapprochement between two polarized camps of incompatible ideology over COVID vaccination may seem remote. Yet AIDS provides an example of how opposing groups came together in the 1990s during a period of contention about the necessity to conduct clinical trials. At the time, TAG, a splinter group of AIDS activists, worked together with the medical establishment to develop new classes of more potent drugs and help evaluate them by promoting conventional studies. The seemingly unlikely rapprochement between the two groups occurred in the context of drug development.[242] This circumstance provides precedence for fostering communication and solidarity between two opposing groups—an approach that could improve public health outcomes if applied to COVID in the context of vaccine distribution.[243]

Public health officials have pointed out that trust and a communitarian ethic are necessary to stop pandemics—that people must learn to cooperate and act in solidarity. This has been the case in Denmark, for example, where most of the population voluntarily supported social distancing (90 percent) and vaccines (85 percent), thereby avoiding the need for mandates during COVID.[244] Countries like Denmark, some have pointed out, have greater adherence to measures like social distancing and vaccine uptake due to the country's higher level of social and institutional trust compared with other countries. Denmark shows how social solidarity and widespread public confidence can improve vaccine confidence and rates.[245] To effectively manage pandemics, social scientists argue for a sense of unity that promotes care among people, without those who are vaccinated stigmatizing the unvaccinated. This ingredient is necessary for community cohesiveness, a communitarian ethic, and a trust in scientist expertise—key elements for improving public health outcomes during epidemics.[246]

In the United States, by contrast, historian David Rosner has noted that the emphasis during the twentieth century was on individualism.[247] Rosner has observed a shift in public health from managing the nineteenth-century infectious diseases of urbanization to a more individualized approach focused on addressing chronic noninfectious diseases like heart disease and cancer.[248] With COVID (during which mandates became necessary), the country was not well versed in emphasizing collective responsibilities. According to Rosner, Americans have embraced individual rights over collective responsibilities—a trend undercutting the notion of a social contract in which people work together to achieve a greater good, even one so basic as maintaining public health during times of infectious disease threats.

At the heart of the issue is how to live as humans during a pandemic. During such times, community cohesiveness and a concern for survival of the community should be the top priority over individual desires. This indeed occurred during the early phase of the HIV epidemic, when gay activists advocated for the survival of the collective and the viability of their community.[249] By restricting their sexual activities to practices that were safe, the gay community made a tacit pact to protect the uninfected.[250] Gay activists saw it as their obligation to take social responsibility for protecting the health of the community through a normative process: leaders of the Gay Men's Health Crisis defined standards of safe behavior.[251] Leadership within the group encouraged concern for the collective so that the community norm balanced what the individual might want against a concern for the health of the group.[252] As discussed earlier in the book, this did not come without a fight, as the community was heterogeneous and demonized with internal politics during the sexual revolution and the new gay rights movement.[253]

The major challenges for public health experts managing COVID today include how to rectify the socioeconomic issues that have driven the pandemic, undermined efforts to eliminate it, and left an uneven distribution of disease. Additional challenges include how to reduce the mistrust in science, medicine, and government that has led to inadequate social-distancing measures and vaccine rates. The most enduring legacy of COVID may be our need to develop a communitarian ethos and collaborative work ethic in times of crisis. These skills will be useful when the next pandemic appears, whatever it may be, as human behavior and activities place us at risk for new emerging diseases—the exact origins of which remain elusive despite scientific attempts to apprehend them.

Syphilis, AIDS, and COVID reveal another limitation of scientific medicine: the failure to elucidate the exact origins of these diseases. Despite the attempts of scientists to identify how these diseases began, and the great public interest in this inquiry, the origins of these epidemics remain mysterious. The debate over the pre-Colombian versus Columbian origin of syphilis remains unresolved.[254] Regardless of how syphilis emerged, its spread via migrating populations (due to war and overseas expansion), the disbanding of mercenary armies, urbanization, income inequality (leading to a rise in brothels), and social habits (communal baths, shared drinking cups) implicates broad swaths of human behaviors. Similarly, with regard to the origin of AIDS, historical events changed the environment so that it became vulnerable to HIV.[255] Infectious disease doctor Jacques Pepin postulates that HIV jumped from chimpanzees to African hunters, then was amplified during mid-century disease-eradication campaigns that used (and reused) improperly sterilized needles during a time when European nations did not adequately invest in the health infrastructure of their colonies. The disease then spread widely following the road building, urbanization, and prostitution that characterized colonialized Africa. Specific historical circumstances—tropical disease eradication campaigns, brothels, colonization, and civil wars—enabled HIV and syphilis to become pandemics.

Although the exact nature and timeline of these events remains unknown, theories surrounding the origin of HIV and syphilis illustrate how humans, through their customs, habits, work, and conquests, change the environment in ways that cannot be anticipated. These activities may unleash an organism from the host in which it evolved (e.g., chimpanzees) into a new species, where it can become pathogenic (e.g., humans). Or they may create an environment that can amplify an epidemic (e.g., migrating populations, urbanization, prostitution, shared needles). The theory of environmental susceptibility to explain the origin of the HIV epidemic removes the blame of initiating the epidemic from a specific individual, such as the spurious idea proposed in the 1980s that early spread was the fault of "Patient Zero," Gaëtan Dugas.[256] Indeed, the inclination to blame an individual or group for a disease has also occurred in the cases of syphilis (blaming sinful sailors from other nations) and COVID (blaming the "Chinese" virus brought to the United States by maligned outsiders). Instead, the theory of environmental susceptibility situates the origins of syphilis and AIDS in human activities that perturb the natural environment, facilitating the emergence and spread of new epidemics.

The discourse surrounding the origins of syphilis and HIV is consistent with René Dubos's idea that epidemics will continue to occur due to the many ways in which humans have manipulated the physical and social environments throughout civilizations. New, unforeseen consequences, he predicted, will be unleased because of human attempts to shape the environment through their habits and customs, including science.[257] These attempts, he maintains, will trade one problem for another and trigger unpredictable consequences.

Since Dubos's prediction, a succession of epidemics have indeed emerged after 1981, following the AIDS epidemics. Population migration resulting from war, commerce, leisure travel, or unstable governments, for example, led to the emergence of SARS, Ebola, Zika, COVID, and Mpox, just as they enabled the spread of syphilis and HIV. Similarly, in medieval times, new modes of transportation that caused deforestation, urbanization, and construction of roads facilitated the dissemination of plague, just as they have done in modern times with Ebola, HIV, and Lyme. Humankind's Enlightenment-based zeal to master nature and become free of disease can release uncontrollable dangers.[258] Epidemics that were once strict zoonoses (e.g., Mpox) have now spilled over to humans, among whom they are contagious (e.g., SARS, COVID, Ebola, HIV, avian influenza). Human activities change our relationship with microbes by causing microbes to escape the environment in which they have co-evolved with their host.[259] As civilizations have evolved, the number of epidemics that have emerged or resurged has increased proportionately, along with public health programs designed to eliminate them.

The origin of COVID, like that of syphilis and AIDS, remains speculative. Most scientists favor the hypothesis of a spillover from human exposure to an intermediate host, but the possibility of a laboratory leak has not been excluded.[260] Scientists struggle to identify the origin of each epidemic, and the result is unsettling. Without the ability to pinpoint exactly how and why these epidemics emerged, society can never fully prepare for future occurrences. This inability underscores the limitations of scientific medicine to reassure humans about how to avoid future epidemics.

Besides AIDS and COVID, a multitude of epidemics have caught an unprepared world by surprise since 1981. The appearance of SARS, three strains of influenza (H5N1, H1N1, and H7N9), Zika, and Ebola demonstrate that epidemics have never been conquered and in fact are becoming more numerous.[261] More recently, a disease caused by the same family as SARS (Middle East respiratory syndrome, or MERS) developed in Saudi Arabia, and new cases continue.[262] Furthermore, the re-emergence of yellow fever in Brazil poses a widespread threat given the extensive prevalence of the vector in tropical nations.[263] Outbreaks of measles have occurred due to undervaccinated populations and widespread air travel.[264] And the devastating COVID pandemic arose and was spread due to commercial practices and travel during holiday seasons.[265] The population density resulting from urbanization and poverty has facilitated the spread of COVID, as well as older diseases like tuberculosis. Indeed, the diverse array of epidemics that have surfaced in response to human activities and their societal consequences since 1981 surpasses any other time in history.

Conclusion

COVID, syphilis, and AIDS share similar patterns. Each appeared suddenly and led to a period of confidence in the promise of biomedicine to eliminate the disease, only to be tempered by the reality that there is no definitive end. Diseases remain with us, and so do our efforts to eliminate them. This defies a narrative that promises any notion of a return to normal pre-epidemic patterns of living. The characterization of an epidemic as having a discrete beginning with a "drift towards closure" was introduced by Charles Rosenberg in 1989.[266] Indeed, the patterns of COVID, syphilis, and AIDS show how these epidemics have defied biomedical attempts to end them. The reality supports historian Guillaume Lachenal's idea that epidemics contain "unsettling . . . periods, during which life has to be recomposed."[267] This book adds to such characterizations by showing that as epidemics mature, they lose public attention and fall from priority, leading to reduced preparedness efforts to prevent future epidemics.

Samuel Cohn points out that not all epidemics follow a prescribed pattern.[268] Some, like tuberculosis, share similarities with syphilis, AIDS, and COVID. Selman Waksman, who discovered the antitubercular drug streptomycin, envisioned a "final eradication" of tuberculosis when multidrug regimens became available in 1964.[269] The disease, however, rages today amid public complacency as socioeconomic factors have undermined biomedically based elimination efforts.[270] On the other hand, the definitive endings of smallpox and Rinderpest, and the specter of eradicating guinea worm and chagas disease, underscore the fact that epidemics do not conform to any uniform pattern.

The arcs of syphilis, AIDS, and COVID also shed light on the unfolding narrative of biomedicine. In the mid-twentieth century, people believed in the limitless potential of biomedicine to eliminate epidemic diseases. Syphilis, AIDS, and COVID, however, reveal the limits of biomedicine by showing that science can neither exactly explain how the epidemics began nor meet the goal of eliminating them. Humans today, consequently, live in a polyepidemic era that is more diverse than in the nineteenth century. The age of the great nineteenth-century epidemics has not ended; their cultural imprint remains significant. However, the focus has shifted from an era characterized by massive deaths to one that requires perpetual calls to regulate our day-to-day behaviors.

Living with epidemics and the biomedical attempts to eliminate them permeates our everyday existence and negates the idea of a complete return to pre-epidemic normalcy. With COVID, previously innocuous activities like going to a crowded performance, attending school, or gathering as a family now entail consciously adopting habits to avoid the potentially dangerous virus. Decisions regarding how to evade the virus have become part of our daily consciousness—regardless of how cavalierly or vigilantly one chooses to behave. For AIDS, syphilis, and Mpox, the at-risk behaviors are more specific than they are for COVID. Nonetheless, the same principle applies: engaging in certain activities (e.g., sexual activity outside a committed relationship) places one at risk. For other infections, the requirement for behavioral change—like cancelling outdoor gatherings to avoid mosquito-borne viral encephalitis, or avoiding travel to Zika-endemic areas during pregnancy—is less frequent. These adjustments underscore the cumulative burden of epidemics on our lives, necessitating behavioral changes that restrict freedoms without abrogating civil liberties. In the next chapter, we will expand on individual behavioral changes and address how humans have attempted to modify their environments to reduce collective vulnerability to AIDS, syphilis, and COVID.

Chapter 6

Vulnerable Environments

Historical Roots

Public health efforts in the nineteenth century focused on rectifying filthy environments that made people vulnerable to the spread of infection. The introduction of the germ theory, however, promised to change the focus of public health. By the early twentieth century, scientific public health campaigns utilized specific strategies devised in bacteriology laboratories to disrupt microbes' contact with their human hosts. The change in focus from the environment to the individual was ushered in with the introduction of bacteriology. The efficacy of biomedical solutions made public health's pre–germ theory focus on rectifying vulnerable environments seem outdated to early twentieth-century public health reformers. A study of syphilis, AIDS, and COVID, however, shows that elimination campaigns must also target social and environmental structures that confound biomedically based campaigns. Studying these diseases and the efforts to eradicate them shows that biomedical public health approaches must include a structural component designed to change susceptible environments. The nineteenth-century focus on environmental vulnerability remains viable today.

Syphilis and AIDS

During the test-and-treat syphilis campaigns of the 1930s to the 1970s (chapters 1 and 3), public health officials and physicians asked patients to cooperate with instructions to be tested, receive treatment, name sexual contacts, and avoid extramarital or commercial sex.[1] But their interviewing techniques failed to consider the cultural and economic characteristics of the differing populations and therefore did not reach prisoners, migrant workers, teenagers, and male homosexuals. Because physicians' methods to target individual behavior did not work for all groups, treatment remained the major focus of campaigns to eliminate syphilis and STIs.[2] Public health methods in the 1970s, as outlined in chapter 3, addressed socioeconomic factors but emphasized primarily a biomedical approach, including treatment with effective antibiotics to cure the disease and prevent transmission.[3]

The limits of the biomedical approach, however, revealed themselves when HIV appeared in the early 1980s. Early diagnosis of HIV was of little benefit to infected patients when there were no effective treatments. At the time, the only way to control the epidemic was through behaviorally based preventive efforts, an approach founded on the idea that providing knowledge about a disease would change behavior. Public health officials advocated the adoption of "knowledge, attitude, perception" (KAP) and "abstinence, be faithful, condom" (A, B, C) programs.[4] These programs assumed that sexual risk and protective behavior result from conscious decision-making processes, that risk for HIV is based on unwise personal choices, and that behaviors are under cognitive control.[5]

Behavioral programs based on moderating individual behavior to reduce HIV transmission have had variable success. In the San Francisco in the 1980s, for example, the "Stop AIDS in SF" movement changed behavior in MSM by mobilizing the local gay community to provide risk-reduction information to individuals.[6] But in other situations, KAP messages have been less effective. Encouraging female sex workers to use condoms in South Africa failed, for example, as doing so would have risked their only source of income, and the disadvantaged social status of women did not allow the workers to negotiate with male clients.[7]

These cognitive approaches targeting individuals fail, social scientists claim, because people may be unable to change their behavior despite being aware of how HIV is spread. The weakness of KAP and ABC programs lies in the assumption that people can make rational choices about sexual risk and protection. People may be knowledgeable about safe-sex practices yet still be unable to change risky behavior.[8] Because human sexuality may not be subject to cognitive control, preventive approaches targeted at the individual may have a limited ability to produce behavior change.[9] Approaches at the individual level neglect broader determinants at the societal level that prompt risky behavior and create environmental susceptibility.[10]

Social Determinants and Structural Programs

Given the limited success of behavioral prevention changes, public health officials and social scientists have addressed the need to target social determinants that underlie risky behavior and create susceptibility at the environmental level.

The social determinants of risk behavior assume behavior is influenced by so-cial, cultural, and economic factors. Public health interventions can target a range of socioeconomic structures to change the context in which high-risk behaviors occur, and they can include changes in policy or legal mandates.[11] Unlike KAP programs, structural-level changes can affect populations and vulnerable environments that lead to risky behaviors.[12]

Many socioeconomic factors create vulnerable environments in develop-ing and industrialized nations. Areas of vulnerability can include the social, economic, and physical makeup of environments marked by chronic poverty, unemployment, and little opportunity for education. Limited job options in communities with chronic unemployment can breed fatalism that can encour-age exaggerated risk-taking behaviors (e.g., drug use, crime, violence).[13] Lack of access to education may limit women's employment opportunities and force them into risky work (e.g., prostitution).[14] This is especially true in regions where gender disparities may discourage female workers from negotiating con-dom use with clients. In some developing countries, men who travel long dis-tances for work (e.g., migrant workers, truck drivers, soldiers, refugees) may adopt risky behaviors, including the frequenting of prostitutes, while being uprooted from family.[15] In Africa, the practice of having concurrent sexual partners allows a person's infection to spread through groups.[16] In developed countries, undereducated minorities in poor urban neighborhoods may find involvement in the illicit drug trade one of their few economic options.[17] Social scientists insist that public health approaches cannot neglect these socioeco-nomic constraints.

Social scientists and public health officials assert that conventional preven-tion programs fail because they overestimate the degree of agency that people can exercise and underestimate the extent to which people may be constrained by socioeconomic factors they cannot control.[18] Campaigns fail when they require workers to relinquish their livelihoods to prevent spread of disease. They have little success in overriding well-established cultural practices. Attempts to change behavior in African communities where individuals may have concurrent partners will not be effective without acknowledging local val-ues regarding long-term relationships in which trust may impede routine con-dom use.[19] Asking drug users to avoid sharing needles will be ineffective unless safe facilities are available and repressive laws that inhibit drug users from using the facilities are modified.[20] The only hope of changing behavior, social scien-tists and policy experts maintain, is to address underlying societal and legal factors that constrain individual agency, propel groups into risky situations, and create vulnerable environments.[21]

Structural programs can target HIV risks at the environmental level. The physical environment can be targeted by upgrading street lights to reduce the likelihood of rape. Structural programs can include the passage of health and safety legislation to improve the working environment of sex workers (e.g., worker registration, brothel inspection to ensure compliance with regulations, licensing workers who have been cleared medically, and mandating that customers use condoms). They can involve expanding clinical services (e.g., needle exchange programs, access to drug substitution therapy for dependence), or changing laws that criminalize use of certain drugs or sex work.[22] They can empower sex workers through peer counseling to establish norms of responsible behavior within a community.[23] They can include cash-transfer programs to provide women with capital to start less-risky income-generating activities.[24] They can remove barriers to retention of care by poor people (e.g., vouchers for travel, telemedicine), and provide messages on the importance of safe practices by peer-group leaders (e.g., clergy in African American communities, female sex workers to negotiate condom use with male clients).[25]

Effective structural programs must be adapted to specific locales.[26] Peer education strategies must be customized to the social makeup of targeted vulnerable groups (e.g., female sex workers, female bar workers in truck stops, and male transport workers), who may be alienated from uniform prevention messages by virtue of their marginalized social status.[27] Customized approaches involve accessing social networks through key individuals and asking them to disseminate risk reduction messages throughout their networks.[28] Customized programs may focus on reducing needle exchange in some Eastern European countries, reducing monogamous couple's concurrent sexual partners in rural South Africa, or using peer education to reduce high-risk behaviors among gay men, including African American gay men, in urban American settings.[29] Messages delivered in group settings at social institutions—including the workplace, prisons, military facilities, faith-based organizations, and schools—are examples of context-specific community mobilization efforts. The most effective strategy depends on knowing the profile of the local at-risk population and customizing the structural program to the environment.

Public health experts, including Michael Merson from the Duke Global Health Institute, and Joep Lange, former president of the International AIDS Society, have emphasized that HIV control programs must combine biomedical strategies with these sorts of structural strategies.[30] Anthropologist João Biehl used the Brazilian AIDS Control Program (BACP) to exemplify this point. Biehl claims that BACP failed because it was too narrow in its focus of supplying ART to all HIV-infected citizens while ignoring the social disparities that gave rise to and fueled the epidemic, including demands for adequate housing and employment, and provision of social support infrastructure. Biehl argued that the BACP neglected to provide a comprehensive plan that addressed socioeconomic structural issues while delivering biomedical treatment.[31]

Both developed countries and LMICs have implemented comprehensive biomedical and structural HIV-control programs sporadically. Philippines and Thailand have created programs that make ART accessible to patients and have endorsed tailored, structural approaches to HIV prevention aimed at groups with elevated risks.[32] These nations have regulated the health of sex workers within a legally sanctioned framework whereby workers are provided with diagnostic screening tests and treatment services, and are required to be medically cleared in order to continue working.[33] They have enlisted the cooperation of sex-establishment owners and sex workers to encourage clients to use condoms, and have implemented multimedia campaigns for school education on AIDS.[34] Canada has encouraged drug users to protect themselves against HIV by implementing needle exchange programs and providing sites where injection can take place under the watch of healthcare personnel.[35] But these measures have not been adopted on a widespread basis. Noting this, the director of HIV prevention at the CDC, Kevin Fenton, advocated broadening the scope of individual prevention programs in the United States to include a wider range of structural programs.[36]

Comprehensive public health campaigns currently include structural components in contexts other than STIs. To counteract diarrheal illnesses, for example, programs have been launched to improve sanitation problems that had led to water supply contamination.[37] They have also included community education to address the stigmatization that prevent persons with leprosy and Chagas disease from seeking health care.[38] Despite these efforts, some have viewed public health programs that address structural factors as being too inefficient, expensive, and imprecise. There is concern that the programs take too long to make any meaningful change and attempt to address factors that may lack relevance to controlling a disease.[39] In addition, it is difficult to measure the effectiveness of broad structural strategies that seek to change society-level factors. For these reasons, public health programs have gravitated toward more efficient proximal epidemic control by employing approaches that target the causative microbe—as advocated by early twentieth-century scientific public health proponents.[40]

Structural interventions, nonetheless, have been used on occasion throughout the twentieth century. During the 1930s, for example, Pholela Community Health Centers were created in South Africa to overcome societal barriers to delivering health care there.[41] Clinics built in rural areas made efforts to change social norms to reduce syphilis among diamond and gold miners.[42] Similarly, public health campaigns from the 1930s to today have attempted to address the social issues that drove the syphilis epidemic while focusing on biomedical testing and treating.[43] Internationally, structural interventions were implemented from the 1960s through the 1980s to provide clean water and adequate housing.[44] The use of structural interventions expanded following the 1978 WHO/UNICEF Alma Ata Declaration, which linked health to the reform of social and economic conditions.[45] This sparked an expansion of existing programs that targeted access to clean water, reduction of tobacco use, and implementation of clean air standards.[46]

Structural factors contributing to the spread of HIV were occasionally addressed during the first decade of the epidemic.[47] As discussed in chapter 2, grassroots changes in social norms led to reduced sexual risk in gay communities, policy changes at the governmental level, and physical alterations such as the closure of bathhouses in San Francisco.[48] In addition, a program in Thailand to ensure 100 percent condom usage by commercial sex workers and their clients involved policy change, condom distribution, and change in the physical environment through the monitoring of brothels.[49] By 1995, structural interventions for HIV prevention that altered the legality of selling sex were in place in several LMICs.[50]

Other structural interventions to promote STI control were addressed during the 1990s. A 1995 Institute of Medicine (IOM) report on HIV prevention encouraged policymakers to use social and behavioral methods to curb the spread of the virus.[51] In 2000, the journal *AIDS* advocated control programs to address laws, policies, norms, institutions (e.g., schools, media), and health and social services (e.g., via improvements in accessibility and location) to reduce HIV spread.[52] They defined a risk environment as a social or physical space in which a variety of factors interact to increase the chances of disease transmission.[53] This framework has been used to characterize other HIV high-risk environments—for example, among drug users, women, and sex workers and in gay communities in Australia.[54] Public health expert King Holmes stressed the importance of structural interventions in high-risk neighborhoods in both the United States and LMICs to reduce syphilis, HIV, and STI transmission. Holmes noted that factors such as poor educational opportunities for women, increasing urban prostitution, injection drug use, war, migration, and the growing number of teenagers and young adults no longer under the regulatory influence of a family created vulnerable environments that drove risky behaviors. He proposed policy changes to access clean needles, media campaigns to increase condom availability, and street outreach programs in high-risk communities.[55]

From the 1990s to the present, structural interventions have continued to be implemented for STD prevention internationally and domestically. Policy changes that increased access to clean syringes were implemented in Australia, European nations, and some U.S. cities to reduce HIV transmission risk among injecting drug users.[56] Public policy interventions were implemented for bathhouses.[57] Media campaigns, initially used in the 1990s to increase condom distribution, have persisted, although their emphasis today is on PrEP advocacy.[58]

Structural interventions to reduce disease among injection drug users include legislation and policy changes to promote needle exchange programs and enable pharmacies to release clean needles and syringes.[59] Street outreach programs conducted by local peers involve interacting with persons in high-incidence neighborhoods to reduce the spread of HIV by eliminating needle sharing.[60] These have been coupled with community mobilization campaigns, which involve personal contacts by peer educators to change norms of risky behavior.[61] Regulation or closure of shooting galleries—where people engage in sex or injection drug use—reduces the number of sexual contacts, increases condom use, and reduces syringe sharing.[62]

Structural interventions have been used to reduce STIs in MSM. Gay activists created media campaigns using posters and fliers to make condoms socially acceptable and desirable, and to increase condom availability in bars serving high-risk individuals.[63] Bathhouses were required to enforce condom use during sex, or otherwise be closed.[64] MSM community leaders sought to change risky sexual norms and behaviors by advocating reforms.[65] Their messages have been incorporated in STD community-level interventions.[66] The variable success of these programs, however, has led to a switch in the emphasis of public health campaigns away from condoms and toward PrEP.[67] Some experts have become concerned about "risk compensation," or increased sexual risk-taking behavior because of a perceived decrease in HIV susceptibility when taking PrEP.[68] Nonetheless, the HIV prevention strategies adopted by a new generation of gay male activists have used social media to lobby for access to global generic markets to make PrEP affordable and increase its use.[69] Popular discourses today portray gay men as complacent about HIV, with their activism targeting global distribution of ART to patients who were left behind in the early 2000s. In fact, however, activists continue to take up the cause of HIV prevention.[70]

Some public health experts have distinguished superstructural factors from the structural-level factors discussed above. Gender inequality, poverty, income inequality, and racial disparities are superstructural factors that drive HIV infection and impede HIV prevention programs.[71] The superstructural drivers of HIV infection are the most difficult to rectify.[72] In the interim, the question is whether it may be most valuable to identify small to modest changes in structural factors to impact HIV control. For example, interventions such as microcredit, cash transfers, and microenterprises (providing loans to female sex workers for startup businesses, e.g., making and selling jewelry), can reduce HIV risk behavior by providing an income that liberates women from engaging in sex work.[73] Public health efforts may be unable to end poverty among all women (a superstructural issue), but they may be able to alleviate poverty among at-risk groups of female sex workers (at the structural level).[74]

Other structural factors leading to vulnerable environments, including inadequate housing and homelessness in developed countries and LMICs, have been targeted in the context of HIV. Unstable housing, along with frequent evictions, is associated with higher HIV risk.[75] Homelessness and housing instability among HIV-infected persons are associated with poorer access to health care, lower ART adherence, higher use of illicit drugs, and exchanging sex for money.[76] HIV risk and poor health outcomes among the homeless are driven by comorbidities (e.g., substance use and psychiatric disorders) that increase HIV risk and challenge ART adherence. Structural interventions targeting the associations between homelessness and HIV risk have included housing subsidies and public housing.[77] In addition, there has been attention to improving the physical character of neighborhoods based on an assumption that community cohesion will reduce HIV disparities.[78] Examples include converting vacant lots and abandoned buildings where drugs are sold and sex exchanges might occur into community gardens.[79]

Food insecurity is another socioeconomic factor linked with HIV risk and outcome. Lack of food security is a predictor of sexual risk behavior (e.g., transactional sex in exchange for money or food). Food insecure patients experience worse medical outcomes: they are less likely to access HIV treatment, remain in care, and adhere to ART.[80] Thus, structural programs designed to rectify food insecurity in developed countries, such as the Ryan White Treatment Program in the United States, aim to improve HIV outcomes by providing nutritious food.[81] Interventions in LMICs, such as the Shamba Maisa Program in Kenya, are designed with similar goals.[82] Furthermore, food programs can enable retention of HIV-infected individuals in clinical care if they are linked with the healthcare system.[83]

Structural interventions aimed at achieving alternative sources of income for female sex workers have been used to improve financial security, particularly in LMICs.[84] Strategies have included microenterprise programs, vocational

training, income-generative activities, and cooperative banking and savings programs.[85] In addition to reducing HIV risk, these programs can promote the
empowerment of workers by confronting the economic exclusion they experience as marginalized communities. Other structural interventions for workers
are aimed at reducing gender inequality and economic vulnerability by decrim-
inalizing sex work and promoting access to safer-sex work venues.[86] With these
interventions, the focus is on empowering and mobilizing sex workers and
reducing environmental vulnerability.[87]

Medication-assisted treatment (MAT) for opioid use disorders and HIV are
other examples of structural interventions. Opioid use leads to an increase in
injection drug use and thereby an increase in HIV infection rates, and it also
serves as a barrier to accessing and staying in HIV care.[88] Health policy experts
note that solutions to structural barriers to linkage, testing, and treatment need
to address substance use and HIV infection, including incorporating MAT with
specific agents (e.g., buprenorphine and suboxone) in primary care settings.[89]
Interventions include changes in legal constraints that discourage primary care
physicians from prescribing MAT, thereby improving adherence to and retention in care, and improving HIV treatment outcomes.[90] Healthcare experts argue
that MAT needs to be integrated with HIV treatment.

Community mobilization is another important component of various HIV
structural strategies, as exemplified by the Brazilian rights-based approach that
empowered key affected populations. During the 2000s in Brazil, a coalition of
MSM-rights activists confronted HIV stigma, demanding that the rights of people
with AIDS be respected by their government and their fellow citizens.[91] AIDS
advocacy groups developed legal programs that focused on an expanded drug
formulary and laboratory testing used to monitor HIV treatments.[92] They
attempted to break down stigma surrounding homosexuality and HIV.[93] Sex
workers have also organized to protect themselves as workers—for example,
Brazil's National Network of Prostitutes. These groups have been able to attain
retirement benefits and health and social services assistance.[94] This progress
stems from a multidimensional intervention focused on community mobilization to prevent HIV infection, empowering gay communities in the process.

In summary, successful control programs are possible if they address environmental susceptibilities at the structural level in addition to using biomedical approaches. Public health programs must target socioeconomic factors by,
for example, improving housing, expanding access to education, ameliorating
poverty, rectifying social inequalities, and ensuring food security. These factors
all have the unfortunate potential to worsen disease spread.[95] Elimination programs must target environmental causes of disease more broadly, rather than

solely targeting individual risk factors or combating the responsible microbe.[96] Charles Chapin's hope in 1902 to focus public health efforts on the microbe and its interaction with the host, while ignoring broader environmental vulnerabilities, is insufficient to manage today's epidemics. Strategies must address social, cultural, and economic issues that create environmental vulnerability and are obstacles to achieving goals. The principles of nineteenth-century public health campaigns to rectify vulnerable environments remain important today.

As is the case with syphilis and AIDS, COVID elimination campaigns must address socioeconomic issues (chapter 5). Beyond relying on a vaccine, public health strategies for dealing with COVID must address housing stability, food security, educational equity, and pathways to economic opportunities.[97] Control strategies must include structural approaches targeted at providing universal health care, housing reform (to allow essential workers to safely isolate at home), universal worker protection, and an increase in minimum wage to reverse long-standing racial inequalities. They need to enlist messages from peer groups to advocate for vaccination and address mistrust in science and the government, and to mitigate stigmas that prevent people from wearing face masks.[98] Structural strategies at the governmental level must also address how to mass distribute a limited supply of vaccines to the people who need them, such as disadvantaged populations living in vulnerable environments—inner-city areas, homeless shelters, crowded jails, and remote Native American Indian reservations.[99]

To date, COVID, AIDS, and syphilis show that attempts to eliminate disease solely through biomedical strategies have been insufficient. These efforts must be accompanied by structural programs to address environmental vulnerabilities. The elimination programs of AIDS, syphilis, and COVID demonstrate that although the nineteenth-century public health emphasis on sanitizing the environment to control infectious diseases is no longer a major priority, the era's focus on rectifying vulnerable environments remains relevant.

Historical Roots of Today's Structural Programs

Efforts to control disease through manipulation of the environment or changes in policy are long-standing. Attempts to ensure a clean water supply, for example, date back to antiquity, when the Romans developed aqueducts for sewerage.[100] The Paris School in 1348 made efforts to control plague through environmental cleanup, offal removal, and discarding belongings of deceased plague victims from their homes.[101] These sanitation efforts later became key elements of public health practice during a period of increasing urbanization and population density in the mid-nineteenth century, coinciding with industrial expansion and urban growth.

The nineteenth-century idea that preventive efforts needed to take social responsibility into account is the historical analog for implementing structural measures to address HIV and syphilis today. These efforts must be directed toward rectifying environmental factors of disease spread. The nineteenth-century public health movement was based on the notion that living environments were the major determinant of physical disease. The considerable death and destruction caused by cholera, tuberculosis, smallpox, and yellow fever in American cities prompted public health measures to control them. Consequently, much of the work during that era was based on the prevailing theory that dirt caused disease, and that social conditions influenced a person's susceptibility to an unhealthful life.

In the nineteenth century, the dire social conditions of the growing masses in urban centers of England and the United States stirred reform in the field of community health.[102] Cities in Britain became medically dangerous (due, e.g., to cholera). Reformers like Edwin Chadwick proposed a goal for the state to remove filth through civil engineering—through the building of sewers, and through waste removal, street cleaning, and improved housing.[103] Chadwick believed that health was affected by the state of the physical and social environment. He illustrated how poor wages, disease prevention, environmental causes, and governmental action were intimately related. Chadwick's report declared that communicable disease was related to environmental conditions, lack of drainage, water supply, and inadequate, crowded housing, and he advocated a solution of removing refuse from houses and streets. Chadwick's focus on public health in the 1840s was to provide better dwellings for the poor and to promote sanitary reform. The same was true in the United States, where industrial expansion resulted in an influx of immigration, resulting in congested urban areas. A growing awareness of widespread poverty, malnutrition, and disease caused socially minded citizens, physicians, clergy, social workers, and government officials in the United States to rally around issues they sought to correct. They emphasized general hygiene for disease prevention, dietary improvement, higher wages, and housing reform.[104]

In Germany, Rudolf Virchow addressed the importance of changing the social environment in addition to the physical environment. Virchow saw the causes of ill health as resulting from social problems—low wages, inadequate diet, unregulated factories, poor clothing, lack of education, unhealthful working conditions, sweatshops, mines and factories, and overcrowded housing. He viewed disease not strictly as a biological event, but also as a social phenomenon.[105] Whereas Chadwick had focused on rectifying unsanitary environments through technological measures (e.g., drains, sewers, water pipes, etc.), Virchow emphasized changing the social environment to include reforms in education, wages, and housing. In the pregerm era, both were paying attention to improving susceptible environments—the physical (Chadwick) and the social (Virchow)—to promote health and control disease.

In the latter half of the nineteenth century, European scientists expanded on public health interventions to reduce risky environments. During a cholera outbreak in London from 1854 to 1856, John Snow changed the structures of water pumps to provide clean water.[106] During the Crimean War, from 1854 to 1898, Florence Nightingale implemented changes to the physical structure of the hospital at Scutari and procedural changes for patient care and the hospital's cleanliness.[107] Following her return to England, she worked to improve health care and disease prevention for British soldiers through structural and policy changes to improve institutional sanitation.

Similar efforts took place in the United States.[108] Health officers developed a range of responses, including urban sanitation projects to bring clean water into cities, regulating tenement housing, improving working environments to prevent tuberculosis, and regulating slaughterhouses. Additional strategies involved social and economic reforms designed to raise the low wages of workmen to reduce unhealthy behaviors such as excessive alcohol use.[109] Nineteenth-century public health officials believed unhealthy behaviors were rooted in environmental defects, and they considered efforts to change environmental factors necessary to correct these behavioral issues.[110]

Officials such as Henry Bowditch, of the Massachusetts Department of Public Health, also focused on changing the environment to prevent the spread of disease. Bowditch pointed out that social and environmental conditions created disease susceptibility—specifically, that the growth of cities post–Civil War led to overcrowded tenements that were conducive to illness. He focused on correcting the economic and social injustices that deprived the poor of their opportunity for health. He proposed preventing the sale of adulterated food, improving tenement life, improving exhausting workplace conditions (by providing sunlight and ventilation), facilitating the abatement of nuisances (e.g., encouraging butchers to dispose of waste material), and cleaning streets. These efforts stressed the physical and social conditions—rather than personal inadequacies—that led to dependency and disease. The key to restoring health was to correct structural issues (e.g., high prices and low wages) that created a vulnerable environment and risky behavior. Bowditch believed that improving the physical and social environments that predestined the poor to a life of destitution and disease was the best way to restore public health.[111]

Thus, public health efforts prior to widespread adoption of the germ theory, like the structural interventions targeting syphilis, AIDS, and COVID today, were focused on correcting the social and physical environments that lie at the root of risky behavior and disease. Nineteenth-century reformers like Chadwick and Bowditch stressed the importance of achieving health by changing a vulnerable environment rather than through individual instruction. Chadwick's emphasis on structural changes is mirrored today by reform efforts that focus on, for example, redesign of inner-city neighborhoods, improvement in urban street lighting, and repair of streets. Likewise, Bowditch stressed environmental changes that are echoed in public health programs for syphilis and AIDS today: remedying poverty, improving housing, and reducing unhealthy working conditions.[112] In the nineteenth century, disease was seen as resulting from the irresponsibility of society.[113]

But the focus of public health shifted following adoption of the germ theory. The doctrine that claimed that absence of filth was a sufficient barrier against contagion was challenged as scientists identified microbes that caused specific diseases. The development of chemical and medical methods, along with specialized bacteriological techniques, for reducing mortality from diphtheria in the 1890s contributed to a shift in responsibility for health from the layperson to the trained scientist, engineer, chemist, or biologist. With the advent of medical bacteriology and postulation of the germ theory, the focus of public health programs shifted from environmental control to targeting specific communicable diseases.[114] Historians Barbara Rosenkrantz, John Duffy, and Judith Walzer Leavitt have identified the 1880s through the early twentieth century as a transitional period for public health departments.[115]

Nineteenth-century public health campaigns also assumed that freedom from disease depended on individuals accepting a social and moral obligation to behave with personal moderation to protect society.[116] Thus, there is historical precedent for public health measures from the late 1900s until today that emphasize the assumption of personal moderation to protect one's own health and promote the health of the general population—a social contract. In liberal-democratic societies, it is the responsibility of the infected person to behave responsibly, to restrict their behavior while maintaining their liberty to protect the uninfected and insure the survival of the community. Certain well-established behaviors—for example, bathing, breastfeeding, refraining from spitting in public, avoiding alcoholism—are guided by such community morals and norms.

By the mid-1890s, health departments began to utilize bacteriology laboratories to perform diagnostic tests on individuals to determine whether it was appropriate to administer preventive vaccine or therapeutic serum.[117] By the early twentieth century, public health authorities argued that a scientific understanding of the elements involved in the transmission of communicable diseases permitted greater discrimination in implementing disease control measures than had been previously possible. In 1901, Chapin was a leader in using bacteriology to move the focus of public health work away from environmental sanitation and toward scientific testing of individuals (chapter 1).[118] Chapin argued to replace sanitation programs with methods using bacteriologic tools to identify infection, then choosing the practice that logically followed—vaccination, isolation, or treatment with serum.[119] He advocated tailoring these specific interventions on an individual basis, as determined by bacteriologic testing. Chapin hoped to make public health campaigns more efficient by focusing on the microbe and its interaction with the individual host and veering away from indiscriminate environmental concerns.[120] This approach was furthered by Milton Rosenau, who argued for surveillance of cases utilizing bacteriology laboratories and customizing interventions to prevent contact between the pathogen and the human host.[121]

Later in the twentieth century, physicians and medical historians expanded on Chapin's view that bacteriology allowed for the development of more targeted public health measures than had been possible before. In 1921, Stephen Smith, an officer in the New York Metropolitan Board of Health, concluded that knowledge of specific disease transmission among individuals was an advance over environmental approaches.[122] Howard Kramer, a medical historian, reinforced this idea in 1948, claiming that a bacteriological knowledge of methods of transmission allowed for precision in diagnosis and treatment.[123] The medical historian George Rosen stated in 1958 that the microbiology laboratory made the empirical sanitation of an earlier day more precise.[124] John Duffy, a professor of history, argued in 1990 that accurate microbiological methods of preventing disease spread enabled the use of effective vaccines.[125] These comments from physicians and historians both echo Chapin's arguments and show that as medical prophylaxes and therapies were introduced, the emphasis of public health shifted away from social reform and environmental improvement toward interventions that emphasized germ prevention or individual cure.[126]

The faith in science that began to replace the nineteenth-century public health focus on vulnerable environments was reinforced in the 1950s by the successes of antibiotics and vaccines in handling a variety of bacterial and viral infections. Confidence grew that cures and preventive vaccines that targeted specific diseases could be developed. The need for social reform and environmental changes seemed remote following the successes of the biomedical model in managing the polio and smallpox epidemics during the decades immediately preceding the AIDS pandemic.

But as the AIDS, syphilis, and COVID epidemics have evolved, public health authorities and social scientists have insisted on implementing structural measures targeted at the environment to accompany the biomedical approach. Science and microbiology have not displaced the need for a comprehensive approach to public health to correct environmental risks that are not necessarily related to specific pathogens. The AIDS, syphilis, and COVID pandemics show that policies aimed at social and environmental issues—together with biomedical therapeutic and preventive strategies—remain an important component of a public health campaign against epidemics. The new treatment and public health policies introduced for HIV illustrate that structural reforms addressing risky social and physical environments and biomedical approaches targeting individuals are complementary rather than binary. For AIDS, public health measures that emphasize personal responsibility and incorporate social factors to address the environment remain as relevant as they were in late nineteenth-century America.

Conclusion

AIDS, syphilis, and COVID illustrate the need for public health programs to incorporate structural changes targeted at the environmental level. But they are not the only diseases to do so. Structural interventions continued to be important internationally through the turn of the twentieth century, highlighted by yellow fever eradication efforts led by Walter Reed and others in Cuba and Panama, and malarial control efforts in the United States and abroad. These efforts aimed to rectify elements of the physical environment that were conducive to the spread of disease by draining low-lying swamps, eliminating areas of stagnant water buildup, and implementing other mosquito control measures.[127] In addition, tuberculosis control, as mentioned, relies on structural programs to address crowded and poorly ventilated home and work environments that facilitate disease spread. AIDS, syphilis, COVID, and other diseases show that nineteenth-century efforts to address socioeconomic factors that create environmental vulnerabilities remain an important component of public health strategies, even after the adoption of the germ theory.

Conclusion

In 1959, René Dubos contested a widespread belief that biomedicine would render epidemics obsolete.[1] A series of new epidemics appearing from the 1970s to today has substantiated his prediction that epidemic diseases will continue to occur. Public health officials, nonetheless, have remained confident that biomedicine has the power to end each new epidemic. However, despite the implementation of scientific campaigns to eliminate syphilis, AIDS, and COVID, each of these epidemics persists, with the highest burden in disadvantaged populations.[2] Outcomes show that effective campaigns cannot address biomedical solutions exclusively. Structural proposals need to be included to rectify socioeconomic conditions that lead to risky behavior, create vulnerable environments, and hinder the success of elimination programs. Addressing environmental vulnerabilities and socioeconomic issues, which was the focus of public health measures prior to the germ theory, remains an essential component of public health campaigns. Living with these diseases and the attempts to eliminate them is a part of human existence, even for those who deny, and hence defy, public health recommendations.

People who choose not to adhere to public health guidance have framed government and medical recommendations as impingements on individual rights and liberties. Syphilis and AIDS illustrate how, indeed, there have been instances when the government has deprived people of civil liberties in the name of public health—ranging from the detention of sex workers (to control syphilis during World War I), to discussions about quarantine and denial of insurance, housing, and work (to control AIDS in the 1980s). In contrast, in most nations, the restrictions recommended during COVID are temporary inconveniences rather than

permanent deprivations of livelihoods. The framing of COVID public health recommendations as a threat to civil liberty underscores two forms of problematic
denial. It evades the idea that citizens could avoid acquiring a serious disease by
following recommended behaviors, and is blind to the tenet that failure to adopt
public health recommendations can threaten the health of others.

Pandemics are not merely occurrences of past centuries, whether the
fourteenth (Black Death), the nineteenth (cholera), or the twentieth (1918 influenza). The number of new infectious epidemics in more recent times has grown
significantly, as have campaigns to eliminate them. These campaigns require
cooperation among citizens and a commitment by all to behave according to
what benefits society collectively, rather than merely pursuing one's individual
desires. During COVID, however, society has remained divided. Conflicts have
ensued between those who accept public health recommendations—grudgingly
or willingly—and those who do not, thereby further impeding strategies to
eliminate the disease. The challenge of public health campaigns for future pandemics will be how to engage all citizens, even those on opposing political sides,
to act in solidarity with a mutual goal of preventing harm and keeping the population healthy.

The implications of fostering a social obligation during epidemics goes
beyond preserving population survival. As authors throughout history have
pointed out, it involves preserving our humanity. During the plague of 430 B.C.E.,
for example, Thucydides noted how the panicked healthy abandoned the sick
to die in solitude without the comforting presence of others.[3] During the Black
Death in the thirteenth century, Boccaccio referred to those who disregarded
their friends and family members as inhuman, and Guy de Chuliac reminded
physicians to honor their duty to care for the ill, even though they could not
alter the course of plague.[4] Daniel Defoe concurred when he noted that wealthy
Londoners escaped their city during a plague outbreak in 1665 and left their
relatives to die alone.[5] Albert Camus, in his 1947 novel *The Plague*, depicted
Bernard Rioux, a banal physician who decides not to flee the town of Oran during a fictional outbreak of plague in order to continue his professional duties,
even though he could not change the trajectory of the disease.[6] Together, these
authors remind us of our obligations to behave with compassion, solidarity, and
empathy toward one another during epidemic times.

While addressing the undeniable necessity of mutual care, authors have also
acknowledged the risk this entails. Katherine Anne Porter addressed the tragic
consequences of tending to one another during the 1918 influenza. In her 1939
novel *Pale Horse, Pale Rider*, a soldier, Adam, dies of influenza that he likely
caught while tending to his lover, Miranda, who had the disease and recovered.[7]

Similarly, Sinclair Lewis in his 1925 novel *Arrowsmith* writes about how a young medical researcher, Martin Arrowsmith, discovers a potential cure during an outbreak of plague. While Martin tests the product's efficacy in the population, he loses his wife, Leora, who received a placebo to help determine whether the drug might be helpful to others.[8] Tending to one another's needs during epidemics, these authors suggest, is necessary to preserve humanity, despite the potential for steep personal costs.

These personal and fictional accounts of epidemics were written before scientific products to alter their course became available. Nonetheless, their themes—of the essential importance of elements that create mutual reliance in society (empathy, duty to others, solidarity)—remain true even though biomedical products to treat and prevent many diseases are now available. Furthermore, these principles that make society worthwhile transcend moments of crisis and disruption (e.g., pandemics, natural disasters) and apply to everyday life. Pandemics, as this book shows, remain part of our lives today. To maintain our humanity, the authors suggest that we must define ourselves by honoring our obligations to one another, even during times of disaster. Today, depending on the disease, this means getting tested, and, if positive, treated, wearing masks, avoiding crowds, getting vaccinated, and providing personal support to citizens who are ill.

These themes are important as we continue to live through epidemics. During the early years of AIDS, some healthcare workers continued to provide care for patients with AIDS, while others who were worried about catching a lethal virus refused to do so. Likewise, during COVID, prior to the availability of preventive vaccines or antiviral drugs, healthcare workers continued their work even though they risked endangering themselves during PPE shortages. Important social obligations that protect the population's health and preserve our humanity are not merely a theme of fictional stories. Their meanings are applicable to all members of society—healthcare workers and the general population alike—during pandemic and nonpandemic times.

Complying with social contracts had been an expectation of several public health movements. George Rosen pointed out there have been mandates in the past to comply with general sanitary measures or targeted interventions to protect public health. Colonists issued quarantine laws and fines for disobeying them in the 1700s, and public health departments delivered vaccines to halt smallpox in the twentieth century.[9] During World War I, public health officials issued widespread mandates over masks and business closures, though in response San Francisco antimask leagues were formed, motivated by concerns about civil liberty violations.[10] More recently, as David Rosner has argued, the focus on keeping Americans healthy turned increasingly toward individualized treatments for diseases like heart disease and cancer, and the need for such mandates declined during the mid-twentieth century.[11] Public health programs to eliminate AIDS and syphilis have been implemented during this era, but they have been based entirely on voluntarism. COVID, however, showed that mandates—for masks and vaccines—have become necessary again, at a time when citizens are not familiar with mandatory public health measures.

Today, liberal Western democracies have prioritized individual rights over social obligations and collective responsibilities. This trend undercuts the notion of a social contract in which people work together to keep the population healthy. During the early course of the HIV/AIDS epidemic, however, gay activists demonstrated how individuals can honor a social contract and work together for the health of the collective by advocating for restraints in behavior.[12] Community leaders insisted that gay men forsake newly found individual freedoms of behavior to protect the survival of their collective. Their argument was that to live in solidarity with fellow humans takes precedence over individual rights and desires. The implication of their activism has relevance today. In this era, when there are cumulatively a greater number of infectious diseases compared with any time in history, there is a heightened need to reinforce the idea that individuals must act for the greater good to keep the population healthy.

Living with restraints to protect public health is in some ways part of our existing everyday routine. Nancy Tomes, for example, has noted that the germ theory changed day-to-day existence and posed restrictions on collective behaviors.[13] While microbe-based public health policies brought improvements in health, they also placed new constraints on behavior, because safety from contagion requires the constant discipline of bodies (e.g., no spitting in public) and households (e.g., washing vegetables), which required a shared social contract to enact. Those same restraints remain important today given the cumulative number of infections we live with. Working in solidarity remains essential to stemming epidemics like COVID—wearing masks, accepting vaccines, social distancing. But in today's politically polarized society, it has become challenging for those with opposing ideologies to act in solidarity in the name of public health.

It is tempting to consider how the history of AIDS and syphilis might serve as an avenue for communication between people who are on opposite sides of the COVID vaccine issue today. Acknowledgment of the limitations of scientific medicine—an issue that is at the root of some of today's vaccine hesitation—may establish common ground that could serve as a platform to inform the unvaccinated. Vaccinated individuals could acknowledge the legitimacy of some people's concerns for safety, especially given past instances when vaccines were unsafe (e.g., the Parks-Brodie polio vaccine in the 1930s, Cutter polio vaccines in the 1950s, the dengue virus vaccine, and Dengvaxia, in Philippines, 2015). Health experts and others could emphasize that today's COVID vaccines, unlike some vaccines in the past, meet rigorous safety-testing standards. It remains entirely speculative whether the unvaccinated, if approached in this fashion, would be receptive, or whether histories of syphilis and AIDS could be used to help those who are vaccine hesitant to get shots.

The appearance of AIDS, syphilis, and COVID and the obstacles encountered by public health programs to eliminate them, of course, were not the only developments to confound the triumphant view of biomedicine since it reached its apogee in the 1950s. The English physician Thomas McKeown contested the confident view of biomedicine in the 1970s. McKeown pointed out that the reduction in childhood diseases and killer epidemics had preceded the introduction of vaccines and chemotherapy, and biomedicine therefore received an undue amount of credit for their decline.[14] Furthermore, the medical writer Lewis Thomas described the ways in which germs can thrive despite antibiotics, underscoring that the limitations of antimicrobials had not been addressed by those who predicted that infections would be conquered with biomedicine.[15] Furthermore, by the 1970s, there were episodes where biomedicine had not provided effective tools to handle potential epidemic threats (e.g., swine flu, 1976), or prevent newly described infections (Legionnaire's disease, 1976; Lyme disease, 1978).

Since the 1970s, sequential epidemics have emerged and persisted in a low-level fashion or recurrent patterns. Their occurrence underscores how humans, through their activities, create environments that are susceptible to unleashing epidemic threats. Displacement of humans through travel, war, commerce, poverty, or unstable governments, for example, have led to the emergence of SARS, Ebola, Zika, and COVID, and to the resurgence of syphilis and tuberculosis. New modes of transportation that have accompanied globalization, urbanization, and construction of roads and air-travel routes have facilitated the dissemination of Ebola and HIV. Also, as Thomas has pointed out, efforts to free humans from disease have themselves led to the emergence of MDROs, multidrug-resistant tuberculosis, and HIV (complicating campaigns to eradicate tropical diseases by reusing syringes).[16] Moreover, through entertainment, travel, deforestation, and urbanization, microbes that had once been strictly confined to animals have now spilled over to humans, becoming contagious epidemics (e.g., monkeypox, West Nile virus, eastern equine encephalitis [EEE], SARS, MERS, Lyme, COVID, Ebola, HIV, Nipah virus, and influenza [avian H5N1, swine H1N1, and reassortment H7N9]). These epidemics have all emerged since Dubos's hypothesis that human activities accompanying civilization will change our relationship with microbes by enabling them to escape the environmental niche in which they co-evolved with their host.

The fact that we now live with collective pandemics, along with efforts to eliminate them, refutes any narrative that the great nineteenth-century infectious diseases (e.g., cholera, smallpox) have been eradicated with sanitation, nutrition, biomedical advances (e.g., polio vaccine, smallpox vaccine), or public health measures (e.g., upgraded water systems), and have been entirely replaced by chronic ailments like heart disease and cancer. Emerging diseases prove not only that epidemics have not been conquered, as hoped in the 1950s, but that humans are now dealing with more pandemics cumulatively than at any time in the past. New epidemics show that the same conditions that have fueled gains in health and wealth—increased trade, travel, and labor migration—have made humans increasingly vulnerable to pandemics.[17]

Not only do humans in the twenty-first century have to deal with a greater array of epidemics than their nineteenth-century forebearers, but the range of behaviors they must adopt to protect themselves from harm is greater than in the past. Although most of the present-day epidemics are not as lethal as the great nineteenth-century diseases, they cause individual distress, disrupt families and communities, and impact the economy and strength of nations. In fact, to avoid the spread of new infections, humans must learn to alter their daily behaviors in myriad ways—including masking, covering coughs, and avoiding crowds (COVID); avoiding summer activities during dusk or twilight to prevent mosquito bites (Zika, EEE); refraining from hiking without proper clothing to prevent tick bites (Lyme); avoiding certain meats and quarantining if exposed to an infected person (Ebola, Nipah); avoiding undercooked fish or meats (tapeworms, salmonella); washing all foods well (typhoid, salmonella); and avoiding promiscuous sex if so inclined (syphilis, AIDS, monkeypox). The array of behavioral changes and how they have become part of the fabric of our day-to-day lives underscores the widespread footprint of current infectious diseases and the voluntary public health measures put in place to control them. This is how we experience pandemics in the biomedical era.

Undoubtedly, the trends of civilization that make environments vulnerable to pandemics cannot be reversed. Turning back the clock is not a realistic option. In fact, some public health experts predict the opposite—that pandemics will occur with increasing frequency, primed by globalization, intercontinental travel, ecological changes in distribution of disease-carrying mosquitoes and other vectors that accompany climate change, and human migration to live closer to different species of animals, thereby increasing the chance of spill-over.[18] With the array of epidemics that have emerged since 1981, and the specter of more to come due to continued human activities and enhanced pathogen-recognition procedures, public health officials have addressed how to prevent the next epidemic from occurring.

The most realistic expectation public health officials have is to be able react as quickly as possible to an epidemic once it has been unleashed. Their best hope is to manage an epidemic when it is most containable: before it has become widespread. This can best be accomplished using modern communication. ProMED and HealthMap are two online reporting systems run by the International Society for Infectious Diseases that are designed to track, store data, and network with multiple institutions to provide quick information on possible outbreaks.[19] The U.S. government has begun to pay independent groups, such as EcoHealth Alliance, to search for pathogens that spill over from animals to humans—often in areas where human development disrupts natural animal habitats.[20] Use of whole genome sequencing has permitted a greater understanding of how microbes mutate, evolve, and can be contained.[21] These technologies are indispensable components of today's approach to contain a newly occurring epidemic by better detecting evolving pathogens, identifying new diseases, and responding to them as quickly as possible. Nonetheless, the public health system's data collection system has become outdated due to deprioritization of preparedness efforts and neglect. Updating this infrastructure with standards that can integrate information critical to monitoring and fighting public health threats (e.g., for COVID, recording the number of hospitalizations and deaths according to vaccine status) is crucial to suppressing outbreaks early in their course.

It will be important to use these strategies to connect public health agencies with hard-to-reach populations. At beginning of the COVID epidemic, much public engagement was passive (standing in line for vaccines, requesting reimbursement from insurers, developing rapid diagnostic testing). This excluded many people who were disabled or older. Likewise, earlier employment of these programs during the 2022 monkeypox pandemic (e.g., streamlined testing, vaccine rollout in high-risk populations, and removing barriers to accessing effective therapies) could have avoided unnecessary morbidity and global spread of the disease, particularly among MSM.[22] More proactive outreach will be important in future emergencies—whether pandemics (COVID, Mpox, or others), hurricanes, wildfires, or other disasters. Otherwise, underserved or marginalized groups will be left out, thereby further widening disparities in care and outcomes.[23]

At the end of the day, however, these remarkable scientific approaches cannot absolutely prevent new epidemics from occurring. The most hopeful scenario is that employing programs as early as possible will avoid unnecessary spread and thereby limit the suffering, death, and destruction that widespread epidemics cause. Regardless of how creative the approaches may be, they can only contain diseases before transmission becomes widespread. Other efforts to contain the spread of epidemics early include developing biomedical products that work quickly, including the rapid testing needed for surveillance and vaccines. With regard to vaccines, the Coalition for Epidemic Preparedness Innovations aims to develop next-generation vaccines to manage future epidemics.[24] Their goal is to produce a library of prototype vaccines against representative pathogens from critical viral types, and to build a vaccine against a viral family that could be applied rapidly to a new disease once it emerges.[25] This strategy of building a prototype vaccine against twenty families of virus, albeit still reactive in nature, could yield a vaccine more quickly than was possible with the novel coronavirus. To prevent an epidemic from spreading quickly, rapid vaccine development would need to be accompanied by timely development of rapid diagnostic testing—a key step in preparedness that was delayed in both COVID in 2020 and Monkeypox in 2022.

Today's interest in the origins of diseases, and how syphilis, AIDS, and COVID became widespread, is an indirect indicator of our interest in prevention and preparedness. The exact origins of these diseases remain speculative, despite decades of investigation and keen public interest. It could be argued that apprehending their origins would not provide any useful inroads into their management or prevention. Nonetheless, knowing how a disease started and what was responsible for its amplification may provide clues for how to avoid the next infectious epidemic.

Despite interest in preventing disease, when epidemics mature and begin to wane, society tends to forget about them. Newspapers, magazines, and TV news shows lose interest in following up on them because the media outlets perceive them to no longer be newsworthy—even though the epidemics persist. This is part of the cycle of epidemics like syphilis, HIV/AIDS, and COVID. The amnesia can be detrimental to epidemic control programs for several reasons. Complacency can lead to deprioritizing disease elimination programs and withdrawal of sustained funding that is needed while epidemics still pose a problem. In addition, complacency can lead to lack of funding of preparedness programs that are needed for early detection and response to future epidemics. The cycle of panic during an epidemic and neglect after its peak compromises preparedness and control programs alike. Ideally, world leaders would abandon complacency and commit to a new framework of prevention, detection, and sustained response to strengthen national, regional, and global institutions and scale up development of the public health workforce.

Syphilis, AIDS, and COVID illustrate the powers and limitations of biomedicine. Each disease has bolstered the confident narrative of biomedicine with the promise that it can be managed through laboratory-generated insights and the spectacular products of medical science. These cases illuminate the question of why the public trusts science—in part because it has come to rely on the ability of science to deliver remarkable products that can heal serious diseases in individuals and prevent disease spread in the population. But at the same time, this book reveals the limitations of science; its inabilities to apprehend the precise origins of epidemics and its hopes of eliminating disease have fallen short. A study of syphilis, AIDS, and COVID therefore illustrates the impressive advances of science while exposing its shortcomings. The histories of these diseases provide insight into the accomplishments and limitations of biomedicine and, as a corollary, enable insight into the circumstances under which science is trusted and mistrusted.

The expectations surrounding biomedicine today remain powerful, although more measured than they were in mid-twentieth-century America. Today, few realistically adhere to that era's certainty that biomedicine can conquer all epidemics. Nonetheless, public health officials remain confident that scientifically based public health campaigns can ultimately end epidemics like AIDS and syphilis. Today's measured expectations of biomedicine involve a comprehensive approach that combines scientifically based surveillance and treatment programs with structural strategies targeting vulnerabilities in the social and physical environments. A combined public health approach is necessary to control epidemics. However, because structural programs are not easy to design, fund, and implement quickly, epidemics will endure, particularly in vulnerable environments. Epidemic narratives, unlike the celebratory narrative that public health officials envisioned in the middle of the last century, will rarely have discrete endings to bookend their abrupt beginnings. Rather, epidemic diseases, along with efforts to contain them, will continue to be an inescapable part of our existence.

Acknowledgments

This book is derived from two courses that I have taught in the history department at the University of Michigan: the History of Sexually Transmitted Infections (History 233) and the History of Epidemics (History 376). I gratefully acknowledge my students, whose enthusiasm, questions, and input have been invaluable. I also acknowledge my colleagues in the history department who made this book possible. I was fortunate to obtain input from Martin Pernick, Joel Howell, John Carson, and Howard Markel, whose feedback has strengthened the depth of my scholarship. I would also like to acknowledge the input of historians Harold Cook and Ethan Pollock from Brown University. Their critical comments and suggestions have added a depth to my work that I aspired toward but would have been unable to achieve otherwise.

I would like to thank my colleagues in the Division of Infectious Diseases and the Department of Microbiology and Immunology at the University of Michigan Medical School for their helpful scientific input, particularly Adam Lauring. I thank my colleagues in the Department of Epidemiology at the University of Michigan School of Public Health, particularly Laura Power for her insights into public health issues. I wish to thank individual experts with whom I have spoken during my research, including scientists who developed and tested anti-HIV drugs in the 1980s and 1990s (Samuel Broder, James Keirns, and Emilio Emini), and immunology and gene editing today (Carl June). I also thank Greg Gonsalves, a patient representative; Peter Marks, a key regulator during COVID; and physicians who have managed HIV patients in impoverished regions in the United States since the 1990s (Wendy Armstrong, Claire Pomeroy) and abroad (Paul Farmer).

I thank the staff of the Bentley Historical Library at the University of Michigan for the guidance and help they provided during my research. I also thank the staff of the Archives of the Venereal Disease Branch of the Centers for Disease Control and Prevention for their guidance. I thank Jessica Sciberras for her invaluable help in checking references and in formatting and preparing the manuscript and notes. I also thank Megan Orringer for carefully reading the monograph and providing editorial input. I thank the Division of Infectious Disease at the medical school for their understanding while I wrote this book.

Finally, I am most grateful to my wife, Sahira, and my children, Powel III, Louisa, and Sarine, for their love and encouragement during the time I spent researching and writing this book.

Notes

Introduction

1. Allan M. Brandt, *No Magic Bullet: A Social History of Venereal Disease in the United States since 1880* (New York: Oxford University Press, 1987). See also Elizabeth Fee and Daniel M. Fox, eds., *AIDS: The Burdens of History* (Berkeley: University of California Press, 1988).
2. Allan M. Brandt, "AIDS: From Social History to Social Policy," in *AIDS*, ed. Fee and Fox, 147–168.
3. Fee and Fox, *AIDS*. See also Brandt, *No Magic Bullet*.
4. Fee and Fox, *AIDS*; Brandt, *No Magic Bullet*. See also John Parascandola, *Sex, Sin, and Science: A History of Syphilis in America* (London: Praeger Press, 2008).
5. Harvey V. Fineberg, "The Social Dimensions of AIDS," *Scientific American* 259, no. 4 (1988): 111–121. See also Patrick Buchanan, "Editorial," *Seattle Times*, July 31, 1993; "LaRouche Initiative Stopped Dead," *New York Native*, November 17, 1986.
6. Frederick T. Roberts, *A Handbook on the Theory and Practice of Medicine* (Philadelphia: Lindsay and Blakiston, 1876). See also Rudolf Virchow, *Ueber die Natur der Consititutionnell Syphilitischen Affectionem* (Berlin, 1859).
7. Fritz Schaudinn and Erich Hoffmann, "Vorläufiger Bericht über das Vorkommen von Spirochaeten in Syphilitischen Krankheitsprodukten und bei Papillomen," *Arbeiten aus dem Kaiserlichen Gesundheitsamte* 22 (1905): 527–534.
8. Paul Ehrlich, "Ueber die Behanklung der Syphilis mit dem Praparate '606'," *Allg Wien Med Zeit* 55 (1910): 457–458 and 469–470.
9. Roy M. Gulick, John W. Mellors, Diane Havlir, Joseph J. Eron, Charles Gonzalez, Deborah McMahon, Douglas D. Richman, et al., "Treatment with Indinavir, Zidovudine, and Lamivudine in Adults with Human Immunodeficiency Virus Infection and Prior Antiretroviral Therapy," *New England Journal of Medicine (NEJM)* 337, no. 11 (1997): 734–739. See also Randy Shilts, *And the Band Played On* (New York: St. Martin's Press, 1987), 34–90.
10. Merle Sande and Paul Volberding, *The Medical Management of AIDS* (Philadelphia: Saunders, 1999).
11. Julie Marquis, "Antiviral Cocktail: The Toast of HIV Researchers Medicines," *Los Angeles Times*, March 14, 1995. See also Harold Varmus and Neal Nathanson, "Science and the Control of AIDS," *Science* 280, no. 5371 (1998): 1815.
12. Milton Rosenau, "Syphilis," in *Preventive Medicine and Hygiene* (New York: Appleton, 1913), 50–62.
13. Parascandola, *Sex, Sin, and Science.*
14. Thomas Parran, "Why Don't We Stamp Out Syphilis?," *Reader's Digest*, July 1936, 65–73.
15. Myron S. Cohen, Ying Q. Chen, Marybeth McCauley, Theresa Gamble, Mina C. Hosseinipour, Nagalingeswaran Kumarasamy, James G. Hakim, et al., "Prevention of HIV-1 Infection with Early Antiretroviral Therapy," *NEJM* 365 (2011): 493–495.
16. Charles V. Chapin, "History of State and Municipal Control of Disease," in *A Half Century of Public Health*, ed. Mazyck P. Ravenal (New York: American Public Health Association, 1921), 133–161.

17. C.E.A. Winslow, *The Conquest of Epidemic Disease* (Madison: University of Wisconsin Press, 1943), 380. See also Berton Roueche, "Something Extraordinary," in *Eleven Blue Men*, ed. Berton Roueche (New York: Berkley Publishing, 1958), 147.

18. John D. Ratcliff, "Yellow Magic of Penicillin," *Reader's Digest*, July 1943, 47–51. See also Allan Chase, *Magic Shots* (New York: William Morrow and Company, 1982); "Penicillin the Wonder Drug," *Time*, June 7, 1943, 31–32.

19. Samuel Rapport and Helen Wright, *Great Adventures in Medicine* (New York: Dial Press, 1952), 766.

20. William Bolton, "Pneumonia's Waterloo," *Hygeia* (1948): 21, 22–31. See also Chase, *Magic Shots*, 272–293.

21. N. Tomes, *Gospel of Germs: Men, Women, and the Microbe in American Life* (Cambridge, MA: Harvard University Press, 1988).

22. R. Gibbons, "End of Syphilis in Sight?," *Science Digest*, January to June 1951, 48.

23. Naomi Oereskes, *Why Trust Science* (Princeton, NJ: Princeton University Press, 2021).

24. Jo A. Valentine and Gail A. Bolan, "Syphilis Elimination: Lessons Learned Again," *Sexually Transmitted Diseases* 45, no. 9S (September 2018): S80–S85. See also UNAIDS, "Success in Reaching '15 by 15' Shows That We Can End the AIDS Epidemic," Press Release, UNAIDS, accessed November 22, 2019, https://www.unaids .org/en/resources/presscentre/pressreleaseandstatementarchive/2015/july/20150719 _15x15_PR.

25. See World Health Organization, *Global Health Sector Strategy on Sexually Transmitted Infections 2016–2021* (Geneva, Switzerland: WHO Document Production Services, 2016). See also Patrick Sullivan, David W. Purcell, Jeremy A. Grey, Kyle T. Bernstein, Thomas L. Gift, Taylor A. Wimbly, Eric Hall, and Eli S. Rosenberg, "Patterns of Racial/Ethnic Disparities and Prevalence in HIV and Syphilis Diagnoses among Men Who Have Sex with Men, 2016: A Novel Data Visualization," *American Journal of Public Health* 108 (2018): S266–S273.

26. Noah Kojima and Jeffrey D. Klausner, "An Update on the Global Epidemiology of Syphilis," *Current Epidemiology Reports* 5, no. 1 (March 2018): 24–38.

27. Jon Cohen, "Ending AIDS Movement Falters," *Worldwide Science* 361 (2018): 438. See also Linda Gail Bekker, George Alleyne, Stefan Baral, Javier Cepeda, Demetre Daskalakis, David Dowdy, Mark Dybul, et al., "Advancing Global Health and Strengthening the HIV Response in the Era of the Sustainable Development Goals: The International AIDS Society," *Lancet* 392 (2018): 312–364.

28. Sullivan et al., "Patterns of Racial/Ethnic Disparities and Prevalence."

29. Anish P. Mahajan, Jennifer N. Sayles, Vishal A. Patel, Robert H. Remien, Sharif R. Sawires, Daniel J. Ortiz, Greg Szekeres, and Thomas J. Coates, "Stigma in the HIV/ AIDS Epidemic: A Review of the Literature and Recommendations for the Way Forward," *AIDS* 22, no. 2 (August 2008): S67–S79.

30. N. El-Bassel, P. L. Marotta, L. Gilbert, E. Wu, S. Springer, D. Goddard-Eckrich, and T. Hunt, "Integrating Treatment for Opioid Use Disorders and HIV Services into Primary Care Solutions for the 21st Century," in *Structural Interventions for HIV Preventions*, ed. Richard Crosby and Ralph DiClemente (Oxford, UK: Oxford University Press, 2019), 221–255. See also R. A. Crosby, R. J. DiClemente, and J. P. Sims, "Social Conditions and the AIDS Pandemic: A Proposed Framework for Structural-Level Interventions," in *Structural Interventions for HIV Preventions*, ed. Crosby and DiClemente, 377–391.

31. Judith Wasserheit and Sevgi O. Aral, "The Dynamic Topology of Sexually Transmitted Disease Epidemics: Implications for Prevention Strategies," *Journal of Infectious Diseases* 174, no. 2 (1996): S201–S213.

32. Kevin A. Fenton and Frederick R. Bloom, "STD Prevention with MSM: Examples of Structural Interventions," in *Behavioral Interventions for Prevention and Control of Sexually Transmitted Diseases*, ed. Sevgi O. Aral, John M. Douglas, and Judith Lipshutz (New York: Springer, 2007), 325–354.

33. J. Cohen, *Shots in the Dark: The Wayward Search for an AIDS Vaccine* (New York: Norton, 2001). See also William J. Clinton, "Commencement Address at Morgan State University in Baltimore, Maryland," May 18, 1997, American Presidency Project, www.presidency.ucsb.edu/documents/commencement-address-morgan-state -university-baltimore-maryland; UNAIDS, "Success in Reaching '15 by 15.'"

34. William Brown, "Talk Delivered at Venereal Disease Conference," University of Oklahoma, November 6, 1965, *CDC Records*, Acc 70A470.

35. R. G. Petersdorf, "The Doctors' Dilemma," *NEJM* 299 (1978): 628–634.

36. T. Kingston, "Death by Placebo: The Sacrificial Lambs of Protocol 019," *Coming Up!*, September 1988, 10–11. See also S. Epstein, *Impure Science, AIDS, Activism, and the Politics of Knowledge* (Berkeley: University of California Press, 1996).

37. Kiran van Rijn, "The Politics of Uncertainty: The AIDS Debate, Thabo Mbeki and the South African Government Response," *Social History of Medicine* 19, no. 3 (2006): 521–538.

38. Gerald H. Friedland, Brian R. Saltzman, Martha F. Rogers, Patricia A. Kahl, Martin L. Lesser, Marguerite M. Mayers, and Robert S. Klein, "Lack of Transmission of HTLV-III/LAV Infection to Household Contacts of Patients with AIDS or AIDS-Related Complex with Oral Candidiasis," *NEJM* 314, no. 6 (1986): 344–350.

39. German Lopez, "The Reagan Administration's Unbelievable Response to the HIV/ AIDS Epidemic," *Vox*, 2016, www.vox.com/2015/12/1/9828348/ronaldreagan-hiv -aids. See also D. Gould, "Rock the Boat, Don't Rock the Boat, Baby: Ambivalence and the Emergence of Militant AIDS Activism," *Passionate Politics: Emotions and Social Movements*, ed. Jeff Goodwin, James M. Jasper, and Francesca Polletta (Chicago: University of Chicago Press, 2001), 135–157.

40. Susan Reverby, *Tuskegee's Truths: Rethinking the Tuskegee Syphilis Study* (Chapel Hill: University of North Carolina Press, 2000). See also Susan Reverby, "Ethical Failures and History Lessons: The U.S. Public Health Service Research Studies in Tuskegee and Guatemala," *Public Health Reviews* 34, no. 1 (2012): 1–19.

41. Dwayne T. Brandon, Lydia A. Isaac, and Thomas A. LaVeist, "The Legacy of Tuskegee and Trust in Medical Care: Is Tuskegee Responsible for Race Differences in Mistrust of Medical Care?," *Journal of the National Medical Association* 97, no. 7 (July 2005): 951–956.

42. "Controversial Chinese Experiment to Edit 'Anti-HIV' Gene May Have Actually Failed," *Science*, The Wire, May 12, 2019, https://science.thewire.in/health/he -jiankui-genetically-edit-embryos-ccr5-hiv-crispr-cas9-ethics/.

43. Scott W. Stern, *The Trials of Nina McCall: Sex, Surveillance, and the Decades-Long Government Plan to Imprison Promiscuous Women* (Boston: Beacon Press, 2018).

44. William F. Buckley Jr., "Identify All the Carriers," *New York Times*, March 18, 1986. See also Robert Steinbrook, "The Times Poll: 42% Would Limit Civil Rights in AIDS Battle," *Los Angeles Times*, July 31, 1987, 1.

45. Sharon LaFraniere, Katie Thomas, Noah Weiland, David Gelles, Sheryl Gay Stolberg, and Denise Grady, "Politics, Science, and the Remarkable Race for a Viable Vaccine," *New York Times*, November 22, 2020.

46. Sheryl Gay Stolberg, "Biden Declares 'Independence' from the Virus to Some Dismay," *New York Times*, July 3, 2021. See also "Curing Covid-19," *Lancet Infectious Diseases* 20, no. 10 (October 2020): 1101.

47. Josh Holder, "Tracking Coronavirus Vaccination around the World," *New York Times*, March 12, 2022, A1.

48. Sarah Jacoby, "Three Years into the Pandemic, Should I Still Worry about COVID?," *Today*, March 20, 2023, https://www.today.com/health/coronavirus/should-i-worry-about-covid-rcna74918.

49. Roni Caryn Rabin, "Leading New Task Force, Yale Doctor Takes Aim at Racial Gaps in Care," *New York Times*, January 12, 2021.

50. Thomas Fuller, "Isolation Helps Homeless Who Avoid the Shelters," *New York Times*, December 24, 2020.

51. Harald Schmidt, Parag Pathak, Tayfun Sonmez, and M. Utku Unver, "Covid-19: How to Prioritize Worse-Off Populations in Allocating Safe and Effective Vaccines," *British Medical Journal* 371 (2020): 1–4.

52. Noah Weiland, "How the CDC Lost Its Voice under Trump," *New York Times*, December 17, 2020, A8. See also Donald McNeil, "Claims of Herd Immunity Called Nonsense, as Well as Dangerous," *New York Times*, September 30, 2020, A1 and A7.

53. Apoorva Mandavilli, "Experts Seek More Data as They Weigh the Need for Another Virus Booster," *New York Times*, March 24, 2023, A20.

54. Anne Gearan and John Wagner, "Trump Expresses Support for Angry Anti-Shutdown Protesters as More States Lift Coronavirus Lockdowns," *Washington Post*, May 2, 2020, www.wdbj7.com/2020/09/12/dakotas-lead-us-in-virus-growth-as-both-reject-mask-rules/.

55. Philip Rucker, Josh Dawsey, Ashley Parker, and Robert Costa, "Invincibility Punctured by Infection: How the Coronavirus Spread in the Trump White House," *Washington Post*, October 2, 2020, www.washingtonpost.com/politics/trump-virus-spread-white-house/2020/10/02/38c5b354-04cc-11eb-b7ed-141dd88560ea_story.html.

56. Editorial, "A Powerful Display of Dissent in China," *New York Times*, December 4, 2022, SR 9.

57. "Achievements in Public Health, 1900–1999: Control of Infectious Diseases," CDC, July 30, 1999, www.cdc.gov/mmwr/preview/mmwrhtml/mm4829a1.htm. See also D. L. Hoyert, K .D. Kochanek, and S. L. Murphy, "Deaths: Final Data for 1997," *National Vital Statistics Reports* 47, no. 19 (June 1999); David Rosner, "Moral Virtue in the Time of Cholera," *Foreign Affairs*, November 18, 2020, www.foreignaffairs.com/articles/united-states/2020-11-18/moral-virtue-time-cholera.

58. Donald Moynihan and Gregory Porumbescu, "Trump's 'Chinese Virus' Slur Makes Some People Blame Chinese Americans. But Others Blame Trump," *Washington Post*, September 22, 2020.

59. Yingyi Ma and Ning Zhan, "To Mask or Not to Mask amid the COVID-19 Pandemic: How Chinese Students in America Experience and Cope with Stigma," *Chinese Sociological Review* 54, no. 1 (October 20, 2020), https://doi.org/10.1080/21620555.2020.1833712.

60. Editorial Board, "Congress, Test Thyself," *New York Times*, August 3, 2020.

Chapter 1 Syphilis

1. Alfred Crosby, "The Early History of Syphilis: A Reappraisal," in *The Columbian Exchange* (Westport, CT: Praeger, 2003), 122–164.

2. Crosby, "The Early History of Syphilis."

3. G. Fracastoro, *Syphilis or the French Disease* (1530), trans. H Wynne-Finch (London: G. P. Putnam and Sons, 1930).

4. Fracastoro, *Syphilis or the French Disease*.

5. Ruy Díaz de Isla, *Tractado llamado fructo de todos los auctos: Contra el mal Serpentino. Venido de la ysla Española* (Al fin: Seuilla: Por Andres de burgos, 1542). See also Crosby, "The Early History of Syphilis," 123.

6. Crosby, "The Early History of Syphilis," 122–164. See also C. E. A. Winslow, "Fracastorius," in *The Conquest of Epidemic Disease*, ed. C. E. A. Winslow (Madison: University of Wisconsin Press, 1980), 129.

7. Thucydides, *Book II, History of the Peloponnesian War* (430 B.C.E.), trans. B. Jowett (Oxford, UK: Clarendon Press, 1881), 135–136. See also Guy de Chauliac, "Bubonic Plague," (1368) in *A Source Book in Medieval Science, Medical Practice*, trans. Michael McVaugh (Cambridge, MA: Harvard University Press, 1974), 773–774.

8. Crosby, "The Early History of Syphilis," 122–164.

9. Kerttu Majander, Saskia Pfrengle, Arthur Kocher, Judith Neukamm, Louis du Plessis, Marta Pla-Diaz, Natasha Arora, et al., "Ancient Bacterial Genomes Reveal a High Diversity of *Treponema pallidum* Strains in Early Modern Europe," *Current Biology* 30, no. 19 (October 5, 2020): 3788–3803.

10. Fracastoro, *Syphilis or the French Disease*. See also Girolamo Fracastoro, *Contagion, Contagious Diseases, and Their Treatment* (1546), trans. W. C. Wright (New York: B. P. Putnam and Sons, 1930).

11. "Fracastorius," 129.

12. Ulrich von Hutten, *De Morbo Gallico* [About French Disease], trans. Thomas Paynell (London: Thomas Berthelet, 1533), 143–144.

13. Gilbert the Englishman, "General Symptoms of Leprosy" (1250), in *A Source Book in Medieval Science*, ed. Edward Grant (Cambridge, MA: Harvard University Press, 1974), 752.

14. Richard Palmer, "The Church, Leprosy and Plague in Medieval and Early Modern Europe," in *The Church and Healing: Papers Read at the Twentieth Summer Meeting and the Twenty-first Winter Meeting of the Ecclesiastical History Society*, ed. W. J. Shields (Oxford, UK: B. Blackwell, 1982), 83.

15. Saul Nathaniel Brody, *The Disease of the Soul: Leprosy in Medieval Literature* (Ithaca, NY: Cornell University Press, 1974), 96.

16. Gilbert the Englishman, "General Symptoms of Leprosy," 753.

17. Fracastoro, *Contagion, Contagious Diseases, and Their Treatment*, 73.

18. Von Hutten, *De Morbo Gallico*, 143–144.

19. "Fracastorius," 129, 131.

20. "Report of the Paris Medical Faculty" (1348), in *The Black Death*, trans. and ed. Rosemary Horrox (Manchester, UK: Manchester University Press, 1994), 158–163 and 773–774.

21. "Transmission of Plague" (1348), in *The Black Death*, trans. and ed. Horrox, 182–194.

22. Crosby, "The Early History of Syphilis," 122–164.

23. Ruth Mazo Karras, "The Regulation of Brothels in Later Medieval England," *Signs: Journal of Women in Culture and Society* 14, no. 2 (1989): 399–433. See also J. M. Bennett, "Working Together in the Middle Ages: Perspectives on Women's Communities," *Signs: Journal of Women in Culture and Society* 14 (Winter 1989): 255–260.

24. Palmer, "The Church, Leprosy and Plague in Medieval and Early Modern Europe," 79–101. See also Gilbert the Englishman, "General Symptoms of Leprosy," 752–759.

25. Francis Bacon, *The New Organon: or True Directions Concerning the Interpretation of Nature* (1620), Early Modern Texts, accessed March 25, 2024, www .earlymoderntexts.com/assets/pdfs/bacon1620.pdf.

26. John Locke, *An Essay Concerning Human Understanding* (1689) (London: T. Tegg and Son, 1836).

27. G. G. Meynall, "John Locke and the Preface to Thomas Sydenham's Observationes Medicae," *Medical History* 50, no. 1 (2006): 93–110.

28. J. F. Payne, *Thomas Sydenham* (London: T .F. Unwin, 1900), 158–182.

29. Janet Doe, "Jean Astruc (1694–1766): A Biographical and Bibliographical Study," *Journal of the History of Medicine* 15, no. 2 (1960): 184–197.

30. John Lane, *Portraits of Robert Willan* (Chicago: American Medical Association, 1929).

31. Benjamin Bell, *Treatise on Gonorrhoea Virulenta and Lues Venerea* (Edinburgh: James Watson, 1793), 1–44.

32. Claude Quetel, *History of Syphilis*, trans. Judith Braddock (Baltimore, MD: Johns Hopkins University Press, 1990).

33. John Hunter, *Treatise on the Venereal Disease* (London, 1786), 324–327. See also Jean Francois Hernandez, *Essai analytique sur la non-identite de virus gonorrhoique et syphilitique* (Toulon, 1812).

34. Giovanni Morgagni, *De Sedibus et causis morborum per anatomen indagatis* (Padua, Italy, 1771).

35. Edward Adams, "Founders of Modern Medicine: Giovanni Battista Morgagni (1682–1771)," *Medical Library and Historical Journal* 1, no. 4 (October 1903): 270–277.

36. Antonio Benivieni, *On the Hidden and Marvelous Causes of Disease and Healing* (1502), trans. Charles Singer (Oxford, UK: Blackwell Publications, 1954), 111–120. See also Théophile Bonet, *Sepulchretum: Sive anatomia practicea ex cadaveribus morbo denatis* (Geneva: Cramer and Perachon, 1700).

37. Adams, "Founders of Modern Medicine: Giovanni Battista Morgagni."

38. Erwin Ackerknecht, *Medicine at the Paris Hospital 1794–1848* (Baltimore, MD: Johns Hopkins University Press, 1967).

39. Michael Titford, "A Short History of Histopathology Technique," *Journal of Histotechnology* 29, no. 2 (2006): 99–110.

40. Knud Faber, *Nosography in Modern Medicine* (New York: Paul Hoeber, 1928).

41. John Harley Warner, *Against the Spirit of System: The French Impulse in Nineteenth Century American Medicine* (Princeton, NJ: Princeton University Press, 1998).

42. Robley Dunglison, *The Practice of Medicine: Treatise on Special Pathology and Therapeutics* (Philadelphia: Lea and Blanchard, 1848).

43. John Bristowe, *A Treatise on the Theory and Practice of Medicine* (Philadelphia: H. C. Lea, 1876).

44. Frederick Thomas Roberts, *The Theory and Practice of Medicine* (Philadelphia: Lindsay and Blakiston, 1876).

45. Franz Ebneter, *Die Dermatologie in Paris von 1800–1850* (Zurich: Juris, 1964). See also Ackerknecht, *Medicine at the Paris Hospital 1794–1848*, 175.

46. John Thorne Crissey and David A. Denenholz, "Development of the Modern Forms and Concepts of Syphilis," *Clinics in Dermatology* 2, no. 1 (1984): 1–10.

47. Chief editor, "Editorial," *AMA Archives of Dermatology* 71, no. 1 (1955): 1.

48. W. Erb, "Tabes und syphilis," *Centralblt Med Wissenschft* 19 (1881): 195–198, 213–215.

49. J. Hutchinson, "An Address on Syphilis as an Imitator," *British Medical Journal* 1 (1879): 499–501, 541–542.

50. A. Fournier, *De l'ataxie locomotrice d'origine syphilitique* (Paris: Masson, 1876).

51. Hippocrates, "Of the Epidemics," in *The General works of Hippocrates*, trans. Francis Adams (London: Printed for the Sydenham Society, 1849).

52. P. Ricord, *Traité pratique des maladies vénériennes: ou, Recherches critiques et expérimentales sur l'inoculation appliquée à l'étude de ces maladies, suivies d'un résumé thérapeutique et d'un formulaire spécial* (Paris: Rouvier et Le Bouvier, 1838).

53. P. L. A. Cazenave and H. E. Schedel, *A Practical Synopsis of Cutaneous Diseases* (Philadelphia: Carey, Lea, and Carey, 1829), 336–367.

54. B. B. Beeson, "Philippe Ricord 1800–1889," *AMA Archives of Dermatology and Syphilology* 22 (1930): 1061–1068. See also "Editorial," *Lancet* 1 (1869): 164.

55. Hutchinson, "An Address on Syphilis as an Imitator," 499–501, 541–542.

56. A. Fournier, "Syphilis and General Paresis," in *Selected Essays and Monographs* (London: New Sydenham Society, 1897), 375–392.

57. Juan Rosai, *Guiding the Surgeon's Hand: The History of American Surgical Pathology* (Washington, DC: Armed Forces Institute of Pathology, 1997).

58. Rudolf Virchow, *Ueber die Natur der Consititutionnell Syphilitischen Affectionem* (Berlin, 1859). See also Aldred Scott Warthin, "Virchow's Conception of Constitutional Syphilis," *Annals of Clinical Medicine* 5, no. 6 (December 1926): 570–574.

59. Virchow, *Ueber die Natur der Consititutionnell Syphilitischen Affectionem.*

60. Virchow, *Ueber die Natur der Consititutionnell Syphilitischen Affectionem.* See also Fournier, "Syphilis and General Paresis."

61. Adolf Strumpell, *A Text-Book of Medicine for Students and Practitioners* (New York: D. Appleton, 1887).

62. Hutchinson, "An Address on Syphilis as an Imitator," 499–501, 541–542.

63. William Osler, "Syphilis," in *The Principles and Practice of Medicine*, 9th ed. (New York: Appleton, 1921), 268–283.

64. Sebastian Ruhs, "Avoiding the 'Great Imitator': Syphilis Facts and Prevention," blog, Chase Brexton Health Care, January 18, 2019, https://chasebrexton.org/blog/avoiding-%E2%80%9Cgreat-imitator%E2%80%9D-syphilis-facts-and-prevention.

65. J. Henle, "Von den Miasmen und Contagien und von den Miasmatisch contagiösen Krankheiten," in *Pathologische Untersuchungen* (Berlin: August Hirschwald Verlag, 1840), trans. Thomas Brock, Milestones in Microbiology (Washington, DC: ASM Press; 1999), 1–82.

66. G. Fracastoro, *De sympathia et antipathia rerum, liber unus, De contagione et contagiosis morbis et curatione et contagiosis morbis et curatione, lib. iii* (Venice, 1546), trans. Wilmer C. Wright (New York: G. P. Putnam's Sons, 1930).

67. Antony van Leeuwenloek, "Microscopic Observations about Animals in the Scurf of the Teeth," *Philosophical Transactions of the Royal Society of London* 14, no. 159 (May 1684): 568–574.

68. Theodore Schwann, "Vorläufige Mittheilung, betreffend Versuche über die Weingährung und Fäulnis," *Annalen der Physik und Chemie* 41 (1837): 184–193. See also Charles Cagniard-Latour, "Mémoire sur la Fermentation Vineuse," *Annales de chimie et de physique* 68 (1838): 206–222, trans. Thomas Brock, in *Milestones in Microbiology 1546 to 1940* (Washington, DC: ASM Press, 1999), n. 28, 16–24.

69. Henle, "Von den Miasmen und Contagien und von den Miasmatisch contagiösen Krankheiten," 1–82, esp. 76–79.

70. William Ford, "Development of Our Early Knowledge Concerning Magnification," *Science* 79 (1934): 578–581.

71. William Bulloch, *The History of Bacteriology* (New York: Dover Publications, 1938), 79, 578–581.

72. Christian Gram, "Ueber die isolirte Färbung der Schizomyceten in Schnitt-und Trock-enpräparaten," *Fortschritte der Medicin* 2 (1884): 185–189, trans. Thomas Brock, in *Milestones in Microbiology*, n. 30, 215–218.

73. Robert Koch, "Die Aetiologie der Milzbrand-Krankheit, begründet auf die Entwick-lungesgeschichte des Bacillus Anthracis," *Beiträge zur Biologie der Pflanzen*, 2 (1876): 277–310, trans. Thomas Brock, in *Milestones in Microbiology*, n. 30, 89–95, 109–115.

74. Wesley W. Spink, *Infectious Diseases: Prevention and Treatment in the Nineteenth Century* (Minneapolis: University of Minnesota Press, 1978).

75. Howard D. Kramer, "The Germ Theory and the Early Public Health Program in the United States," *Bulletin of the History of Medicine* 22 (1948): 233–247. See also George Rosen, *A History of Public Health* (Baltimore, MD: Johns Hopkins University Press, 1993).

76. Rosen, *A History of Public Health*, 286, 289–291.

77. C. E. A. Winslow, *The Life of Hermann M. Biggs, M.D., D.Sc., LLD: Physician and Statesman of the Public Health* (Philadelphia: Lea and Febiger, 1929), 237.

78. Bulloch, *History of Bacteriology*.

79. William W. Ford, *Bacteriology* (New York: Paul B. Hoeber, Medical Book Department of Harper and Brothers, 1939).

80. Robert W. Taylor, *The Pathology and Treatment of Venereal Diseases* (Philadelphia: Lea Brothers, 1895). See also Strumpell, *A Text-Book of Medicine for Students and Practitioners*.

81. H. M. Malkin, "Rudolf Virchow and the Durability of Cellular Pathology," *Perspectives in Biology and Medicine* 33, no. 3 (1990): 431–443.

82. Klaus Lange, "Rudolf Virchow, Poverty and Global Health: From 'Politics as Medicine on a Grand Scale' to 'Health in All Policies,'" *Global Health Journal* 5, no. 3 (2021): 149–154.

83. Adolf Strumpell, "Tabes Dorsalis," in *A Text-Book of Medicine for Students and Practitioners*, 960–980.

84. Cazenave and Schedel, *A Practical Synopsis of Cutaneous Diseases*, 336–367. See also Robley Dunglison, "Syphilides," in *The Practice of Medicine: A Treatise on Special Pathology and Therapeutics*, vol. 2 (Philadelphia: Lea and Blanchard, 1848). See also Langston Parker, *The Modern Treatment of Syphilitic Disease, Both Primary and Secondary, Comprising the Treatment of Constitutional and Confirmed Syphilis by a Safe and Successful Method; with Numerous Cases, Formulae, and Clinical Observations.* (Philadelphia: Blanchard and Lea, 1854).

85. Roberts, *The Theory and Practice of Medicine*.

86. Eduard Reich, *Ueber den Einfluss der Syphilis auf das Familienleben*, 2nd ed. (Amsterdam: Dieckmann, 1887).

87. Adolf Lostorfer, "Ueber die Moglichkeit der Diagnose der Syphilis Mittelst der Mikroskopischen Blutuntersuchung," in *Medizinische Jahrbucher*, ed. K. K. Gesellschaft Der Arzte (Vienna, 1872), 96–105.

88. Strumpell, *A Text-Book of Medicine for Students and Practitioners*.

89. E. Bruusgaard, "Ueber das Schicksal der nicht Spizifisch behandelen Leukiter," *AMA Archives of Dermatology and Syphilology* 157 (1929): 309–332.

90. T. Gjestland, "The Oslo Study of Untreated Syphilis: An Epidemiologic Investigation of the Natural Course of the Syphilitic Infection Based upon a Re-study of the Boeck-Bruusgaard Material," *Acta Dermato-Venereologica* 35, no. 4 (1955). See also E. Gurney Clark and Niels Danbolt, "The Oslo Study of the Natural Course of Untreated Syphilis," *Medical Clinics of North America* 48, no. 3 (1964): 613–623.

91. Warthin, "Virchow's Concentration of Constitutional Syphilis." See also Virchow, *Ueber die Natur der Consititutionnell Syphilitischen Affectionem.*

92. Strumpell, *A Text-Book of Medicine for Students and Practitioners.* See also William Osler, *The Principles and Practice of Medicine,* 1st ed. (New York: Appleton, 1893).

93. F. W. Baeslack, "Experimental Syphilis," *Urologic and Cutaneous Review* 4, no. 1 (1916).

94. E. Metchnikoff and E. Roux, *Annales de L'Institut Pasteur* (Paris: Masson et Cie, 1903, 1904, and 1905).

95. Frederick Novy to Fritz Schaudinn, March 18, 1905, Frederick Novy Papers, Box 1, Bentley Historical Library, University of Michigan.

96. Fritz Schaudinn and Erich Hoffmann, "A Preliminary Note upon the Occurrence of Spirochaetes in Syphilitic Lesions and in Papillomata," in *Selected Essays on Syphilis and Small Pox* (London: New Sydenham Society, 1906), 3–15.

97. Schaudinn believed that *Spirocheta ziemannini* in the owl could develop into trypanosomes, a theory called heterogeneisis. See Frederick Novy to Fritz Schaudinn, February 4, 1905, Frederick Novy Papers.

98. Schaudinn and Hoffmann, "A Preliminary Note."

99. K. Landsteiner and V. Mucha, "Zur Technik Der Spirochaetenuntersuchung," *Wiener Klinische Wochenschrift* 19 (1906): 1349–1350.

100. Udo Wile, "The Spirochaeta *pallida;* Its Easy Demonstrability, and a Brief Review of Its History," *Journal of Cutaneous Diseases* 27 (1909): 296–303.

101. Jules Bordet, "Les Leucocytes et les proprieties actives du serum chez les caccines," *Annales de L'Institut Pasteur* 9 (1895): 462–506. See also A. Wassermann, A. Neisser, and C. Bruck, "Eine serodiagnostische Reaktion bei Syphilis," *Dtsch Med Wochenschr* 32 (1906): 746.

102. Osler, "Syphilis," 268–283. See also A. Wassermann and F. Plaut, "Ueber das Verhandensein syphilitischer Antisitoffe in der Cerebrospinalflussigkeit von Paralytikern," *Deutsche Medizinische Wochenschrift* 32 (1906): 1769–1772.

103. J. Citron, "Die Serodiagnostik der Syphilis," *Berliner Klinische Wochenschrift* 44 (1907): 1370–1373.

104. The term "regain" (reacts) was used to refer to substances that fix complement.

105. H. Boas, "Die Wassermannsche Reaktion beiaktiven und inaktiven Sera," *Berl Klin Wochenschr* 46 (1908): 400–402.

106. M. Levaditi, "Sur la coloration du *Spirochaete pallida* Schaudin dans les Coupes," *Comptes Rendus des Seances* 2 (1905): 326–327.

107. Aldred Scott Warthin, "A More Rapid and Improved Method of Demonstrating Spirochetes in Tissues," *American Journal of Syphilis, Gonorrhea, and Venereal Diseases* 4 (1920): 97–103.

108. Aldred Scott Warthin, "The Persistence of Active Lesions and Spirochetes in the Tissues of Clinically Active or 'Cured' Syphilis," *American Journal of Medical Sciences* (1916): 508–521. See also "Pathological Studies, Syphilis," n.d., Aldred Warthin Papers, Box 2, Call number 86199, Bentley Historical Library, University of Michigan.

109. H. Noguchi and J. W. Moore, "A Demonstration of Treponema Pallidum in the Brain in Cases of General Paralysis," *Journal of Experimental Medicine* 17, no. 2 (1913): 232–238.

110. Hobart Amory Hare, *A Text-Book of the Practice of Medicine for Students and Practitioners* (Philadelphia: Lea and Fibiger, 1915). See also James M. Anders, *A Text-Book of the Practice of Medicine,* 11th ed. (Philadelphia: W. B. Saunders, 1913).

111. Baeslack, "Experimental Syphilis." See also Hare, *A Text-Book of the Practice of Medicine for Students and Practitioners.*

112. Louis Pasteur, "Sur les virus-vaccins du cholera des poules et du charbon," *Comptes rendus des travaux du Congres international des directeurs des stations agronomiques, session de Versailles,* June 1881.

113. Christoph Gradmann, *Laboratory Disease,* trans. Elborg Forster (Baltimore, MD: Johns Hopkins University Press, 2009), 176–182.

114. Emil von Behring and S. Kitasato, "Ueber das Zustandekommen der Diphtherie-Immunität und der Tetanus-Immunität bei Thieren," *Deutsche Medizinische Wochenschrift* 16 (1890): 1113–1119, trans. Thomas Brock, in *Milestones in Microbiology,* n. 30, 138–44.

115. F. G. Novy, "Bacterial Toxins and Anti-toxins," *Medical and Surgical Reporter* 74, no. 12 (March 21, 1896): 351–359. See also F. G. Novy, "Practical Benefits of Bacteriology," in *First Report of the Michigan Academy of Science,* ed. Walter B. Barrows (Lansing, MI: Robert Smith Printing, 1894).

116. Brock, *Milestones in Microbiology,* 184.

117. Dobson, "The History of Antimalarial Drugs," in *Antimalarial Chemotherapy: Mechanisms of Action, Resistance, and New Directions in Drug Discovery,* ed. Philip J. Rosenthal (Totowa, NJ: Humana Press, 2001), 15–25.

118. John Parascandola, "The Theoretical Basis of Paul Ehrlich's Chemotherapy," *Journal of the History of Medicine* 16 (1981): 19–43.

119. Paul Ehrlich, "Ueber modern Chemotherapie," in *Beitrage zur experimentellen Pathologie und Chemotherapie* (Leipzig: Akademische Verlagsgesellschaft, 1909), 167–202. See also Brock, *Milestones in Microbiology,* 176–184.

120. Marguerite Marks, "Paul Ehrlich, the Man and His Work," *McClure's Magazine* 36, no. 2 (1910): 184.

121. Paul Ehrlich, "Ueber die Behanklung der Syphilis mit dem Praparate '606,'" *Allgemeine Wiener medizinische Zeitung* 55 (1910): 457–458 and 469–470.

122. Paul Ehrlich, "Ueber modern Chemotherapie. Vortrag gehalten," in *Der X. Tagung der Deutschen Dermatologischen Gesellschaft. Beitrage zur experimentellen Pathologie und Chemotherapie* (Leipzig: Akademische Verlagsgesellschaft, 1909), 167–202.

123. Parascandola, "Theoretical Basis of Paul Ehrlich's Chemotherapy," 19–43.

124. Ehrlich, "Ueber modern Chemotherapie. Vortrag gehalten," 167–202. Brock, *Milestones in Microbiology,* 177, 178.

125. Marks, "Paul Ehrlich," 184.

126. Frederick Novy to Fritz Schaudinn, February 4, 1905, Frederick Novy Papers.

127. Paul Ehrlich and S. Hata, "Versuche bei Syphilis an Kaninchen," in *Die experimentelle Chemotherapie der Spirillosen* (Berlin: Julius Springer, 1910), 58–85.

128. Ehrlich, "Ueber die Behanklung der Syphilis mit dem Praparate '606,'" 457–458 and 469–470.

129. "The Ehrlich-Hata Preparation for Syphilis," *American Journal of Urology* 6, no. 11 (November 1, 1910): 503.

130. Martha Marquardt, *Paul Ehrlich* (New York: Schuman, 1951), 163–175.

131. J. P. Bull, "The Historical Development of Clinical Therapeutic Trials," *Journal of Chronic Diseases* 10, no. 3 (1959): 218–248.

132. Laura E. Bothwell and Scott H. Podolsky, "The Emergence of the Randomized, Controlled Trial," *New England Journal of Medicine* 275, no. 6 (2016): 501–504.

133. See "Ehrlich and His Discovery," *American Druggist and Pharmaceutical Record* 57 (December 12, 1910): 333. See also "The Ehrlich-Hata Preparation for Syphilis," 503.

134. "The Ehrlich-Hata Preparation for Syphilis," 503.

135. Marks, "Paul Ehrlich," 184.

136. Marquardt, *Paul Ehrlich*, 163–206.

137. A. L. Thorburn, "Paul Ehrlich: Pioneer of Chemotherapy and Cure by Arsenic (1854–1915)," *British Journal of Venereal Diseases* 59, no. 6 (1983): 404.

138. "Ehrlich and His Discovery," 333

139. Bull, "The Historical Development of Clinical Therapeutic Trials," 218–248.

140. "Ehrlich and His Discovery," 333.

141. Marquardt, *Paul Ehrlich*, 163–206.

142. "The Ehrlich-Hata Preparation for Syphilis," 503.

143. Wilhelm Wechselmann, "The Treatment of Syphilis with Ehrlich's Dioxydiamido-arsenobenzol," *Lancet* 176, no. 4548 (October 29,1910): 1295–1297.

144. M. S. Kakels, "Preliminary Report on the Ehrlich-Hata Preparation for the Cure of Syphilis," *Medical Record* 78, no. 13 (September 1910): 517.

145. "Ehrlich and His Discovery," 333.

146. H. Elsner, "The New Treatment of Syphilis (Ehrlich Hata): Observations and Results," *JAMA* 55, no. 24 (December 10, 1910): 2052.

147. Kakels, "Preliminary Report on the Ehrlich-Hata Preparation," 517.

148. Our Regular Correspondent, "Our Berlin Letter: Ehrlich's Theory of Chemotherapy of Infectious Diseases," *Medical Record* 77, no. 10 (March 5, 1910): 416.

149. Our Regular Correspondent, "Our Berlin Letter."

150. Mrs. Marks, "Professor Ehrlich's Discoveries," *McClure's Magazine* 35, no. 6 (October 1910): 713.

151. Steven Diner, *A Very Different Age: Americans of the Progressive Era* (New York: Hill and Wang, 1998).

152. Murray Rothbard, *The Progressive Era* (Auburn, AL: Mises Institute, 2017).

153. Paul de Kruif, *Microbe Hunters* (New York: Harcourt Brace, 1926), esp. 319, 331.

154. William Allen Pusey, *The History and Epidemiology of Syphilis* (Springfield, IL: Charles C Thomas, 1933), 74.

155. Marks, "Paul Ehrlich," 184, 187, 189.

156. "Paul Ehrlich's Career as the Conqueror of the Cell," *Current Literature* 50, no. 1 (1911): 56.

157. "Paul Ehrlich's Career," 53–57.

158. Wilhelm Wechselmann, *The Treatment of Syphilis with Salvarsan* (New York: Rebman, 1911), 55, 67, 152, 161.

159. "Paul Ehrlich Obituary," *The Times* (London), August 20, 1916.

160. Marquardt, *Paul Ehrlich*, 163–206.

161. John T. Crissey, *The Dermatology and Syphilology of the Nineteenth Century* (New York: Praeger, 1981), 359–366.

162. K. J. Williams, "The Introduction of 'Chemotherapy' Using Arsphenamine: The First Magic Bullet," *Journal of the Royal Society of Medicine* 102, no. 8 (2009): 343–348.

163. T. W. Gibbard and L. W. Harrison, "The Treatment of Syphilis with Salvarsan and Neo-Salvarsan," *British Medical Journal (BMJ)* 2, no. 2702 (1912): 953–955.

164. Lloyd Jones and A. J. Gibson, "Salvarsan Treatment of Syphilis: An Analysis of Two Hundred Cases," *BMJ* 1, no. 2927 (1917): 152–154.

165. Hobart Amory Hare, "Syphilis," in *A Text-Book of the Practice of Medicine for Students and Practitioners* (Philadelphia: Lea and Fibiger, 1915), 302–316.

166. Suzanne White Junod, "FDA and Clinical Drug Trials: A Short History," archive, press announcements, U.S. Food and Drug Administration, last updated February 1,

2008, www.fda.gov/media/110437/download#:~:text=Efficacy%20Under%20the%20 1962%20Drug%20Amendments&text=This%20provision%20required%20 controlled%20trials%20that%20could%20indeed%20support%20claims%20of %20efficacy.

167. Ehrlich, "Ueber die Behanklung der Syphilis mit dem Praparate '606,'" 457–458 and 469–470.

168. C. F. Marshall, "Salvarsan ('606')," *BMJ* 1, no. 2613 (1911): 226.

169. Warthin, "The Persistence of Active Lesions and Spirochetes," 508–532.

170. Anders, *A Text-Book of the Practice of Medicine.*

171. "Some Toxic Effects of Salvarsan," *BMJ* 1, no. 2665 (1912): 205–206. See also Ehrlich and Hata, "Versuche bei Syphilis an Kaninchen," 58–85; John Adams, "Salvarsan Treatment of Syphilis," *BMJ* 1, no. 2929 (1917): 244.

172. Hare, "Syphilis," 302–316.

173. Adams, "Salvarsan Treatment of Syphilis," 244. See also Osler, "Syphilis," 283–288.

174. J.E.R. McDonagh, "The Action of Salvarsan and Neo-Salvarsan on the Wassermann Reaction," *BMJ* 1, no. 2684 (1912): 1287–1289.

175. Julius Bernstein, "The Action of Salvarsan," *BMJ* 1, no. 2687 (1912): 1513.

176. Osler, "Syphilis," 283–288.

177. "Parenchymatous Syphilis," *BMJ* 1, no. 2822 (1915): 215–216.

178. C. L. Williams, "Neosalvarsan in Brain Syphilis: A Report of a Case of Brain Syphilis Treated with Neosalvarsan, with Recovery," *Public Health Reports* 28, no. 46 (1913): 2405–2407. See also Kakels, "Preliminary Report on the Ehrlich-Hata Preparation," 517.

179. Parker, *The Modern Treatment of Syphilitic Disease*, 136–149, 258.

180. Charles V. Chapin, "Dirt, Disease and the Health Officer," *Public Health Papers and Reports* 28 (1902): 296–299.

181. Charles V. Chapin, "History of State and Municipal Control of Disease," in *A Half Century of Public Health*, ed. Mazyck P. Ravenal (New York: American Public Health Association, 1921), 133–161. See also James H. Cassedy, *Charles V. Chapin and the Public Health Movement* (Cambridge, MA: Harvard University Press, 1962), 94–112.

182. Chapin, "Dirt, Disease and the Health Officer," 296–299.

183. Hibbert Winslow Hill, "The Old Practice and the New," in *The New Public Health* (Minneapolis, MN: Press of the Journal Lancet, 1913), 42.

184. William T. Sedgwick, "The Origin, Scope and Significance of Bacteriology," *Science* 13, no. 317 (1901): 121–128.

185. Amy L. Fairchild, David Rosner, James Colgrove, Ronald Bayer, and Linda P. Fried, "The EXODUS of Public Health: What History Can Tell Us about the Future," *American Journal of Public Health* 100, no. 1 (January 2010): 54–63.

186. Milton J. Rosenau, *Preventive Medicine and Hygiene* (New York: D. Appleton, 1913), 42–63, esp. 55.

187. Rosenau, *Preventive Medicine and Hygiene*, ix, x.

188. Rosenau, *Preventive Medicine and Hygiene*, 49–50.

189. Rosenau, *Preventive Medicine and Hygiene*, 49–50.

190. Rosenau, *Preventive Medicine and Hygiene*, 50–51.

191. Rosenau, *Preventive Medicine and Hygiene*, 56, 58.

192. Rosen, *A History of Public Health*, 107–166. See also "Prevention of Syphilis by the State," *American Journal of Public Health* 17, no. 10 (1927): 1042–1043.

193. John Parascandola, *Sex, Sin, and Science: A History of Syphilis in America* (London: Praeger Press, 2008). See also Allan M. Brandt, *No Magic Bullet: A Social History of*

Venereal Disease in the United States since 1880 (New York: Oxford University Press, 1987), 144.

194. Scott W. Stern, *The Trials of Nina McCall: Sex, Surveillance, and the Decades-Long Government Plan to Imprison Promiscuous Women* (Boston: Beacon Press, 2018).

195. Thomas Sternberg, E. B. Howard, L. H. Dewey, and P. Padget, "Venereal Diseases," in *Medical Department, United States Army Preventive Medicine in World War II*, vol. 5, *Communicable Diseases Transmitted through Contact or by Unknown Means*, ed. John Boyd Coates Jr. (Washington, DC: Office of the Surgeon General Department of the Army, 1960), 137–139.

196. G. F. Blandy, "Nation's Danger," *The Survey* 40 (1918): 407. See also "Syphilis: The Scourge of Society," *The Survey* 34, no. 25 (1915): 547; "Prevention of Syphilis by the State," 1042–1043.

197. Charles E. Miner, "Social Hygiene and Venereal Disease Control," *American Journal of Public Health* 16, no. 4 (1926): 386–388.

198. Milton Rosenau, T. Salmon, J. Trask, J. Whipple, and G. Chandler, *Preventive Medicine and Hygiene*, 4th ed. (New York: D. Appleton and Company, 1921).

199. Milton Rosenau, "Syphilis," in *Preventive Medicine and Hygiene*, 4th ed., 117.

200. Parascandola, *Sex, Sin, and Science*.

201. Thomas Parran, *Shadow on the Land: Syphilis* (New York: Reynal and Hitchcock, 1937), 85, 131.

202. Miner, "Social Hygiene and Venereal Disease Control," 386–388.

203. "Thomas Parran, Jr. (1936–1948)," Previous Surgeons General, U.S. Department of Health and Human Services, accessed April 15, 2024, archived at https://wayback .archive-it.org/3929/20171201191739/https://www.surgeongeneral.gov/about /previous/bioparran.html.

204. Thomas Parran, "The Eradication of Syphilis as a Practical Public Health Objective," *JAMA* 97, no. 2 (1931): 73–77.

205. Parran, "The Eradication of Syphilis as a Practical Public Health Objective."

206. Thomas Parran, "The Next Great Plague to Go," *Survey Graphic* 25, no. 7 (1936): 405–411.

207. Parran, *Shadow on the Land*, 7, 29, 48, 205, 221, 254, 255.

208. Parran, *Shadow on the Land*, 7, 26, 48, 205, 221, 255.

209. 163, 283, 289.

210. Parran, *Shadow on the Land*, 47, 245.

211. Parran, *Shadow on the Land*, 267.

212. Parran, "The Next Great Plague to Go."

213. Henry Christian, "Syphilis," in *Principles and Practice of Medicine*, 13th ed., ed. William Osler, Henry Christian, and Thomas McRae (New York: Appleton, 1936), 344–369.

214. For example, Russell Cecil, *A Textbook of Medicine* (Philadelphia: W. B. Saunders, 1937), 361–382.

215. Thomas Parran, "Why Don't We Stamp Out Syphilis?," *Reader's Digest*, July 1936, 65–73.

216. "Medicine: Venereal Disease Campaign," *Time*, January 11, 1937, 38–39.

217. Parran, "The Next Great Plague to Go."

218. "Medicine: Venereal Disease Campaign."

219. Parran, *Shadow on the Land*, 267.

220. Parran, *Shadow on the Land*, 25, 56, 96–97, 131.

221. Parran, *Shadow on the Land*, 209–223.

222. "Medicine: Venereal Disease Campaign."
223. "Medicine: Venereal Disease Campaign." See also "Syphilis: Conference in Washington Hits Taboos and Insufficient Funds," *Newsweek*, January 9, 1937, 40; "The War on Syphilis," *Newsweek*, February 20, 1939, 35; Thomas Parran, "Eradication of Syphilis Possible," *Scientific American* 154, no. 5 (May 1936): 277; Paul de Kruif, "Can We Now Fight Syphilis?," *Ladies' Home Journal*, November 1937, 29.
224. Parran, "The Next Great Plague to Go," 405–411.
225. Parran, *Shadow on the Land*, 56.
226. U.S. Treasury Department Public Health Service, *Proceedings of the Conference on Venereal Disease Control Work, Washington, D.C., December 28–30, 1936, Supplement No. 3* (Washington, DC: United States Government Printing Office, 1937).
227. Parran, "Why Don't We Stamp Out Syphilis?"
228. "Syphilis: Conference in Washington Hits Taboos and Insufficient Funds."
229. Committee on Commerce, *Investigation and Control of Venereal Diseases: Hearings before a Subcommittee of the Committee on Commerce, United States Senate, Seventy-Fifth Congress, Third Session on S.3290* (Washington, DC: United States Government Printing Office, 1938).
230. Odin Anderson, *Syphilis and Society: Problems of Control in the United States, 1912–1964*, Research Series 22 (Chicago: University of Chicago Press, 1965), 1–49.
231. Brandt, *No Magic Bullet*, 144.
232. Parascandola, *Sex, Sin, and Science*, 95.
233. Ibid, Parran, *Shadow on the Land*, 159, 267, 287, 296.
234. Louis Galambos and Jane Sewell, *Networks of Innovation: Vaccine Development at Merck, Sharp & Dohme, and Mulford, 1895–1995* (Cambridge, UK: Cambridge University Press, 1995).
235. Erin Wuebker, "Taking the Venereal Out of Venereal Disease: The 1930s Public Health Campaign against Syphilis and Gonorrhea," *Notches* (blog), May 31, 2016, https://notchesblog.com/2016/05/31/taking-the-venereal-out-of-venereal-disease-the-1930s-public-health-campaign-against-syphilis-and-gonorrhea/.
236. "Medicine: Venereal Disease Campaign." See also "The War on Syphilis"; de Kruif, "Can We Now Fight Syphilis?"
237. Parran, "The Eradication of Syphilis as a Practical Public Health Objective."
238. Parran, "Why Don't We Stamp Out Syphilis?" See also "Medicine: Venereal Disease Campaign"; "The War on Syphilis"; Parran, "Eradication of Syphilis Possible"; de Kruif, "Can We Now Fight Syphilis?"
239. Parran, *Shadow on the Land*.
240. Frank Snowden, "Lecture 12. Syphilis: From the 'Great Pox' to the Modern Version," Open Yale Courses, accessed March 26, 2024, https://oyc.yale.edu/history/hist-234/lecture-12.
241. E. R. Squibb & Sons, "About Penicillin," Squibb Advertisement, 1944, https://digital.sciencehistory.org/works/jd472w56b.
242. Edward P. Abraham, E. Chain, C. M. Fletcher, A. D. Gardner, N. G. Heatley, M. A. Jennings, and H. W. Florey, "Further Observations on Penicillin," *Lancet* 238, no. 6155 (August 1941): 177–189.
243. "News of Science," *New Republic*, December 14, 1942, 791–792.
244. "Life Story of a Miracle," *Newsweek*, March 19, 1945, 86–87.
245. "Medicine: Penicillin's Progress," *Time*, June 7, 1943, 68–69.
246. Samuel Napier, "The Magic of Penicillin," *Contemporary Review* 165 (1944): 303–304.

247. Chester S. Keefer, Francis G. Blake, E. Kennerly Marshall Jr., John S. Lockwood, and W. Barry Wood Jr., "Penicillin in the Treatment of Infections: A Report of 500 Cases," *JAMA* 122, no. 18 (1943): 1209–1217.

248. Daniel Kevles, *The Physicists: The History of a Scientific Community in Modern America* (Cambridge, MA: Harvard University Press, 1995), 22–34.

249. J. F. Mahoney, R. C. Arnold, and Ad Harris, "Penicillin Treatment of Early Syphilis," *Venereal Disease Information* 24, no. 12 (1943): 355–357.

250. J. F. Mahoney, R. C. Arnold, Burton L. Sterner, Ad Harris, and M. R. Zwally, "Penicillin Treatment of Early Syphilis," *JAMA* 126, no. 2 (1944): 63–67.

251. Christian, "Syphilis," 366.

252. R. Gibbons, "End of Syphilis in Sight?," *Science Digest* 29 (1951): 48.

253. John Pfeiffer, "A New Magic Bullet Ends an Old Disease," *Popular Science Monthly*, September 1953, 58.

254. Rudolph Kampmeier, *Essentials of Syphilology* (Philadelphia: Lippincott, 1943).

255. See G. Boudin, *Neurologie: La fin de la syphilis nerveuse* (Paris: Masson, 1955).

256. Paul Le Van, "The Story of Syphilis," *Hygeia* 27, no. 4 (1949): 238–239.

257. Russell L. Cecil and Robert F. Loeb, *A Textbook of Medicine*, 9th ed. (Philadelphia: Saunders, 1955). See also Russell L. Cecil and Robert F. Loeb, *A Textbook of Medicine*, 7th ed. (Philadelphia: Saunders, 1947).

258. "Syphilis," in *Cecil-Loeb Textbook of Medicine*, ed. Russel Cecil and Walsh McDermott (Philadelphia: Saunders, 1947), 358–408. See also "Syphilis," in *Cecil-Loeb Textbook of Medicine*, 11th ed., ed. Paul Beeson and Walsh McDermott (Philadelphia: Saunders, 1963), 349–376.

259. Marquardt, *Paul Ehrlich*, 163–175. See also Paul de Kruif, "Paul Ehrlich, the Magic Bullet," in *Microbe Hunters*, 314–337.

260. Elizabeth Fee, "Sin vs. Science," in *AIDS: The Burdens of History*, ed. Elizabeth Fee and Daniel Fox (Berkeley: University of California Press,1988), 121–146.

261. R. Dubos, *Mirage of Health: Utopias, Progress, and Biological Change* (Garden City, NY: Anchor Books, 1959), 113–181.

Chapter 2   AIDS

1. Anthony S. Fauci, "The Acquired Immune Deficiency Syndrome: The Ever-Broadening Clinical Spectrum," *JAMA* 249, no. 17 (1983): 2375–2376.

2. Jean L. Marx, "New Disease Baffles Medical Community," *Science* 217, no. 4560 (1982): 618.

3. For example, Jerry Falwell, "Jerry Falwell Quotes," Think Exist, 2010, http://thinkexist.com/quotes/jerry_falwell. See also Patrick Buchanan, "Editorial," *Seattle Times*, July 1993.

4. Elizabeth Fee and Daniel M. Fox, eds., *AIDS: The Burdens of History* (Berkeley: University of California Press, 1988), 12–66.

5. Allan Brandt, "Plagues and Peoples: The AIDS Epidemic," in *No Magic Bullet: A Social History of Venereal Disease in the United States since 1880* (New York: Oxford University Press, 1987), 183–204.

6. "LaRouche Initiative Stopped Dead," *New York Native*, November 17, 1986.

7. Fee and Fox, *AIDS*, 12–66.

8. Allan M. Brandt, "AIDS: "From Social History to Social Policy,'" in *AIDS*, ed. Fee and Fox, 147–171.

9. Marx, "New Disease Baffles Medical Community."

10. CDC, "Pneumocystis Pneumonia—Los Angeles," in *Morbidity and Mortality Weekly Report* 30, no. 21 (June 5, 1981): 250–252.

11. Robert C. Gallo, *Virus Hunting: AIDS, Cancer, and the Human Retrovirus: A Story of Scientific Discovery* (New York: Basic Books, 1991), 44–162.

12. Anders Vahlne, "A Historical Reflection on the Discovery of Human Retroviruses," *Retrovirology* 6, no. 40 (2009), https://doi.org/10.1186/1742-4690-6-40.

13. Bernard J. Poiesz, Francis W Ruscetti, Adi F. Gazdar, P. A. Bunn, J. D. Minna, and Robert Gallo, "Detection and Isolation of Type C Retrovirus Particles from Fresh and Cultured Lymphocytes of a Patient with Cutaneous T-Cell Lymphoma," *PNAS* 77, no. 12 (1980), https://doi.org/10.1073/pnas.77.12.7415.

14. Bernard J. Poiesz, Francis W. Ruscetti, Marvin S. Reitz, V. S. Kalyanaraman, and Robert C. Gallo, "Isolation of a New Type C Retrovirus (HTLV) in Primary Uncultured Cells of a Patient with Sezary T-Cell Leukaemia," *Nature* 294, no. 5838 (1981): 268–271.

15. L. Montagnier, J. Gruest, S. Chamaret, C. Dauguet, C. Axler, D. Guetard, M. T. Nugeyre, et al., "Adaptation of Lymphadenopathy Associated Virus (LAV) to Replication in EBV-Transformed B Lymphoblastoid Cell Lines," *Science* 225, no. 4657 (1984): 63–66.

16. Robert C. Gallo, Syed Z. Salahuddin, Mikulas Popovic, Gene M. Shearer, Mark Kaplan, Barton F. Haynes, Thomas J. Palker, et al., "Frequent Detection and Isolation of Cytopathic Retroviruses (HTLV-III) from Patients with AIDS and at Risk for AIDS," *Science* 224, no. 4648 (1984): 500–503.

17. Jay A. Levy, Anthony D. Hoffman, Susan M. Kramer, Jill A. Kandis, Joni M. Shimabururo, and Lyndon S. Oshiro, "Isolation of Lymphocytopathic Retroviruses from San Francisco Patients with AIDS," *Science* 225, no. 4664 (1984): 840–842.

18. Jonathan N. Weber and Robin A. Weiss, "HIV Infection: The Cellular Picture," *Scientific American* 259, no. 4 (1988): 100–109.

19. Jay A. Levy, "Human Immunodeficiency Viruses and the Pathogenesis of AIDS," *JAMA* 261, no. 20 (1989): 2997. See also William L. Heyward and James W. Curran, "The Epidemiology of AIDS in the U.S.," *Scientific American* 259, no. 4 (1988): 72–81.

20. Vahlne, "A Historical Reflection on the Discovery of Human Retroviruses."

21. J. Cohen, *Shots in the Dark: The Wayward Search for an AIDS Vaccine* (New York: Norton, 2001), 3–15, 11.

22. Gallo, *Virus Hunting*, 44–162.

23. Richard A. Kaslow, David G. Ostrow, Roger Detels, John P. Phair, B. Frank Polk, and Charles R. Rinaldo Jr., "The Multicenter AIDS Cohort Study: Rationale, Organization, and Selected Characteristics of the Participants," *American Journal of Epidemiology* 126, no. 2 (1987): 310–318.

24. Paul Volberding and P.T. Cohen, "Natural History, Clinical Spectrum and General Management of HIV Infection," in *The AIDS Knowledge Base*, ed. P. T. Cohen, Merle Sande, and Paul Volberding (Waltham, MA: Medical Publishing Group, 1990), 4.1.1–4.1.4.

25. Michael Saag, "The Natural History of HIV-1 Infection," in *Textbook of AIDS Medicine*, ed. Samuel Broder, Thomas Merigan, and Dani Bolognesi (Baltimore, MD: Williams and Wilkins, 1994), 45–54.

26. Margaret Fischl, "An Introduction to the Clinical Spectrum of AIDS," in *Textbook of AIDS Medicine*, ed. Broder, Merigan, and Bolognesi, 149–160. See also John L. Fahey, Jeremy M. G. Taylor, Roger Detels, Bo Hofmann, Raphael Melmed, Pari Nishanian, and Janis V. Giorgi, "The Prognostic Value of Cellular and Serologic Markers in

Infection with Human Immunodeficiency Virus Type 1," *New England Journal of Medicine (NEJM)* 322, no. 3 (1990): 166–172.

27. Robert Yarchoan, David J. Venzon, James M. Pluda, Jill Lietzau, Kathleen M. Wyvill, Anastasios A. Tsiatis, Seth M. Steinberg, and Samuel Broder, "CD4 Count and the Risk for Death in Patients Infected with HIV Receiving Antiretroviral Therapy," *Annals of Internal Medicine* 115, no. 3 (1991): 184–189.

28. Diana Finzi and Robert F. Siliciano, "Viral Dynamics in HIV-1 Infection," *Cell* 93, no. 5 (1998): 665–671.

29. "LaRouche Initiative Stopped Dead."

30. Julia Smith, "Europe's Shifting Response to HIV/AIDS," *Health and Human Rights* 18, no. 2 (2016): 145–156.

31. Brandt, "AIDS: "From Social History to Social Policy."

32. David Musto, "Quarantine and the Problem of AIDS," in *AIDS*, ed. Fee and Fox, 67–85.

33. *Jacobson v. Massachusetts*, 197 U.S. 11 (1905).

34. Brandt, "AIDS: "From Social History to Social Policy." See also Mary Dunlap, "AIDS and Discrimination in the United States: Reflections on the Nature of Prejudice in a Virus," *Villanova Law Review* 34 (1989): 909.

35. Gerald M. Oppenheimer and Ronald Bayer, "The Rise and Fall of AIDS Exceptionalism," *American Medical Association Journal of Ethics* 11, no. 12 (2009): 988–992.

36. Randy Shilts, *And the Band Played On: Politics, People, and the AIDS Epidemic* (New York: St. Martin's Press, 1987).

37. David France, *How to Survive a Plague: The Inside Story of How Citizens and Science Tamed AIDS* (New York: Knopf, 2016).

38. Patrick Strudwick, "These Posters Show What AIDS Meant in the 1980s," *BuzzFeed News*, December 1, 2015, www.buzzfeednews.com/article/patrickstrudwick/these-1980s-aids-posters-show-the-desperate-fight-to-save-li.

39. Ronald Bayer, "Public Health Policy and the AIDS Epidemic: An End to HIV Exceptionalism?," *NEJM* 324, no. 21 (1991): 1500–1504.

40. Ronald Bayer, *Private Acts, Social Consequences: AIDS and the Politics of Public Health* (New Brunswick, NJ: Rutgers University Press, 1991).

41. "AfrAIDs," *New Republic* 193, no. 16 (1985): 7–9.

42. Powel Kazanjian, personal interviews with HIV-infected persons, Ann Arbor, Michigan, 2011–2021.

43. Ronald Bayer and Gerald M Oppenheimer, *AIDS Doctors: Voices from the Epidemic* (Oxford, UK: Oxford University Press, 2000), 63–118.

44. Fee and Fox, *AIDS*, 1–11. See also Virginia Berridge and Philip Strong, *AIDS and Contemporary History* (New York: Cambridge University Press, 1993), 1–14.

45. Mirko D. Grmek, *History of AIDS: Emergence and Origin of a Modern Pandemic* (Princeton, NJ: Princeton University Press, 1990).

46. Susan Maizel Chambre, *Fighting for Our Lives: New York's AIDS Community and the Politics of Disease, Critical Issues in Health and Medicine* (New Brunswick, NJ: Rutgers University Press, 2006), 57–110.

47. German Lopez, "The Reagan Administration's Unbelievable Response to the HIV/AIDS Epidemic," *Vox*, updated December 1, 2016, www.vox.com/2015/12/1/9828348/ronaldreagan-hiv-aids.

48. Mark Joseph Stern, "Listen to Reagan's Press Secretary Laugh about Gay People Dying of AIDS," *Outward* (blog), December 1, 2015, www.slate.com/blogs/outward/2015/12/01/reagan_press_secretary_laughs_about_gay_people_dying_of_aids.html.

49. Shilts, *And the Band Played On*, 34–90.
50. Fee and Fox, *AIDS*, 12–66. See also Bruce Lambert, "Kimberly Bergalis Is Dead at 23," *New York Times*, December 9, 1991, D9.
51. L. Duncan Bulkley, *Syphilis in the Innocent (Syphilis Insontium)* (New York: Bailey and Fairchild, 1894).
52. Paul Farmer and Arthur Kleinman, "Politics in the First Part of the AIDS Pandemic: AIDS as Human Suffering," *Daedalus* 118, no. 2 (1989): 135–160.
53. William F. Buckley Jr., "Identify All the Carriers," *New York Times*, March 18, 1986.
54. Chambre, *Fighting for Our Lives*, 57–110.
55. In 1985, Reagan allocated $213 million to AIDS research; in 1984, he had asked Congress for $33 million. See Congress Office of Technology Assessment, *Review of the Public Health Service's Response to AIDS: A Technical Memorandum* (Washington, DC: U.S. Government Printing Office, 1985).
56. Martin Hirsch, "Azidothymidine," *Journal of Infectious Diseases* 157 (1988): 427–431.
57. Frederick Hayden and R. Gordon Douglas, "Antiviral Agents," in *Principles and Practice of Infectious Diseases*, ed. Gerald Mandell (New York: John Wiley and Sons, 1979), 353–370.
58. H. Mitsuya, K. J. Weinhold, P. A. Furman, M. H. St Clair, S. N. Lehrman, R. C. Gallo, D. Bolognesi, D. W. Barry, and S. Broder, "3'-Azido-3'-deoxythymidine (BW A509U): An Antiviral Agent That Inhibits the Infectivity and Cytopathic Effect of Human T-Lymphotropic Virus Type III/Lymphadenopathy-Associated Virus in Vitro," *PNAS* 82, no. 20 (1985): 7096–7100.
59. Robert Yarchoan, Kent J. Weinhold, H. Kim Lyerly, Edward Gelmann, Robert M. Blum, Gene M. Shearer, Hiroaki Mitsuya, et al., "Administration of 3'-azido-3'-deoxythymidine, an Inhibitor of HTLV-III/LAV Replication, to Patients with AIDS or AIDS-Related Complex," *Lancet* 1, no. 8481 (1986): 575–580.
60. S. Epstein, *Impure Science: AIDS, Activism, and the Politics of Knowledge* (Berkeley: University of California Press, 1966).
61. Dominique Lapierre, *Beyond Love* (New York: Warner Books, 1991), 369.
62. Epstein, *Impure Science*, 194–207.
63. Margaret A. Fischl, Douglas D. Richman, Michael H. Grieco, Michael S. Gottlieb, Paul A. Volberding, Oscar L. Laskin, John M. Leedom, et al., "The Efficacy of Azidothymidine (AZT) in the Treatment of Patients with AIDS and AIDS-Related Complex: A Double-Blind, Placebo-Controlled Trial," *NEJM* 317, no. 4 (1987): 185–191.
64. France, *How to Survive a Plague*.
65. Martin S. Hirsch and Richard T. D'Aquila, "Therapy for Human Immunodeficiency Virus Infection," *NEJM* 328, no. 23 (1993): 1686–1695.
66. David J. Rothman and Harold Edgar, "AIDS, Activism, and Ethics," in *AIDS: Problems and Prospects*, ed. Lawrence Corey (New York: Norton Medical Books, 1993), 145–155.
67. Deborah J. Cotton, "Disappointing Assessment of Current Antiretrovirals," *AIDS Clinical Care* 5, no. 12 (1993): 51–53.
68. Gavin X. McLeod and Scott M. Hammer, "Zidovudine: Five Years Later," *Annals of Internal Medicine* 117, no. 6 (1992): 487–501.
69. A. Novick, "Reflections on a Term of Public Service with the FDA Antivirals Advisory Committee," *AIDS and Public Policy Journal* 8 (1993): 55–61.

70. Concorde Coordinating Committee, "Concorde: MRC/ANRS Randomized Double-Blind Controlled Trial of Immediate and Deferred Zidovudine in Symptom-Free HIV Infection," *Lancet* 343, no. 8902 (1994): 871–881.
71. Gregg Gonsalves and Diana Zuckerman, "Commentary: Will 20th Century Patient Safeguards Be Reversed in the 21st Century?," *British Medical Journal (BMJ)* 350 (2015): h1500. See also Powel Kazanjian, personal communication with Greg Gonsalves, February 26, 2019.
72. France, *How to Survive a Plague*.
73. Powel Kazanjian, interview with Emelio Emini, former director of virology, Merck Inc., March 23, 2020.
74. T. Mavromoustakos, S. Durdagi, C. Koukoulitsa, M. Simcic, M. G. Papadopoulos, M. Hodoscek, and S. Golic Grdadolnik, "Strategies in the Rational Drug Design," *Current Medicinal Chemistry* 18, no. 17 (2011): 2517–2530. See also Noel A. Roberts, Joseph A. Martin, Derek Kinchington, Anne V. Broadhurst, J. Charles Craig, Ian B. Duncan, Sarah A. Galpin, et al., "Rational Design of Peptide-Based HIV Proteinase Inhibitors," *Science* 248, no. 4953 (1990): 358–361.
75. Joseph J. Eron, Sharon L. Benoit, Joseph Jemsek, Rodger D. MacArthur, Jorge Santana, Joseph B. Quinn, Daniel R. Kuritzkes, Mary Ann Fallon, and Marc Rubin, "Treatment with Lamivudine, Zidovudine, or Both in HIV-Positive Patients with 200 to 500 CD4+ Cells per Cubic Millimeter," *NEJM* 333, no. 25 (1995): 1662–1669.
76. Jon H. Condra, William A. Schleif, Olga M. Blahy, Lori J. Gabryelski, Donald J. Graham, Juilo C. Quintero, Audrey Rhodes, et al., "In Vivo Emergence of HIV-1 Variants Resistant to Multiple Protease Inhibitors," *Nature* 374, no. 6522 (1995): 569–571.
77. J. H. Condra, D. J. Holder, W. A. Schleif, O. M. Blahy, R. M. Danovich, L. J. Gabryelski, D. J. Graham, et al., "Genetic Correlates of In Vivo Viral Resistance to Indinavir, a Human Immunodeficiency Virus Type 1 Protease Inhibitor," *Journal of Virology* 70, no. 12 (1996): 8270–8276.
78. Ann C. Collier, Robert W. Coombs, David A. Schoenfeld, Roland L. Bassett, Joseph Timpone, Alice Baruch, Michelle Jones, et al., "Treatment of Human Immunodeficiency Virus Infection with Saquinavir, Zidovudine, and Zalcitabine," *NEJM* 334, no. 16 (1996): 1011–1017.
79. Martin Markowitz, Michael Saag, William G. Powderly, Arlene M. Hurley, Ann Hsu, Joaquin M. Valdes, David Henry, et al., "A Preliminary Study of Ritonavir, an Inhibitor of HIV-1 Protease, to Treat HIV-1 Infection," *NEJM* 333, no. 23 (1995): 1534–1539.
80. David A. Katzenstein, Scott M. Hammer, Michael D. Hughes, Holly Gundacker, J. Brooks Jackson, Susan Fiscus, Suraiya Rasheed, et al., "The Relation of Virologic and Immunologic Markers to Clinical Outcomes after Nucleoside Therapy in HIV-Infected Adults with 200 to 500 CD4 Cells per Cubic Millimeter," *NEJM* 335, no. 15 (1996): 1091–1098.
81. John W. Mellors, Charles R. Rinaldo Jr., Phalguni Gupta, Roseanne M. White, John A. Todd, and Lawrence A. Kingsley, "Prognosis in HIV-1 Infection Predicted by the Quantity of Virus in Plasma," *Science* 272, no. 5265 (1996): 1167–1170.
82. Emilio A. Emini, "Protease Inhibitors," in *XI International AIDS Conference* (Vancouver, Canada, July 1996).
83. Frank J. Palella Jr., Kathleen M. Delaney, Anne C. Moorman, Mark O. Loveless, Jack Fuhrer, Glen A. Satten, Diane J. Aschman, and Scott D. Holmberg, "Declining Morbidity and Mortality among Patients with Advanced HIV Infection," *NEJM* 338, no. 13 (1998): 853–860.

84. Merle A. Sande and Paul Volberding, *The Medical Management of AIDS*, 3rd ed. (Philadelphia: W. B. Saunders, 1992. See also Merle A. Sande and Paul Volberding, *The Medical Management of AIDS*, 5th ed. (Philadelphia: W. B. Saunders, 1997.

85. Joe DeCapua, "AIDS: The Lazarus Effect," *VOA*, December 8, 2010, www.voanews.com/a/decapua-aids-lazarus-effect-9dec10-111605079/157017.html.

86. Alan S. Perelson, Avidan U. Neumann, Martin Markowitz, John M. Leonard, and David D. Ho, "HIV-1 Dynamics in Vivo: Virion Clearance Rate, Infected Cell Life-Span, and Viral Generation Time," *Science* 271, no. 5255 (1996): 1582–1586.

87. John W. Mellors, "Viral-Load Tests Provide Valuable Answers," *Scientific American* 279, no. 1 (1998): 90–93.

88. Barney S. Graham, "Science, Medicine, and the Future: Infection with HIV-1," *BMJ* 317, no. 7168 (1998): 1297–1301.

89. Thomas C. Quinn, Maria J. Wawer, Nelson Sewankambo, David Serwadda, Chuanjun Li, Fred Wabwire-Mangen, Mary O. Meehan, Thomas Lutalo, and Ronald H. Gray, "Viral Load and Heterosexual Transmission of Human Immunodeficiency Virus Type 1," *NEJM* 342, no. 13 (2000): 921–929.

90. Vannevar Bush, *Science: The Endless Frontier* (Washington, DC: United States Government Printing Office, 1945).

91. Harold E. Varmus and Neal Nathanson, "Science and the Control of AIDS," *Science* 280, no. 5371 (1998): 1815.

92. Varmus and Nathanson, "Science and the Control of AIDS."

93. D. Stehelin, H. E. Varmus, J. M. Bishop, and P. K. Vogt, "DNA Related to the Transforming Gene(s) of Avian Sarcoma Viruses Is Present in Normal Avian DNA," *Nature* 260, no. 5547 (1976): 170–173.

94. Vannevar Bush Award, 2002, Notable Names Database, accessed March 27, 2024, https://www.nndb.com/honors/278/000099978/.

95. Bush, *Science*.

96. Daniel Greenberg, *The Politics of American Science* (Harmondsworth, UK: Penguin, 1969).

97. Varmus and Nathanson, "Science and the Control of AIDS."

98. Harold Varmus, "Breakthrough of the Year," *Science* 280 (1998): cover.

99. Varmus and Nathanson, "Science and the Control of AIDS."

100. Harold Jaffe, "Whatever Happened to the U.S. AIDS Epidemic?," *Science* 305, no. 5688 (2004): 1243–1244.

101. Jonathan M. Mann and Daniel J. M. Tarantola, "HIV 1998: The Global Picture," *Scientific American* 279, no. 1 (1998): 82–84.

102. Paul Farmer, *Pathologies of Power: Health, Human Rights and the New War on the Poor* (Berkeley: University of California Press, 2005), 1–28. See also Nathan Lachowsky and Julio Montaner, "Foreword," in *Structural Interventions for HIV Prevention*, ed. Richard Crosby and Ralph Diclemente (Oxford, UK: Oxford University Press, 2019), ix–xi.

103. Tae-Wook Chun, Lucy Carruth, Diana Finzi, Xuefei Shen, Joseph A. DiGiuseppe, Harry Taylor, Monika Hermankova, et al., "Quantification of Latent Tissue Reservoirs and Total Body Viral Load in HIV Infection," *Nature* 387, no. 6629 (1997): 183–188.

104. SMART Study Group, "CD4+ Count–Guided Interruption of Antiretroviral Treatment," *NEJM* 355, no. 22 (2006): 2283–2296.

105. Margaret Chesney, "The Elusive Gold Standard: Future Perspectives for HIV Adherence Assessment and Intervention," *Journal of Acquired Immune Deficiency Syndromes* 43, no. 1 (2006): S149–S155.
106. Powel Kazanjian, interview with Paul Farmer, April 7, 2017. See also Milt Freudenheim, "Price of Success in AIDS Treatment: Hospitals Confront New Therapy," *New York Times*, June 7, 2001, C1; and Farmer, *Pathologies of Power*, 1–28.
107. Interview with Paul Farmer.
108. Greg Behrman, *The Invisible People: How the U.S. Has Slept through the Global AIDS Pandemic, the Greatest Humanitarian Catastrophe of Our Time* (New York: Free Press, 2004). See also Mann and Tarantola, "HIV 1998."
109. Freudenheim, "Price of Success in AIDS Treatment." See also Stephen Lewis, *Race against Time: Searching for Hope in AIDS-Ravaged Africa* (Berkeley, CA: House of Anansi Press, 2005), 1–36.
110. Randall Packard, *A History of Global Health* (Baltimore, MD: Johns Hopkins University Press, 2014).
111. Ezekiel Kalipeni, *HIV and AIDS in Africa: Beyond Epidemiology* (Malden, MA: Blackwell, 2004), 175–190.
112. Packard, *A History of Global Health*, 267–304.
113. Kalipeni, *HIV and AIDS in Africa*, 175–190. See also Catherine Campbell, *Letting Them Die: Why HIV/AIDS Intervention Programmes Fail* (Bloomington: Indiana University Press, 2003), 132–196.
114. Farmer, *Pathologies of Power*, 1–28. See also Mann and Tarantola, "HIV 1998"; Behrman, *The Invisible People*, 167–178; Lewis, *Race against Time*, 145–190; interview with Franklin Graham, "The Age of Aids," *Frontline*, January 31, 2005, www.pbs.org/wgbh/pages/frontline/aids/interviews/graham.html.
115. UNAIDS, *World AIDS Day Report*.
116. Jim Yong Kim and Paul Farmer, "AIDS in 2006: Moving toward One World, One Hope?," *NEJM* 355 (2006): 645–647.
117. Ethan B. Kapstein and Josh Busby, "Antiretrovirals as Merit Goods," in *Routledge Handbook of Global Public Health*, ed. Richard Parker and Marni Sommer (London: Routledge, 2011), 461.
118. Packard, *A History of Global Health*, 273.
119. Luke Messac and Krishna Prabhu, "Redefining the Possible: The Global AIDS Response," in *Reimagining Global Health: An Introduction*, ed. Paul Farmer, Arthur Kleinman, Jim Yong Kim, and Matthew Basilico (Berkeley: University of California Press, 2013), 117–119.
120. Interview with Franklin Graham.
121. Victoria Harden, *AIDS at 30: A History* (Washington, DC: Potomac Books, 2012), 185, 227, 232.
122. Powel Kazanjian, "The AIDS Pandemic in Historic Perspective," *Journal of the History of Medicine and Allied Sciences* 69, no. 3 (2014 351–382.
123. Kapstein and Busby, "Antiretrovirals as Merit Goods," 468.
124. Linda Ahdieh-Grant, Traci E. Yamashita, John P. Phair, Roger Detels, Steven M. Wolinsky, Joseph B. Margolick, Charles R. Rinaldo, and Lisa P. Jacobson, "When to Initiate Highly Active Antiretroviral Therapy: A Cohort Approach," *American Journal of Epidemiology* 157, no. 8 (2003): 738–746.
125. Kim and Farmer, "AIDS in 2006." See also Ethan Kapstein, "Making Markets for Merit Goods: The Political Economy of Antiretrovirals," *Global Policy* 1, no. 1 (2010), https://doi.org/10.1111/j.1758-5899.2009.00012.x.

126. Kapstein, "Making Markets for Merit Goods.

127. Packard, *A History of Global Health*, 267–304.

128. UNAIDS, *DOHA+10 Trips Flexibilities and Access to Antiretroviral Therapy: Lessons from the Past, Opportunities for the Future* (2011), www.unaids.org/sites/default/files /media_asset/JC2260_DOHA+10TRIPS_en_0.pdf.

129. United Nations Development Program, *The Doha Declaration Ten Years on and Its Impact on Access to Medicines and the Right to Health* (December 20, 2011), www .undp.org/sites/g/files/zskgke326/files/publications/Discussion_Paper_Doha _Declaration_Public_Health.pdf.

130. Jim Yong Kim, "Scaling Up Access to Care in Resource Constrained Settings: What Is Needed?" (Plenary Address, XV International AIDS Conference, Bangkok, 2004). See also Patrick L. Osewe, Yvonne K. Nkrumah, and Emmanuel Sackey, *Improving Access to HIV/AIDS Medicines in Africa; Trade-Related Aspects of Intellectual Property Rights Flexibilities* (Washington, DC: World Bank, 2008), 1–57.

131. Kapstein and Busby, "Antiretrovirals as Merit Goods," 425.

132. Packard, *A History of Global Health*, 289–304.

133. "The U.S. President's Emergency Plan for AIDS Relief," PEPFAR, U.S. Department of State, accessed March 28, 2024, www.pepfar.gov/documents/organization/80161 .pdf.

134. Eran Bendavid and Jayanta Bhattacharya, "The President's Emergency Plan for AIDS Relief in Africa: An Evaluation of Outcomes," *Annals of Internal Medicine* 150, no. 10 (2009): 688–695.

135. Nathan C. Lo, Anita Lowe, and Eran Bendavid, "Abstinence Funding Was Not Associated with Reductions in HIV Risk Behavior in Sub-Saharan Africa," *Health Affairs* 35, no. 5 (2016), www-healthaffairs-org.proxy.lib.umich.edu/doi/full/10.1377/hlthaff .2015.0828.

136. Eran Bendavid, "Past and Future Performance: PEPFAR in the Landscape of Foreign Aid for Health," *Current HIV/AIDS Reports* 13, no. 5 (2016): 256–262.

137. Kim and Farmer, "AIDS in 2006."

138. "WHO and UNAIDS Unveil Plan to Get 3 Million AIDS Patients on Treatment by 2005," WHO, accessed April 15, 2024, https://www.who.int/news/item/01-12-2003 -world-health-organization-and-unaids-unveil-plan-to-get-3-million-aids-patients -on-treatment-by-2005.

139. Reuben Granich, Brian Williams, and Julio Montaner, "Fifteen Million People on Antiretroviral Treatment by 2015: Treatment as Prevention," *Current Opinion in HIV and AIDS* 8, no. 1 (2013): 41–49.

140. "Global HIV and AIDS Statistics—Fact Sheet," UNAIDS, November 2016, www .unaids.org/en/resources/fact-sheet.

141. "HIV Data and Statistics: 2020 Estimate," Global HIV Programme, World Health Organization, accessed February 15, 2023, www.who.int/teams/global-hiv-hepatitis -and-stis-programmes/hiv/strategic-information/hiv-data-and-statistics.

142. Stephen Resch, Eline Korenromp, John Stover, Matthew Blakley, Carleigh Krubiner, Kira Thorien, Robert Hecht, and Rifat Atun, "Economic Returns to Investment in AIDS Treatment in Low and Middle Income Countries," *PLoS One* 6, no. 10 (2011): 1–9.

143. "Advances on the AIDS Front," editorial, *New York Times*, December 3, 2010, A30.

144. UNAIDS, "Success in Reaching '15 by 15' Shows That We Can End the AIDS Epidemic," press release, accessed July 19, 2015, www.unaids.org/en/resources /presscentre/pressreleaseandstatementarchive/2015/july/20150719_15x15_PR.

145. UNAIDS, *90-90-90: An Ambitious Treatment Target to Help End the AIDS Epidemic* (Geneva, Switzerland, 2014), www.unaids.org/en/resources/documents/2014/90-90-90.

146. Varmus and Nathanson, "Science and the Control of AIDS."

147. "HIV Treatment as Prevention; It Works," editorial, *Lancet* 377, no. 9779 (2011): 1719.

148. Myron S. Cohen, Ying Q. Chen, Marybeth McCauley, Theresa Gamble, Mina C. Hosseinipour, Nagalingeswaran Kumarasamy, James G. Hakim, et al., "Prevention of HIV-1 Infection with Early Antiretroviral Therapy," *NEJM* 365, no. 6 (2011): 493–495.

149. Joep Lange, "Test and Treat: Is It Enough?," *Clinical Infectious Diseases* 52, no. 6 (2012): 801–802.

150. Cohen et al. "Prevention of HIV-1 Infection with Early Antiretroviral Therapy."

151. "Undetectable = Untransmittable: Public Health and HIV Viral Load Suppression," UNAIDS, July 20, 2018, www.unaids.org/en/resources/presscentre/featurestories/2018/july/undetectable-untransmittable.

152. Reuben M. Granich, Charles F. Gilks, Christopher Dye, Kevin M. DeCock, and Brian G. Williams, "Universal Voluntary HIV Testing with Immediate Antiretroviral Therapy as a Strategy for Elimination of HIV Transmission: A Mathematical Model," *Lancet* 373, no. 9657 (2009): 48–57.

153. Oppenheimer and Bayer, "The Rise and Fall of AIDS Exceptionalism."

154. Hillary Clinton, "Remarks on Creating an AIDS-Free Generation," National Institutes of Health, Bethesda, MD, November 8, 2011, https://2009-2017.state.gov/secretary/20092013clinton/rm/2011/11/176810.htm.

155. Clinton, "Remarks on Creating an AIDS-Free Generation."

156. UNAIDS, *90-90-90*.

157. "Sustainable Development Goals," Sustainable Development Goals, United Nations, last modified 2015, accessed March 20, 2017, www.un.org/sustainabledevelopment/sustainable-developmentgoals/

158. UNAIDS, *90-90-90*.

159. Donald Trump, State of the Union Address, Trump White House Archives, February 5, 2019, https://trumpwhitehouse.archives.gov/sotu.

160. Jesse Hellman, "Trump Vows to End AIDS within 10 Years," *The Hill*, February 5, 2019, https://thehill.com/policy/healthcare/428641-trump-vows-to-end-aids-within-10-years.

161. "What Is Ending the HIV Epidemic in the U.S.?," HIV.gov, updated December 4, 2023, www.hiv.gov/federal-response/ending-the-hiv-epidemic/overview.

162. Lawrence Altman, "New York Study Finds Gay Men Using Safer Sex," *New York Times*, June 28, 1999, A1.

163. Mohsen Malekinejad, Andrea Parriott, Janet C. Blodgett, Hacsi Horvath, Ram K. Shrestha, Angela B. Hutchinson, Paul Volberding, and James G. Kahn, "Effectiveness of Community-Based Condom Distribution Interventions to Prevent HIV in the United States: A Systematic Review and Meta-Analysis," *PLoS One* 12, no. 8 (2017), https://doi.org/10.1371/journal.pone.0180718.

164. "Ending the HIV Epidemic in the U.S. (EHE)," Centers for Disease Control and Prevention, accessed January 21, 2023, www.cdc.gov/endhiv/index.html.

165. Alex Azar, "Ending the HIV Epidemic: A Plan for America," HIV.gov, February 5, 2019, www.hiv.gov/blog/ending-hiv-epidemic-plan-america.

166. L. Shan, Kai Deng, Neeta S. Shroff, Christine M. Durand, S. Alireza, Hung-Chih Yang, and Hao Zhang, "Elimination of the Latent Reservoir for HIV-1 Requires Induction

of CTL Responses," paper, 19th Conference on Retroviruses and Opportunistic Infections (CROI), Seattle, WA, March 2012. See also Boris Juelg and Rajesh Gandhi, "HIV Cure Strategies," in *Fundamentals of HIV Medicine 2019*, ed. W. David Hardy (New York: Oxford University Press, 2019), 59–66.

167. Andrew Carr, "Toxicity of Antiretroviral Therapy and Implications for Drug Development," *Nature Reviews Drug Discovery* 2, no. 8 (2003): 624–634.

168. "Guidelines for the Use of Antiretroviral Agents in HIV-1-Infected Adults and Adolescents," Department of Health and Human Services, accessed February 1, 2023, www.who.int/hiv/pub/arv/adult2010/en/index.html.

169. Stephane de Wit, Caroline A. Sabin, Rainer Weber, Signe Westring Worm, Peter Reiss, and Charles Cazanave, "Incidence and Risk Factors for New-Onset Diabetes in HIV-Infected Patients: The Data Collection on Adverse Events of Anti-HIV Drugs (D:A:D) Study," *Diabetes Care* 31, no. 6 (2008): 1224–1229. See also Angelina Gomes, Emily V. Reyes, L. Sergio Garduno, Rita Rojas, Grealdine Mir Mesejo, Eliza Del Rosario, Lina Jose, et al., "Incidence of Diabetes Mellitus and Obesity and the Overlap of Comorbidities in HIV+ Hispanics Initiating Antiretroviral Therapy," *PLoS One* 11, no. 8 (2016), https://journals.plos.org/plosone/article?id=10.1371/journal.pone.0160797.

170. Steven Deeks, Russell Tracy, and Daniel Douek, "Systemic Effects of Inflammation on Health during Chronic UIV Infection," *Immunity* 39, no. 4 (October 2013): 633–645.

171. Anne F. Luetkemeyer, Diane V. Havlir, and Judith S. Currier, "Complications of HIV Disease and Antiretroviral Therapy," *Topics in HIV Medicine* 18, no. 2 (April 2009): 57–67.

172. Shan et al., "Elimination of the Latent Reservoir for HIV-1 Requires Induction of CTL Responses."

173. Lei Xu, Jun Wang, Yulin Liu, Liangfu Xie, Bin Su, Danlei Mou, Longteng Wang, et al., "CRISPR Edited Sem Cells in a Patient with HIV and Acute Lymphocytic Leukemia," *NEJM* 381, no. 13 (2019): 1240–1247.

174. Carl June, "Emerging Use of CRISPR Technology: Chasing the Elusive HIV Cure," *NEJM* 381, no. 13 (2019): 1281–1283.

175. June, "Emerging Use of CRISPR Technology."

176. Powel Kazanjian, interview with Carl June, professor of pathology and laboratory medicine, University of Pennsylvania, January 15, 2021.

Chapter 3   Fate of Elimination Campaigns

1. John J. Wright, "Venereal Disease Control," *JAMA* 47, no. 15 (1951): 1408–1411.

2. Thomas Parran, *Shadow on the Land: Syphilis* (New York: Reynal and Hitchcock, 1937), 298. See also Wright, "Venereal Disease Control."

3. Odin Anderson, *Syphilis and Society: Problems of Control in the United States, 1912–1964*, Research Series 22 (Chicago: University of Chicago Press, 1965), 13. See also Paul Le Van, "The Story of Syphilis," *Hygeia* 27, no. 4 (April 1949): 238–239.

4. John C. Cutler and R. C. Arnold, "Venereal Disease Control by Health Departments in the Past: Lessons for the Present," in *Tuskegee's Truths: Rethinking the Tuskegee Syphilis Study*, ed. Susan M. Reverby (Chapel Hill: University of North Carolina Press, 2000), 495–506.

5. John Parascandola, *Sex, Sin, and Science: A History of Syphilis in America* (London: Praeger Press, 2008), 130. See also "End of Syphilis Seen by Use of Penicillin: Health Agencies Must Give Free Treatment, Dr. Baehr Says," *New York Times*, May 26, 1944.

6. R. Gibbons, "End of Syphilis in Sight?," *Science Digest* 29 (1951): 48.

7. Cutler and Arnold, "Venereal Disease Control by Health Departments in the Past," 503.

8. Luther Terry, "Opening Address," in *Proceedings of World Forum on Syphilis and Other Treponematoses* (Washington, DC: U.S. Government Printing Office, 1962), 4–8.

9. Cutler and Arnold, "Venereal Disease Control by Health Departments in the Past," 504.

10. Malcolm Merrill, "Responsibility of Public Health in a Program for Syphilis Eradication," in *Proceedings of World Forum on Syphilis and Other Treponematoses*, 36.

11. William J. Brown, "The First Step toward Eradication," in *Proceedings of World Forum on Syphilis and Other Treponematoses*, 23, 24.

12. Uriel Foa, "Social Stratification and Venereal Disease," in *Proceedings of World Forum on Syphilis and Other Treponematoses*, 389, 391.

13. "Luther Leonidas Terry (1961–1965)," SurgeonGeneral.gov, accessed March 31, 2024, archived at http://wayback.archive-it.org/3929/20171201191743/https://www.surgeongeneral.gov/about/previous/bioterry.html.

14. "Dr. Leona Baumgartner," Changing the Face of Medicine, last revised June 3, 2015, https://cfmedicine.nlm.nih.gov/physicians/biography_28.html.

15. Leona Baumgartner, Arthur C. Curtis, A. L. Gray, Benno E. Kuechle, and T. Lefoy Richman, *The Eradication of Syphilis: A Task Force Report to the Surgeon General, Public Health Service, on Syphilis Control in the United States* (Washington, DC: U.S. Government Printing Office, 1962), 8.

16. Leona Baumgartner, "Syphilis Eradication: A Plan for Action Now," in *Proceedings of World Forum on Syphilis and Other Treponematoses*, 26–33.

17. Baumgartner, "Syphilis Eradication."

18. Merrill, "Responsibility of Public Health in a Program for Syphilis Eradication," 38.

19. Baumgartner et al., *The Eradication of Syphilis*, 5 and 25.

20. Baumgartner, "Syphilis Eradication," 29.

21. Merrill, "Responsibility of Public Health in a Program for Syphilis Eradication," 37.

22. Baumgartner, "Syphilis Eradication."

23. Leona Baumgartner, "What Parents Must Know about Teenagers and VD," *McCall's*, January 1963, 44, 118.

24. Warren Davis Jr., "Epidemiology: The Key to Venereal Syphilis Control," in *Proceedings of World Forum on Syphilis and Other Treponematoses*, 33–37.

25. Rudolph Kampmeier, "Responsibility of a Physician in a Program for Syphilis Eradication," in *Proceedings of World Forum on Syphilis and Other Treponematoses*, 70–79.

26. Stephen B. Thacker and Ruth L. Berkelman, "Public Health Surveillance in the United States," *Epidemiologic Reviews* 10, no. 1 (1988): 164–190.

27. Baumgartner, "Syphilis Eradication," 31, 32.

28. Luther Terry, "VDs' Alarming Comeback," *Look*, December 4, 1962, 82. See also Baumgartner, "What Parents Must Know about Teenagers and VD."

29. Baumgartner, "Syphilis Eradication," 30.

30. Baumgartner et al., *The Eradication of Syphilis*, 23.

31. Baumgartner, "What Parents Must Know about Teenagers and VD," 118.

32. Brown, "First Step toward Eradication."

33. Baumgartner, "What Parents Must Know about Teenagers and VD," 118.

34. Baumgartner, "Syphilis Eradication," 31, 32.

35. "Medicine: Resurgent Syphilis: It Can Be Eradicated," *Time*, September 21, 1962, 74–75. See also "Syphilis: Social Scourge," *Science News-Letter* 82, no. 15 (October 13, 1962): 238; David Sanford, "The AMA and That Disease," *New Republic*,

September 18, 1965, 10; "Why the Increasing Incidence of Syphilis?," *JAMA* 183, no. 13 (March 30, 1963): 1104; "Syphilis," *Consumer Reports*, October 1963, 498–499; "Spirochete Is Back," *The Nation*, May 11, 1964, 471; "Infectious Diseases: Syphilis and the Young," *Time*, August 13, 1965, 57.

36. Baumgartner, "What Parents Must Know about Teenagers and VD," 118.

37. Baumgartner, "Syphilis Eradication," 31, 32.

38. Baumgartner, "Syphilis Eradication," 28.

39. Terry, "Opening Address," 4–8.

40. Baumgartner et al., *The Eradication of Syphilis*, 19.

41. Anderson, *Syphilis and Society*, 44.

42. Baumgartner et al., *The Eradication of Syphilis*, 21.

43. Baumgartner et al., *The Eradication of Syphilis*, 3, 5.

44. Parascandola, *Sex, Sin, and Science*, 140–142. See also William Brown, "Progress of the Syphilis Eradication Program in the United States," May 26, 1965, CDC Archives, Records of Division and Branches, 70A470, CDC Records Acc 71A1708, VD Manuscript files, 1965–1966, Atlanta, GA. See also John F. Kennedy, "Special Message to the Congress on the Nation's Youth," American Presidency Project, February 14, 1963, www.presidency.ucsb.edu/node/236955.

45. *Hearings before the Subcommittee on Foreign AID Expeditions of the Committee on Government Operations. 89th Cong., 2dsess., S. 1676, A Bill to Reorganize the Department of State and the Department of Health, Education and Welfare* (Washington, DC: U.S. Government Printing Office, 1967), 1354. See also Brown, "Progress of Syphilis Eradication," 1965–1966.

46. Brown, "Progress of Syphilis Eradication," 1965–1966.

47. Baumgartner, "Syphilis Eradication," 27.

48. Leona Baumgartner, "Medicine and Society: New Issues," *Proceedings of the American Philosophical Society* 115, no. 5 (October 15, 1971): 335–340.

49. D. Colligan, "VD–Hush-Hush Epidemic on a New Rampage," *Science Digest*, June 1973, 26–31. See also E. Tramont, "*Treponema pallidum*," in *Principles and Practice of Infectious Diseases*, vol. 1, ed. Gerald Mandell, Robert Douglas, and John Bennett (New York: Wiley, 1979), 1823.

50. "Venereal Disease: This Hazard to Public Health Control Could Be Eliminated; Instead, It Grows Worse," *Consumer Reports*, March 1970, 118–123.

51. Parascandola, *Sex, Sin, and Science*, 140.

52. Cokie Roberts and Steven V. Roberts, "The Venereal Disease Pandemic," *New York Times*, November 7, 1971, SM62. See also J. E. Brody, "VD Is on the Rise Again," *Readers Digest*, November 1970, 181–182; "Medicine: VD: A National Emergency," *Time*, July 27, 1970, 36.

53. Brown, "First Step toward Eradication."

54. Vernal Cave, "The Prevention of Venereal Disease," *Journal of the National Medical Association* 63, no. 1 (January 1971): 67–68.

55. William J. Brown, "The Public Health Service Venereal Disease Program," *Archives of Environmental Health* 13, no. 3 (1966): 372–375.

56. H. Hunter Handsfield and Edward W. Hook III, "Foreword," in *Behavioral Interventions for Prevention and Control of Sexually Transmitted Diseases*, ed. Sevgi O. Aral and John M. Douglas Jr. (New York: Springer, 2007), i–vii.

57. CDC, *The National Plan to Eliminate Syphilis from the United States* (Atlanta: U.S. Department of Health and Human Services, October 1999), www.cdc.gov/stopsyphilis /plan.pdf.

58. CDC, *Syphilis* (Atlanta: U.S. Department of Health and Human Services, October 27, 1999), www.cdc.gov/std/stats16/syphilis.htm.

59. CDC, *National Plan to Eliminate Syphilis from the United States*, 5

60. CDC, *The Syphilis Elimination Program Assessment and Findings Monograph: Lessons Learned* (Atlanta: U.S. Department of Health and Human Services, 2005), 15.

61. CDC, *National Plan to Eliminate Syphilis from the United States*, 5.

62. Institute of Medicine (U.S.) Committee on Prevention and Control of Sexually Transmitted Diseases, *The Hidden Epidemic: Confronting Sexually Transmitted Diseases*, ed. Thomas Eng and William Butler (Washington, DC: National Academy Press, 1997), https://pubmed.ncbi.nlm.nih.gov/25165803/. See also CDC, *National Plan to Eliminate Syphilis from the United States*.

63. CDC, *National Plan to Eliminate Syphilis from the United States*, 73–86.

64. CDC, *National Plan to Eliminate Syphilis from the United States*, 58–60.

65. Jo A. Valentine and Gail A. Bolan, "Syphilis Elimination: Lessons Learned Again," *Sexually Transmitted Diseases* 45, no. 9S (September 2018): S80–S85.

66. James D. Heffelfinger, Emmett B. Swint, Stuart M. Berman, and Hillard S. Weinstock, "Trends in Primary and Secondary Syphilis among Men Who Have Sex with Men in the United States," *American Journal of Public Health* 97, no. 6 (2007): 1076–1083. See also Marc M. Solomon and Kenneth H. Mayer, "Evolution of the Syphilis Epidemic among Men Who Have Sex with Men," *Sexual Health* 12, no. 2 (2015): 96–102.

67. Valentine and Bolan, "Syphilis Elimination."

68. CDC, *Report of the Syphilis Elimination Effort Consultation August 1–2, 2005* (Atlanta: Division of STD Prevention, HHS, October 2005), www.cdc.gov/stopsyphilis/SyphElimConsultationMeeting.pdf.

69. "Syphilis Elimination Effort (SEE)," CDC, accessed April 14, 2024, https://www.cdc.gov/stopsyphilis/default.htm; CDC, *Report of the Syphilis Elimination Effort Consultation August 1–2, 2005*.

70. CDC, *Report of the Syphilis Elimination Effort Consultation August 1–2, 2005*.

71. "New CDC Report: STDs Continue to Rise in the U.S.," press release, CDC, October 8, 2019, www.cdc.gov/nchhstp/newsroom/2019/2018-STD-surveillance-report-press-release.html.

72. Primary and secondary syphilis cases in the United States from 1956 to 2016. "New CDC Report: STDs Continue to Rise in the U.S."

73. "New CDC Report: STDs Continue to Rise in the U.S."

74. Noah Kojima and Jeffrey D. Klausner, "An Update on the Global Epidemiology of Syphilis," *Current Epidemiology Reports* 5, no. 1 (2018): 24–38.

75. HHS, *Sexually Transmitted Infections: National Strategic Plan for the United States 2021–2025* (Washington, DC, 2021), 3, www.hhs.gov/sites/default/files/STI-National-Strategic-Plan-2021-2025.pdf.

76. "New CDC Report: STDs Continue to Rise in the U.S." The STI plan is being developed by partners across the federal government, with input from a variety of stakeholders. See also "Developing the STI Federal Action Plan: What Is Happening with the STI Federal Action Plan?," HHS, content last reviewed October 1, 2019, www.hhs.gov/programs/topic-sites/sexually-transmitted-infections/action-plan-overview/developing-the-sti-federal-action-plan/index.html.

77. Office of Infectious Disease and HIV/AIDS Policy, "Stakeholders and the Public Weigh in on the Nation's First STI Federal Action Plan," HHS, September 25, 2019, www.hhs.gov/hepatitis/blog/2019/09/25/stakeholders-weigh-in-on-nations-first-sti-federal-action-plan.html.

78. "Developing the STI Federal Action Plan."
79. HHS, *Sexually Transmitted Infections: National Strategic Plan for the United States 2021–2025*, 3.
80. UNAIDS, *90-90-90: An Ambitious Treatment Target to Help End the AIDS Epidemic* (Geneva, Switzerland: UNAIDS, 2014), accessed November 30, 2015, 28, www.unaids .org/en/resources/documents/2014/90-90-90.
81. "The Global HIV/AIDS Epidemic," HIV.gov, accessed March 1, 2023, www.hiv.gov /hiv-basics/overview/data-and-trends/global-statistics.
82. "The Global HIV/AIDS Epidemic."
83. "90–90–90: Good Progress, but the World Is Off-Track for Hitting the 2020 Targets," Update, UNAIDS, September 21, 2020, www.unaids.org/en/resources/presscentre /featurestories/2020/september/20200921_90-90-90.
84. "90-90-90: Treatment for All," Topic, UNAIDS, accessed January 31, 2023, www .unaids.org/en/resources/909090.
85. "90–90–90: Good Progress."
86. "Global HIV & AIDS Statistics: Fact Sheet," Resources, UNAIDS, November 2016, www.unaids.org/en/resources/fact-sheet.
87. "Antiretroviral Therapy Coverage among HIV-Infected Pregnant Women for PMTCT," WHO, accessed January 25, 2023, www.who.int/data/gho/indicator-metadata-registry /imr-details/82.
88. Gilles Wandeler, Leigh F. Johnson, and Matthias Egger, "Trends in Life Expectancy of HIV-Positive Adults on ART across the Globe: Comparisons with General Population," *Current Opinion in HIV and AIDS* 11, no. 5 (2016): 492–500.
89. CDC, Global Health, "HIV," updated November 30, 2020, archived at https://archive .cdc.gov/#/details?url=https://www.cdc.gov/globalhealth/newsroom/topics/hiv /index.html.
90. Brian Dunleavy, "Ending the HIV Epidemic by 2030: Is Trump's SOTU Promise Feasible?," Contagion Live, February 13, 2019, www.contagionlive.com/view /ending-the-hiv-epidemic-by-2030-is-trumps-sotu-promise-feasible-public-health -watch-.
91. Amy Goldstein, "Trump Announces Goal of Ending HIV/AIDS Epidemic by End of Next Decade," *Washington Post*, February 5, 2019. See also Kathie Hiers, "Implementing the Trump Administration's 'Ending the HIV Epidemic' Plan in the Southern United States," *American Journal of Public Health* 110, no. 1 (2020): 32–33.
92. Lindsey Dawson and Jennifer Kates, "The U.S. Ending the HIV Epidemic (EHE) Initiative: What You Need to Know," KFF, February 9, 2021, www.kff.org/hivaids/issue -brief/the-u-s-ending-the-hiv-epidemic-ehe-initiative-what-you-need-to-know/. See also *National HIV/AIDS Strategy for the United States 2022–2025*, The White House, accessed February 15, 2023, www.whitehouse.gov/wp-content/uploads/2021/11 /National-HIV-AIDS-Strategy.pdf.
93. Lindsay Smith Rogers, "Ending the HIV Epidemic: A Plan for America," Johns Hopkins Bloomberg School of Public Health, published November 27, 2019, https:// publichealth.jhu.edu/2019/ending-the-hiv-epidemic-a-conversation-with-the -architects-of-the-proposed-federal-plan.
94. "The HIV/AIDS Epidemic in the United States: The Basics," KFF, June 7, 2021, www .kff.org/hivaids/fact-sheet/the-hivaids-epidemic-in-the-united-states-the-basics/.
95. Myron S. Cohen, Ying Q. Chen, Marybeth McCauley, Theresa Gamble, Mina C. Hosseinipour, Nagalingeswaran Kumarasamy, James G. Hakim, et al., "Prevention of HIV-1 Infection with Early Antiretroviral Therapy," *NEJM* 365, no. 6 (2011):

493–495. See also Thomas Parran, "The Eradication of Syphilis as a Practical Public Health Objective," *JAMA* 97, no. 2 (1931): 73.

96. "How Does Smallpox Spread?," CDC, accessed March 21, 2023, www.cdc.gov /smallpox/transmission/index.html.

97. Jon Cohen, *Shots in the Dark: The Wayward Search for an AIDS Vaccine* (New York: Norton, 2001), 3–15. See also Anthony Fauci, "An HIV Vaccine: Mapping Unchartered Territory," *JAMA* 316, no. 2 (2016): 143–144.

98. In some parts of the world where vaccination was unfamiliar, the stigma challenged public health approaches to dealing with smallpox. Global public health policies and practices were contested by local governments, politicians, and medical officials. See Sanjoy Bhattacharya, *Expunging Variola: The Control and Eradication of Smallpox in India, 1947–1977* (Hyderabad, India: Orient Blackswan, 2006).

99. "AIDS: A Threat to Rural Africa," Food and Agriculture Organization of the U.N., accessed February 21, 2023, www.fao.org/focUS/E/aids/aids6-e.htm.

100. "HIV/AIDS in Rural America," HRSA, February 16, 2017, www.hrsa.gov/enews/past -issues/2017/february-16/hiv-aids-in-rural-america.html.

101. Max Blau, "There Aren't Enough Doctors to Treat HIV in the Rural South," Pew, August 5, 2019, www.pewtrusts.org/en/research-and-analysis/blogs/stateline/2019 /08/05/there-arent-enough-doctors-to-treat-hiv-in-the-south.

102. Powel Kazanjian, personal interviews with Wendy Armstrong, AIDS physician at Grady Hospital's Ponce de Leon Center's Infectious Disease Program, Atlanta, GA, and professor of infectious diseases, Emory University Medical School, February 8, 2019, and February 29, 2024.

103. Tara A. Schwetz, Thomas Calder, Elana Rosenthal, Sarah Kattakuzhy, and Anthony S. Fauci, "Opioids and Infectious Diseases: A Converging Public Health Crisis," *Journal of Infectious Diseases* 220, no. 3 (2019): 346–349. See also Patrick Radden Keefe, "The Family That Built an Empire of Pain: The Sackler Dynasty's Ruthless Marketing of Painkillers Has Generated Billions of Dollars—and Millions of Addicts," *New Yorker*, October 23, 2017.

104. Jaimie P. Meyer, Amy L. Althoff, and Frederick L. Altice, "Optimizing Care for HIV-Infected People Who Use Drugs: Evidence-Based Approaches to Overcoming Healthcare Disparities," *Clinical Infectious Diseases* 57, no. 9 (November 2013): 1309–1317.

105. Robert H. Remien, "The Impact of Mental Health across the HIV Care Continuum," *Psychology and AIDS Exchange Newsletter*, January 2019, www.apa.org/pi/aids /resources/exchange/2019/01/continuum.

106. Hongbo Jiang, Yi Zhou, and Weiming Tang, "Maintaining HIV Care during the COVID-19 Pandemic," *Lancet HIV* 7, no. 5 (May, 2020): E308–E309.

107. Bharat Bhushan Rewari, Nabeel Mangadan-Konath, and Mukta Sharma, "Impact of COVID-19 on the Global Supply Chain of Antiretroviral Drugs: A Rapid Survey of Indian Manufacturers," *Southeast Asia Journal of Public Health* 9, no. 2 (2020): 126–133.

108. Allan M. Brandt, *No Magic Bullet: A Social History of Venereal Disease in the United States since 1880* (New York: Oxford University Press, 1987). See also Parascandola, *Sex, Sin, and Science*.

109. Institute of Medicine (U.S.) Committee on Prevention and Control of Sexually Transmitted Diseases, *The Hidden Epidemic*. See also Laura Nyblade, Pia Mingkwan, and Melissa A. Stockton, "Stigma Reduction: An Essential Ingredient to Ending AIDS by 2030," *Lancet HIV* 8, no. 2 (February 1, 2021): E106–E113.

110. Division of HIV/AIDS Prevention, "Internalized HIV-Related Stigma," Medical Monitoring Project, CDC, accessed March 10, 2023, www.cdc.gov/hiv/pdf/statistics /mmp/cdc-hiv-internalized-stigma.pdf.

111. Nyblade, Mingkwan, and Stockton, "Stigma Reduction." See also "Positive Voices: The National Survey of People Living with HIV," Public Health England, accessed February 27, 2023, www.ucl.ac.uk/global-health/research/z-research/positive-voices -national-survey-people-living-hiv.

112. Rose McKeon Olson and Robert Goldstein, "U = U: Ending Stigma and Empowering People Living with HIV," Harvard Medical School, April 22, 2020, www.health .harvard.edu/blog/uu-ending-stigma-and-empowering-people-living-with-hiv -2020042219583.

113. Division of HIV/AIDS Prevention, "Internalized HIV-Related Stigma."

114. Swastika Suvirya, "Stigma Associated with Sexually Transmitted Infections among Patients Attending Suraksha Clinic at a Tertiary Care Hospital in Northern India," *Indian Journal of Dermatology* 63, no. 6 (2018): 469–474.

115. Samuel M. Jenness, Akshay Sharma, Steven M. Goodreau, Eli S. Rosenberg, Kevin M. Weiss, Karen W. Hoover, Dawn K. Smith, and Patrick Sullivan, "Individual HIV Risk versus Population Impact of Risk Compensation after HIV Preexposure Prophylaxis Initiation among Men Who Have Sex with Men," *PLoS One* 12, no. 1 (2017): e0169484. See also Karla D. Wagner, Stephen E. Lankenau, Lawrence A. Palinkas, Jean L. Richardson, Chih-Ping Chou, and Jennifer B. Unger, "The Perceived Consequences of Safer Injection: An Exploration of Qualitative Findings and Gender Differences," *Psychology, Health and Medicine* 15, no. 5 (2010): 560–573. See also Winnie Wing-Yan Yuen, Lynn Tran, Carlos King-Ho Wong, Eleanor Holroyd, Catherine So-Kum Tang, and William Chi-Wai Wong, "Psychological Health and HIV Transmission among Female Sex Workers: A Systematic Review and Meta-Analysis," *AIDS Care* 28, no. 7 (2016): 816–824; Joerg Dreweke, "Promiscuity Propaganda: Access to Information and Services Does Not Lead to Increases in Sexual Activity," *Guttmacher Policy Review* 22 (June 11, 2019): 29–35.

116. Eran Bendavid and Jayanta Bhattacharya, "The President's Emergency Plan for AIDS Relief in Africa: An Evaluation of Outcomes," *Annals of Internal Medicine* 150, no. 10 (2009): 688–695.

117. Alice Forster, Jane Wardle, Judith Stephenson, and Jo Waller, "Passport to Promiscuity or Lifesaver: Press Coverage of HPV Vaccination and Risky Sexual Behavior," *Journal of Health Communication* 15, no. 2 (2010): 205–217.

118. Thacker and Berkelman, "Public Health Surveillance in the United States."

119. Katinka de Wet, *The Normalization of the HIV and AIDS Epidemic in South Africa* (London: Routledge, 2019). See also Richard Crosby and Ralph Diclemente, eds. *Structural Interventions for HIV Prevention* (Oxford, UK: Oxford University Press, 2019).

120. Baumgartner, "Medicine and Society."

121. Paul Farmer, Bruce Nizeye, Sara Stulac, and Salmaan Keshavjee, "Structural Violence and Clinical Medicine," *PLoS Medicine* 3, no. 10 (2006): e449.

122. Guy Harling, S. V. Subramanian, Till Barnighausen, and Ichiro Kawachi, "Socioeconomic Disparities in Sexually Transmitted Infections among Young Adults in the United States: Examining the Interaction between Income and Race/Ethnicity," *Sexually Transmitted Diseases* 40, no. 7 (2013): 575–581.

123. "Global AIDS Strategy 2021–2026: End Inequalities. End AIDS," UNAIDS, March 25, 2021, www.unaids.org/en/resources/documents/2021/2021-2026-global -AIDS-strategy.

124. UNAIDS, "Structural Change," in *Prevention Gap Report* (Geneva: Joint United Nations Programme on HIV/AIDS, 2016), 16–29, www.unaids.org/en/resources /documents/2016/prevention-gap. See also Esther Sumartojo, Lynda Doll, David Holtgrave, Helene Gayle, and Michael Merson, "Enriching the Mix: Incorporating Structural Factors into HIV Prevention," *AIDS* 14, no. S1 (June 2000): S1–S2.

125. Frederick R. Bloom and Deborah A. Cohen, "Structural Interventions," in *Behavioral Interventions for Prevention and Control of Sexually Transmitted Diseases*, ed. Aral and Douglas, 125–141.

126. Deanna Kerrigan, Jessie Mbwambo, Samuel Likindikoki, and Catherine Shembilu, "Economic Strengthening Approaches with Female Sex Workers: Implications for HIV Prevention," in *Structural Interventions for HIV Prevention*, ed. Crosby and Diclemente, 276–357.

127. "Migration and Health: Key Issues," WHO Regional Office for Europe, www.euro.who .int/en/health-topics/health-determinants/migration-and-health/migration-and -health-in-the-european-region/migration-and-health-key-issues.

128. Richard A. Crosby and Ralph J. Diclemente, "Applying Behavioral and Social Science Theory to HIV Prevention: The Need for Structural Level Approaches," in *Structural Interventions for HIV Prevention*, ed. Crosby and Diclemente, 13–31.

129. Anh Phana, Kathryn Seigfried-Spellar, and Kim-Kwang Raymond Choo, "Threaten Me Softly: A Review of Potential Dating App Risks," *Computers in Human Behavior Reports* 3 (January–July 2021): 1–12.

130. Jo A. Valentine, "Impact of Attitudes and Beliefs Regarding African American Sexual Behavior on STD Prevention and Control in African American Communities: Unintended Consequences," *Sexually Transmitted Diseases* 35, no. 12 (December 2008): S23–S29.

131. Dwayne T. Brandon, Lydia A. Isaac, and Thomas A. LaVeist, "The Legacy of Tuskegee and Trust in Medical Care: Is Tuskegee Responsible for Race Differences in Mistrust of Medical Care?," *Journal of the National Medical Association* 97, no. 7 (July 2005): 951–956.

132. Baumgartner, "Syphilis Eradication."

133. UNAIDS, *90-90-90*, 17.

134. Steffanie A. Strathdee and Chris Beyrer, "Threading the Needle: How to Stop the HIV Outbreak in Rural Indiana," *NEJM* 373, no. 5 (2015): 397–399.

135. Mary McFarlane, Sheana S. Bull, and Cornelis A. Rietmeijer, "The Internet as a Newly Emerging Risk Environment for Sexually Transmitted Diseases," *JAMA* 284, no. 4 (2000): 443–446. See also Dita Broz, Neal Carnes, Johanna Chapin-Bardales, Don C. Des Jarlais, Senad Handanagic, Christopher M. Jones, R. Paul McClung, and Alice K. Asher, "Syringe Services Programs' Role in Ending the HIV Epidemic in the U.S.: Why We Cannot Do It without Them," *American Journal of Preventive Medicine* 61, no. 5 (2021): S118–S129.

136. Handsfield and Hook, "Foreword," vii.

137. Laura J. McGough and H. Hunter Handsfield, "History of Behavioral Interventions in STD Control," in *Behavioral Interventions for Prevention and Control of Sexually Transmitted Diseases*, ed. Aral and Douglas, 3–23.

138. Bloom and Cohen, "Structural Interventions."

139. M. D. Sweat and J. A. Denison, "Reducing HIV Incidence in Developing Countries with Structural and Environmental Interventions," *AIDS* 9, no. SA (1995): S251–S257.

140. Bloom and Cohen, "Structural Interventions." See also S. Allinder and M. McCarten-Gibbs, "Challenges to Continued U.S. Leadership Ahead of Global HIV's Next

Phase," Center for Strategic and International Studies, May 28, 2020, https://www
.csis.org/analysis/challenges-continued-us-leadership-ahead-global-hivs-next
-phase.

141. "HIV Funding Key for Sustainable Development," *Lancet HIV* 3, no. 11 (2016): 499.

142. Allinder and McCarten-Gibbs, "Challenges to Continued U.S. Leadership Ahead of
Global HIV's Next Phase."

143. Gerald Friedland, "Marking Time in the Global HIV/AIDS Pandemic," *JAMA* 316,
no. 2 (2016): 145–146.

144. "Combination HIV Prevention," Pan American Health Organization, accessed
March 10, 2023, www.paho.org/en/topics/combination-hiv-prevention.

145. Stefano Bertozzi, Nancy Padian, Jeny Wegbreit, Lisa DeMaria, Becca Feldman, Helene
Gayle, Julian Gold, Robert Grant, and Michael Isbell, "HIV/AIDS Prevention and
Treatment," in *Disease Control Priorities in Developing Countries*, 2nd ed., ed. Dean T.
Jamison, Joel G. Breman, Anthony R. Measham, George Alleyne, Mariam Claeson,
David B. Evans, Prabhat Jha, et al. (New York: Oxford University Press, 2006),
331–371.

146. Sylvia Shangani, Daniel Escudero, Kipruto Kirwa, Abigail Harrison, Brandon Mar-
shall, and Don Operario, "Effectiveness of Peer-Led Interventions to Increase HIV
Testing among Men Who Have Sex with Men: A Systematic Review and Meta-
Analysis," *AIDS Care* 29, no. 8 (August 3, 2017): 1003–1013. See also Karen R. Florez,
Denise D. Payan, Kathryn P. Derose, Frances M. Aunon, and Laura M. Bogart,
"Process Evaluation of a Peer-Driven, HIV Stigma Reduction and HIV Testing Inter-
vention in Latino and African American Churches," *Health Equity* 1, no. 1 (Decem-
ber 2017): 109–117; Jiayu He, Ying Wang, Zhicheng Du, Jing Liao, Na He, and Yuantao
Hao, "Peer Education for HIV Prevention among High-Risk Groups: A Systematic
Review and Meta-Analysis," *BMC Infectious Diseases* 20, no. 1 (2020): 338.

147. Simona A. Iacob, Diana G. Iacob, and Gheorghita Jugulete, "Improving the Adherence to Antiretroviral Therapy, a Difficult but Essential Task for a Successful HIV
Treatment: Clinical Points of View and Practical Considerations," *Frontiers in Phar-
macology* 8, article no. 832 (2017), www.ncbi.nlm.nih.gov/pmc/articles/PMC5703840
/pdf/fphar-08-00831.pdf.

148. John A. Bartlett, "Addressing the Challenges of Adherence," *Journal of Acquired
Immune Deficiency Syndromes* 29, no. S1 (2002): S2–S10.

Chapter 4 Legacies of Mistrust

1. Udo J. Wile, "The Demonstration of the Spirochaeta Pallida in the Brain Substance
of Living Paretics," *JAMA* 61 (1913): 866.

2. Udo Wile, "Experimental Syphilis in the Rabbit Produced by the Brain Substance of
the Living Paretic," *Journal of Experimental Medicine* 23, no. 2 (1916): 199–202.

3. Risks involved with trephining were unknown at the time, as the procedure was not
performed by surgeons. Powel Kazanjian, personal communication with Stephen
Sullivan, MD, professor of neurosurgery, Michigan Medicine, University of Michigan, February 12, 2022.

4. Wile, "Demonstration of the Spirochaeta Pallida." Rabbit inoculation studies were
performed by Paul de Kruif in the laboratory of Frederick Novy, a bacteriology
professor. See Frederick Novy, Laboratory Notebooks, Notebooks 28–32, 1915,
Frederick Novy Papers, Box 6, Bentley Historical Library, University of Michigan,
Ann Arbor.

5. Wile, "Demonstration of the Spirochaeta Pallida."

6. "Vivisections on Human Beings: Experiment by Michigan Professor on Insane Patients Stirs Storm. Finds Paresis Cause," *Chicago Daily Tribune*, April 12, 1916.

7. "Human Vivisection Arouses Protest," *New York Herald*, April 12, 1916. See also Michael J. Franzblau, "The Legacy of Udo Wile," *Medicine at Michigan: A Publication of the University of Michigan Medical School*, Summer 2002, 4–7.

8. "Vivisections on Human Beings."

9. Susan E. Lederer, *Subjected to Science: Human Experimentation in America before the Second World War* (Baltimore, MD: Johns Hopkins University Press, 1995), 95. See also Letter sent to Udo J. Wile and Victor C. Vaughan, April 27, 1916, Victor C. Vaughan Papers, Michigan Historical Collection, University of Michigan.

10. Lederer, *Subjected to Science*, 97.

11. "Vivisections on Human Beings."

12. "Silly Uproar," *Detroit News*, April 13, 1916.

13. *Code of Medical Ethics of the American Medical Association: Originally Adopted at the Adjourned Meeting of the National Medical Convention in Philadelphia, May 1847* (Chicago: American Medical Association Press, 1897), 84. See also Lederer, *Subjected to Science*, 98.

14. Aldred Warthin, "A Biologic Philosophy or Religion a Necessary Foundation for Race Betterment," in *Proceedings of the Third Race Betterment Conference, January 2–6, 1928* (Race Betterment Foundation, 1928), 86–90.

15. Aldred Warthin, *The Creed of a Biologist: A Biologic Philosophy of Life* (New York: P. B. Hoeber, 1930), 16–19, 35.

16. Warthin, *The Creed of a Biologist*, 36. See also Aldred Warthin, *Physician of the Dance of Death: A Historical Study of the Evolution of the Dance of Death Mythus in Art* (New York: Paul Hoeber, 1931).

17. Powel Kazanjian, personal communication with Dr. Charles Parkos, chair, Department of Pathology, University of Michigan, June 8, 2017.

18. Jeffrey Benzing, "Pitt to Remove Dr. Thomas Parran's Name from University Building. Here's Why," Publicsource, March 27, 2018, www.publicsource.org/will-parran -hall-on-pitts-campus-be-stripped-of-its-name-due-to-racist-ugly-legacy-of-dr -thomas-parran/.

19. Susan Reverby, ed., *Tuskegee's Truths: Rethinking the Tuskegee Syphilis Study* (Chapel Hill: University of North Carolina Press, 2000).

20. Allan Brandt, "Racism and Research: The Case of the Tuskegee Syphilis Study," *Hastings Center Report* 8, no. 6 (December 1978): 21–29.

21. James Jones, *Bad Blood: The Tuskegee Syphilis Experiment* (New York: Free Press, 1981).

22. Allan Brandt, "Racism and Research: The Case of the Tuskegee Syphilis Experiment," in *Tuskegee's Truths*, ed. Susan Reverby, 409–420.

23. Jean Heller, "Syphilis Victims in US Study Went Untreated for 40 Years," *New York Times*, July 25, 1972.

24. R. H. Kampmeier, "Final Report on the 'Tuskegee Syphilis Study,'" *Southern Medical Journal* 67 (1974): 1349–1353.

25. P. Frederick Sparling, "Diagnosis and Treatment of Syphilis," *NEJM* 284 (March 25, 1971): 642–672.

26. Dwayne T. Brandon, Lydia A. Isaac, and Thomas A. LaVeist, "The Legacy of Tuskegee and Trust in Medical Care: Is Tuskegee Responsible for Race Differences in Mistrust of Medical Care?," *Journal of the National Medical Association* 97, no. 7 (July 2005): 951–956. See also Vann Newkirk, "A Generation of Bad Blood," *The*

Atlantic, June 17, 2016, www.theatlantic.com/politics/archive/2016/06/tuskegee
-study-medical-distrust-research/487439/.

27. Jesse Singal, "The Tuskegee Experiment Kept Killing Black People Decades After It
Ended," *New York: The Cut*, June 15, 2016, www.thecut.com/2016/06/tuskegee
-experiment-mistrust.html. See also Peter A. Clark, "A Legacy of Mistrust: African-
Americans, the Medical Profession, and AIDS," *Linacre Quarterly* 65, no. 1 (1988):
66–88; Julie Wernau, "History Drives Distrust in Covid-19 Vaccines for Black Americans in Tuskegee," *Wall Street Journal*, February 25, 2021.

28. Susan Reverby, "Ethical Failures and History Lessons: The US Public Health Service
Research Studies in Tuskegee and Guatemala," *Public Health Reviews* 34, no. 1
(2012): 1–19.

29. "The U.S. Public Health Service Syphilis Study at Tuskegee," Research Implications,
Tuskegee Home, CDC, accessed January 22, 2021, www.cdc.gov/tuskegee/clintonp
.htm. See also CNN Wire Staff, "US Apologizes for Infecting Guatemalans with STDs
in the 1940s," CNN, October 1, 2010, www.cnn.com/2010/WORLD/americas/10/01
/us.guatemala.apology/index.html.

30. Dominique Lapierre, *Beyond Love* (New York: Warner Books, 1991), 369. See also
T. Kingston, "Death by Placebo: The Sacrificial Lambs of Protocol 019," *Coming
up!* September 1988, 10–11.

31. Department of Health, Education, and Welfare, *The Belmont Report* (April 18, 1979),
accessed January 15, 2021, https://www.hhs.gov/ohrp/regulations-and-policy
/belmont-report/read-the-belmont-report/index.html. See also David France, *How to
Survive a Plague: The Inside Story of How Citizens and Science Tamed AIDS* (New
York: Knopf, 2016).

32. Steven Epstein, *Impure Science, AIDS, Activism, and the Politics of Knowledge*
(Berkeley: University of California Press, 1966).

33. David Brewster, "Science and Ethics of Human Immunodeficiency Virus/Acquired
Immunodeficiency Syndrome Controversies in Africa," *Journal of Pediatrics
and Child Health* (September 27, 2011), https://doi.org/10.1111/j.1440-1754.2011
.02179.x.

34. The Wire Staff, "Controversial Chinese Experiment to Edit 'Anti-HIV' Gene May Have
Actually Failed," The Wire, May 12, 2019, https://science.thewire.in/health/he
-jiankui-genetically-edit-embryos-ccr5-hiv-crispr-cas9-ethics/.

35. Nicoli Nattrass, "AIDS and the Scientific Governance of Medicine in Post-Apartheid
South Africa," *African Affairs* 107, no. 427 (February 16, 2008): 157–176.

36. Sarah Boseley, "Mbeki in New Row over AIDS," *The Guardian*, July 10, 2000. See
also Peter Duesberg, *Inventing the AIDS Virus* (Washington, DC: Regnery Publishing, 1996).

37. Boseley, "Mbeki in New Row over AIDS."

38. Pride Chigwedere, George R. Seage III, Sofia Gruskin, Tun-Hou Lee, and M. Essex,
"Estimating the Lost Benefits of Antiretroviral Drug Use in South Africa," *Journal of
Acquired Immune Deficiency Syndromes* 49, no. 4 (December 1, 2008): 410–415.

39. Duesberg, *Inventing the AIDS Virus.*

40. Jon Cartwright, "AIDS Contrarian Ignored Warnings of Scientific Misconduct,"
Nature, May 4, 2010, www.nature.com/articles/news.2010.210.

41. Greg Miller, "AIDS Scientist Investigated for Misconduct after Complaint," *Science*,
April 16, 2010.

42. John Parascandola, *Sex, Sin, and Science: A History of Syphilis in America* (London:
Praeger Press, 2008).

43. Eran Bendavid and Jayanta Bhattacharya, "The President's Emergency Plan for AIDS Relief in Africa: An Evaluation of Outcomes," *Annals of Internal Medicine* 150, no. 10 (2009): 688–695.

44. Karla D. Wagner, Stephen E. Lankenau, Lawrence A. Palinkas, Jean L. Richardson, Chih-Ping Chou, and Jennifer B. Unger, "The Perceived Consequences of Safer Injection: An Exploration of Qualitative Findings and Gender Differences," *Psychology, Health and Medicine* 15, no. 5 (2010): 560–573.

45. Parascandola, *Sex, Sin, and Science*, 32–36.

46. Scott W. Stern, *The Trials of Nina McCall: Sex, Surveillance, and the Decades-Long Government Plan to Imprison Promiscuous Women* (Boston: Beacon Press, 2018).

47. "LaRouche Initiative Stopped Dead," *New York Native*, November 17, 1986. See also Patrick Buchanan, "Editorial," *Seattle Times*, July 31, 1993; William F. Buckley Jr., "Identify All the Carriers," *New York Times*, March 18, 1986; Robert Steinbrook, "The Times Poll: 42% Would Limit Civil Rights in AIDS Battle," *Los Angeles Times*, July 31, 1987, 1.

48. France, *How to Survive a Plague*, 267–268.

49. National Center for HIV, STD, and TB Prevention (U.S.), *The National Plan to Eliminate Syphilis from the United States* (Atlanta: CDC, October 1999), 73–86, https://www.cdc.gov/stopsyphilis/plan.pdf.

50. Allan Brandt, "Plagues and Peoples: The AIDS Epidemic," in *No Magic Bullet: A Social History of Venereal Disease in the United States since 1880* (New York: Oxford University Press, 1987), 183–204.

51. Richard Lawson, "The Reagan Administration's Unearthed Response to the AIDS Crisis Is Chilling," *Vanity Fair*, December 1, 2015, www.vanityfair.com/news/2015/11/reagan-administration-response-to-aids-crisis.

52. D. Gould, "Rock the Boat, Don't Rock the Boat, Baby: Ambivalence and the Emergence of Militant AIDS Activism," *Passionate Politics: Emotions and Social Movements* (2001): 135–157. See also U.S. Congress Office of Technology Assessment, *Review of the Public Health Service's Response to AIDS: A Technical Memorandum* (Washington, DC: U.S. Government Printing Office, February 1985).

53. A. Novick, "Reflections on a Term of Public Service with the FDA Antivirals Advisory Committee," *AIDS and Public Policy Journal* 8 (1993): 55–61. See also France, *How to Survive a Plague*.

54. Frank Snowden, "The Paris School of Medicine," in *Epidemics and Society from the Black Death to the Present* (New Haven, CT: Yale University Press, 2019), 168–183. See also Erwin Ackerknecht, *Medicine at the Paris Hospital 1794–1848* (Baltimore, MD: Johns Hopkins University Press, 1967), 129–138, 183–203; John H. Warner, *Against the Spirit of the System: The French Impulse in Nineteenth-Century American Medicine* (Princeton, NJ: Princeton University Press, 1998).

55. Mary Shelley, *Frankenstein* (London: Penguin Classic Series, 2018 [1818]).

56. Nathaniel Hawthorne, *Rappaccini's Daughter* (Whitefish, MT: Kessinger Publishing, 2018 [1844]).

57. Louis Galambos with Jane Eliot Sewell, *Networks of Innovation: Vaccine Development at Merck, Sharp & Dohme, and Mulford, 1895–1995* (Cambridge, UK: Cambridge University Press, 1995), 6–7.

58. Judith Walzer Leavitt, *The Healthiest City: Milwaukee and the Politics of Health Reform* (Madison: University of Wisconsin Press, 1996), 80–85.

59. Galambos and Sewell, *Networks of Innovation*, 11–14.

60. G. Bernard Shaw, *The Doctor's Dilemma* (London: Penguin Books, 1957 [1906]).

61. R. Dubos, *Mirage of Health: Utopias, Progress, and Biological Change* (Garden City, NY: Anchor Books, 1959).

62. T. McKeown, *The Role of Medicine: Dream, Mirage, or Nemesis?* (London: Nuffield Provincial Hospitals Trust, 1976).

63. M. Foucault, *Birth of a Clinic: An Archeology of Medical Perception* (New York: Pantheon Books, 1973).

64. M. Mulkay, "Norms and Ideology in Science," *Social Science Information* 15, no. 4 (1976): 637–656.

65. A. Rawling, "The AIDS Virus Dispute: Awarding Priority for the Discovery of the Human Immunodeficiency Virus (HIV)," *Science, Technology, and Human Values* 19, no. 3 (1994): 342–360.

66. D. Cyronski, "Woo Suk Hwang Convicted, but Not of Fraud," *Nature* 461, no. 7268 (2009): 1181.

67. Reverby, *Tuskegee's Truths*. See also Reverby, "Ethical Failures and History Lessons."

68. Volker Roelcke and Giovanni Maio, *Twentieth Century Ethics of Human Subjects Research* (Stuttgart: Franz Steiner Verlag, 2004).

69. "Historical Vaccine Concerns," Vaccine Safety, CDC, accessed January 23, 2023, www.cdc.gov/vaccinesafety/concerns/concerns-history.html#:~:text=From%201955%20to%201963%2C%20an,polio%20vaccines%20at%20that%20time.

70. A. J. Wakefield, S. H. Murch, A. Anthony, J. Linnell, D. M. Casson, M. Malik, M. Berelowitz, et al., "Ileal-Lymphoid-Nodular Hyperplasia, Non-Specific Colitis, and Pervasive Developmental Disorder in Children," *Lancet* 351 (1998): 637–641.

71. Brent Taylor, Elizabeth Miller, C. Paddy Farrington, Maria-Christina Petropoulos, Isabelle Favot-Mayaud, Jun Li, and Pauline A. Waight, "Autism and Measles, Mumps, and Rubella Vaccine: No Epidemiologic Evidence for a Causal Association," *Lancet* 353, no. 9169 (1999): 2026–2029.

72. Loring Dales, Sandra Jo Hammer, and Natalie J. Smith, "Time Trends in Autism and in MMR Immunization Coverage in California," *JAMA* 285, no. 9 (2001): 1183–1185.

73. Ivan Illich, "Medical Nemesis," *Lancet* 303, no. 7863 (May 1974): 918–921.

74. Brit Trogen, "New Amsterdam Is a Medical Drama That Fails Doctors—and Viewers," *The Atlantic*, November 28, 2018, www.theatlantic.com/entertainment/archive/2018/11/new-amsterdam-nbc-show-physician-distrust-bellevue/576712/.

75. "TV Doctors' Portrayal Evolves from Saintly to Human," *American Medical News*, November 19, 2012, https://amednews.com/article/20121119/profession/311199949/4/. See also Elliott Tapper, "Doctors on Display: The Evolution of Television's Doctors," *Baylor University Medical Center Proceedings* 23 (2010): 393–399.

76. C. E. Rosenberg, "Disease and Social Order in America: Perceptions and Expectations," *Milbank Quarterly* 64 (1986): 34–55.

77. Strategic Advisory Group of Experts on Immunization, *Report of the SAGE Working Group on Vaccine Hesitancy* (Geneva, Switzerland: World Health Organization, 2014).

Chapter 5 COVID

1. David M. Morens, Peter Daszak, and Jeffery K. Taubenberger, "Escaping Pandora's Box: Another Novel Coronavirus," *NEJM* 382, no. 14 (February 26, 2020): 1293–1295.

2. "2019 Novel Coronavirus, Wuhan, China," Information for Healthcare Professionals, CDC, accessed February 14, 2020, www.cdc.gov/coronavirus/2019-nCoV/hcp/index.html.

3. "Novel Coronavirus (2019-nCoV) Technical Guidance," World Health Organization, accessed February 21, 2020, www.who.int/emergencies/diseases/novel-coronavirus-2019/technical-guidance.

4. Berkeley Lovelace, "Why a Coronavirus Vaccine Might Be Ready Early Next Year—and What Could Go Wrong," accessed May 22, 2020, www.cnbc.com/2020/05/21/coronavirus-vaccine-why-it-may-be-ready-early-next-year-and-what-could-go-wrong.html.

5. "Code Red: China Is Using Its High-Tech Methods of Controlling People to Curb an Epidemic," *The Economist*, February 29, 2020, 33–34.

6. Eliot McLaughlin, "CDC Official Warns Americans It's Not a Question of If Coronavirus Will Spread, but When," CNN, accessed February 26, 2020, www.cnn.com/2020/02/25/health/coronavirus-us-american-cases/index.html.

7. "Going Global: The Virus is Coming. Governments Have an Enormous Amount of Work to Do," *The Economist*, February 29, 2020, 8.

8. Caitlyn Oprysko and Quint Forgey, "'Our Country Wasn't Built to Be Shut Down': Trump Pushes Back against Health Experts," *Politico*, March 23, 2020, www.politico.com/news/2020/03/23/trump-coronavirus-lockdown-skepticism-143800.

9. "A Timeline of COVID-19 Developments in 2020," *American Journal of Managed Care*, January 1, 2021, www.ajmc.com/view/a-timeline-of-covid19-developments-in-2020.

10. Chandini Raina MacIntyre, "Case Isolation, Contact Tracing, and Physical Distancing Are Pillars of COVID-19 Pandemic Control, Not Optional Choices," *Lancet Infectious Diseases* 20 (October 2020): 1105–1106.

11. Jessica Newfield, "The Impact of Culture on Covid-19 Responses," Berkeley Public Policy The Goldman School, December 18, 2020, https://gspp.berkeley.edu/faculty-and-impact/news/recent-news/the-impact-of-culture-on-covid-19-responses.

12. J. M. Carethers, "Insights into Disparities Observed with COVID-19," *Journal of Internal Medicine* (November 8, 2020), https://doi.org/10.1111/joim.13199.

13. "Introduction to COVID-19 Racial and Ethnic Health Disparities," Work and School, CDC, updated December 10, 2020, www.cdc.gov/coronavirus/2019-ncov/community/health-equity/racial-ethnic-disparities/index.html.

14. Ruth McCabe, Nora Schmit, Paula Christen, Josh C. D'Aeth, Alessandra Lochen, Dheeya Rizmie, Shevanthi Nayagam, et al., "Adapting Hospital Capacity to Meet Changing Demands During the COVID-19 Pandemic," *BMC Medicine* (October 16, 2020), https://bmcmedicine.biomedcentral.com/articles/10.1186/s12916-020-01781-w.

15. "Tackling the Mental Health Impact of the COVID-19 Crisis: An Integrated, Whole-of-Society Response," OECD, May 12, 2021, www.oecd.org/coronavirus/policy-responses/tackling-the-mental-health-impact-of-the-covid-19-crisis-an-integrated-whole-of-society-response-0ccafa0b/.

16. "Most Americans Say State Governments Have Lifted COVID-19 Restrictions Too Quickly," Pew Research Center, August 6, 2020, www.pewresearch.org/politics/2020/08/06/most-americans-say-state-governments-have-lifted-covid-19-restrictions-too-quickly/.

17. Tariro Mzezewa and Sarah Cahalan, "The U.S. Passes 4 Million Cases in November Alone, Doubling October's Tally," *New York Times*, November 28 2020.

18. Jamie Ducharme, "The U.S. COVID-19 Outbreak Is Worse than It's Ever Been. Why Aren't We Acting Like It?," *Time*, November 30, 2020, https://time.com/5913620/covid-third-wave/.

19. Jon Cohen, "Unveiling 'Warp Speed,' the White House's America-First Push for a Coronavirus Vaccine," *Science*, May 12, 2020, www.science.org/content/article /unveiling-warp-speed-white-house-s-america-first-push-coronavirus-vaccine.

20. David Leonhardt, "A Complete List of Trump's Attempts to Play Down Coronavirus," *New York Times*, March 15, 2020, www.nytimes.com/2020/03/15/opinion/trump -coronavirus.html.

21. Christian Paz, "All the President's Lies about the Coronavirus," *The Atlantic*, November 2, 2020, www.theatlantic.com/politics/archive/2020/11/trumps-lies-about-co ronavirus/608647/.

22. Andre Kalil, "Treating Covid 19: Off-Label Drug Use, Compassionate Use, and Randomized Clinical Trials during Pandemics," *JAMA* 323, no. 19 (May 19, 2020): 1897–1898.

23. Sharon LaFraniere, Katie Thomas, Noah Weiland, David Gelles, Sheryl Gay Stolberg, and Denise Grady, "Politics, Science and the Remarkable Race for a Viable Vaccine," *New York Times*, November 22, 2020.

24. Stephanie Baker and Cynthia Koons, "Inside Operation Warp Speed's $18 Billion Sprint for a Vaccine," *Bloomberg Business Week*, October 29, 2020, www.bloomberg .com/news/features/2020-10-29/inside-operation-warp-speed-s-18-billion-sprint -for-a-vaccine.

25. David Remnick, "A Historian's View of the Coronavirus Pandemic and the Influenza of 1918," *New Yorker*, March 25, 2020, www.newyorker.com/culture/video-dept/a -historians-view-of-the-coronavirus-pandemic-and-the-influenza-of-1918. See also John Barry, *The Great Influenza: The Story of the Deadliest Pandemic in History* (New York: Penguin Books, 2004), 120–129.

26. Howard Markel, Harvey B. Lipman, and J. Alexander Navarro, "Nonpharmaceutical Interventions Implemented by US Cities During the 1918–1919 Influenza Pandemic," *JAMA*, August 8, 2007, https://jamanetwork.com/journals/jama/article-abstract /208354.

27. John Eyler, "The State of Science, Microbiology and Vaccines circa 1918," *Public Health Reports* 125, Suppl. 3 (2010): 27–36.

28. Powel Kazanjian, "Polio, AIDS, and Ebola: A Recurrent Ethical Dilemma," *Clinical Infectious Diseases* 70, no. 2 (2020): 334–337.

29. W. C. Braisted, "The Navy and Its Health Problems," *American Journal of Public Health* 7 (1917): 931.

30. Carol Byerly, "The U.S. Military and the Influenza Pandemic of 1918–1919," *Public Health Reports*, accessed November 10, 2020, www.ncbi.nlm.nih.gov/pmc/articles /PMC2862337/pdf/phr125s30082.pdf.

31. Simon Flexner and James Thomas Flexner, *William Welch and the Heroic Age of American Medicine* (New York: Viking Press, 1941), 376–377.

32. William Carlos Williams, "Sour Grapes," in *The Autobiography of William Carlos Williams* (New York: New Directions, 1967), 159.

33. Barry, *The Great Influenza*, 403.

34. Giovanni Boccaccio, *The Decameron* (1349), trans. Wayne Rebhorn (New York: W. W. Norton, 2013), 88.

35. Guy de Chuliac, "The Bubonic Plague," in *A Sourcebook of Medical Science*, ed. Edward Grant (Cambridge, MA: Harvard University Press, 1974), 773–774.

36. "COVID-19, MERS and SARS," NIAID, accessed October 21, 2021, www.niaid.nih .gov/diseases-conditions/covid-19.

37. Lawrence Wright, "The Plague Year: The Mistakes and Struggles behind an American Tragedy," *New Yorker*, January 4, 2021, 22–59. See also "Code Red."
38. Aishvarya Kavi, "With Supplies Still Scarce, Calls Grow for Greater Use of Wartime Law," *New York Times*, July 23, 2020.
39. "Going Global."
40. David Leonhardt and Lauren Leatherby, "Nations Led by Populists See Fastest Virus Spread," *New York Times*, June 5, 2020.
41. Cohen, "Unveiling 'Warp Speed.'"
42. Manny Fernandez, Campbell Robertson, Mitch Smith, and Will Wright, "As Surge Spreads, No Corner of Nation Is Spared," *New York Times*, November 26, 2020. See also Melanie J. Firestone, Haley Wienkes, Jacob Garfin, Xiong Wang, Kelley Vilen, Kirk E. Smith, Stacy Holzbauer, et al., "COVID-19 Outbreak Associated with a 10-Day Motorcycle Rally in a Neighboring State—Minnesota, August–September 2020," *Morbidity and Mortality Weekly Report* 69, no. 47 (November 2020): 1771–1776.
43. Giorgia Guglielmi, "Coronavirus and Public Holidays: What the Data Say," *Nature* 588 (2020): 549–550.
44. "Dropping the Ball: Covid-19 Is Rapidly Spreading in America," *The Economist*, March 14, 2020, 17–18. See also Michael Corkery, "Wall Street Suffers Its Worst Week Since 2008 as Virus Angst Grows," *New York Times*, February 29, 2020.
45. Sheryl Gay Stolberg, "Opening Too Soon Poses Deadly Risk, Senate Is Warned. Markets Are Rattled as Health Experts Veer from President's Optimism," *New York Times*, May 13, 2020. See also Sheryl Gay Stolberg and Noah Weiland, "Experts Sketch Gloomy Picture of Virus Spread," *New York Times*, June 24, 2020.
46. Robinson Meyer and Alexis C. Madrigal, "A Devastating New Stage of the Pandemic," *The Atlantic*, June 25, 2020, www.theatlantic.com/science/archive/2020/06/second-coronavirus-surge-here/613522.
47. Kobi Cohen and Amir Leshem, "Suppressing the Impact of the COVID-19 Pandemic Using Controlled Testing and Isolation," *Scientific Reports* 11 (2021): 6279. See also Wright, "The Plague Year."
48. The United States and other nations avoided centralized guidelines for widespread testing and remote schooling early in the epidemic. See "Going Global." See also Leonhardt and Leatherby, "Nations Led by Populists See Fastest Virus Spread."
49. Guardian Staff, "Donald Trump Calls Covid-19 'Kung Flu' at Tulsa Rally," *The Guardian*, June 20, 2020, www.theguardian.com/us-news/2020/jun/20/trump-covid-19-kung-flu-racist-language.
50. "Dropping the Ball."
51. Stolberg, "Opening Too Soon Poses Deadly Risk."
52. Stolberg and Weiland, "Experts Sketch Gloomy Picture of Virus Spread."
53. Meyer and Madrigal, "Devastating New Stage." See also Sabrina Tavernise, Frances Robles, and Louis Keene, "Cases Soaring as Leadership on Virus Fails," *New York Times*, June 28, 2020, A1 and A5.
54. See Cohen, "Unveiling 'Warp Speed.'"
55. Noah Weiland, "How the CDC Lost Its Voice under Trump," *New York Times*, December 17, 2020, A8. See also Sonja A. Rasmussen and Denise J. Jamieson, "Public Health Decision Making during Covid-19: Fulfilling the CDC Pledge to the American People," *NEJM* 383, no. 10 (2020): 901–903.
56. Peter Baker, "Trump Scorns Own Scientists over Virus Data," *New York Times*, September 27, 2020, A1 and 19.

57. Christina Morales and Allyson Waller, "A Timeline of Trump's Symptoms and Treatments," *New York Times*, October 5, 2020, www.nytimes.com/2020/10/04/us/trump-covid-symptoms-timeline.html.

58. Sharon LaFraniere, "A Trump Aide's Bizarre Warning of Conspiracies and Hit Squads," *New York Times*, September 15, 2020, A1 and A5.

59. See Donald McNeil, "Claims of Herd Immunity Called Nonsense, as Well as Dangerous," *New York Times*, September 30, 2020, A1 and A7.

60. Mark Mazaetti, Noah Weiland, and Sheryl Gay Stolberg, "Under Pence, Politics Seeped into Coronavirus Response," *New York Times*, October 9, 2020, A9.

61. Javier Hernandez, "Propaganda Machine Muddies Virus's Origin: Misrepresenting Remarks of Experts and Casting Iffy Theories as Science," *New York Times*, December 7, 2020, A5.

62. Misinformation from these websites threatened to reduce the number of people willing to take the vaccine. See Alba Davey and Sheera Frenkel, "Misinformation Peddlers Are Shifting Gears," *New York Times*, December 17, 2020, A8.

63. MacIntyre, "Case Isolation, Contact Tracing, and Physical Distancing Are Pillars." See also Sarah Mervosh, David Goodman, and Julie Bosman, "Deaths Climb Fast as Hurdles Loom for Vaccine Plans. Horrifying Toll Seen in Coming Months," *New York Times*, November 15, 2020, A1 and A9.

64. "Two Billion COVID Vaccine Doses Secured, WHO Says End of Pandemic Is in Sight," United Nation News, December 18, 2020, https://news.un.org/en/story/2020/12/1080422.

65. Marlene Cimons, "Reports of Two Promising Covid-19 Vaccines Don't Mean We 'Magically,' Quickly Return to Normal," *Washington Post*, November 21, 2020, www.washingtonpost.com/health/covid-vaccine-masks-normal-life/2020/11/20/b4ed16c8-2922-11eb-9b14-ad872157ebc9_story.html.

66. Fernando P. Polack, Stephen J. Thomas, Nicholas Kitchin, Judith Absalon, and Alejandra Gurtman, "Safety and Efficacy of the BNT162b2 mRNA Covid-19 Vaccine," *NEJM* 383, no. 27 (December 10, 2020), www.nejm.org/doi/full/10.1056/nejmoa2034577.

67. Elie Dolgin, "The Tangled History of mRNA Vaccines," *Nature* 597 (September 16, 2021): 318–324.

68. "Curing Covid-19," *Lancet Infectious Diseases* 20, no. 10 (October 2020): 1101.

69. Gina Kolata, "Lasker Prizes Recognize Scientists behind Vaccine," *New York Times*, September 24, 2021, A19. See also "Suppression of RNA Recognition by Toll-Like Receptors: The Impact of Nucleoside Modification and the Evolutionary Origin of RNA," *Immunity* 23, no. 2 (August 2005): 165–175.

70. The viruses that mRNA had been tested against included CMV, MERS, and HIV. See Sandhya Vasan and Punnee Pitisuttithum, "Vaccine Development Lessons between HIV and Covid 19," *Lancet Infectious Diseases* 21, no. 6 (June 2021): 759–761.

71. Dolgin, "Tangled History of mRNA Vaccines."

72. Sheryl Stolberg, "Moderna and US at Odds over Vaccine Patent Rights," *New York Times*, September 24, 2021.

73. Sharon LaFraniere, Katie Thomas, Noah Weiland, David Gelles, and Sheryl Gay Stolberg, "Politics, Science, and the Remarkable Race for a Viable Vaccine," *New York Times*, November 22, 2020, A1, A10, and A11.

74. Denise Grady, Abby Goodnough, and Noah Weiland, "Moderna Vaccine is Second to Get Cleared by FDA," *New York Times*, December 19, 2020, A1 and A8.

75. Polack et al., "Safety and Efficacy of the BNT162b2 mRNA Covid-19 Vaccine." See also Eric Rubin and Dan L. Longo, "Sars-CoV-2 Vaccination: An Ounce (Actually Much Less) of Prevention," *NEJM* 383 (December 31, 2020): 2677–2678.

76. Editorial Board, "Prepare for the President to Rush the Vaccine," *Boston Globe*, September 14, 2020, www.bostonglobe.com/2020/09/24/opinion/prepare-president-rush -vaccine/.

77. Michael Gold, "New York Will Review Virus Vaccines, Citing Politicization of Process," *New York Times*, December 3, 2020.

78. Berkeley Lovelace, "The U.S. Has Vaccinated Just 1 Million People Out of a Goal of 20 Million for December," CNBC, December 23, 2020, www.cnbc.com/2020/12/23 /covid-vaccine-us-has-vaccinated-1-million-people-out-of-goal-of-20-million-for -december.html.

79. Sheryl Gay Stolberg, "Biden Unveils National Strategy That Trump Resisted," *New York Times*, January 21, 2021.

80. Sheryl Gay Stolberg, "Biden Declares 'Independence' from the Virus to Some Dismay," *New York Times*, July 3, 2021.

81. Josh Holder, "Tracking Coronavirus Vaccinations around the World," *New York Times*, January 13, 2022.

82. John Elflein, "Percentage of Population in Select Countries and Territories Worldwide That Had Received a COVID-19 Vaccination as of January 12, 2022," Statista, www.statista.com/statistics/1202074/share-of-population-vaccinated-covid-19-by -county-worldwide/.

83. Liz Hamel and Ashley Kirzinger, "KFF COVID-19 Vaccine Monitor: December 2020," KFF, December 15, 2020, www.kff.org/coronavirus-covid-19/report/kff-covid-19 -vaccine-monitor-december-2020/.

84. Ashley Kirzinger, Grace Sparks, Audrey Kearney, Mellisha Stokes, Liz Hamel, and Mollyann Brodie, "KFF COVID-19 Vaccine Monitor: November 2021," KFF, December 2, 2021, www.kff.org/coronavirus-covid-19/poll-finding/kff-covid-19-vaccine -monitor-november-2021/.

85. Christie Aschwanden, "Five Reasons Why COVID Herd Immunity Is Probably Impossible," *Nature* 591 (March 18, 2021): 520–522.

86. Noah Weiland, "High Hopes Fizzle for One-Dose Covid Vaccine," *New York Times*, June 19, 2021.

87. Sarah Mervosh and Amy Harmon, "US Vaccine Rollout Was Big. Could It Have Been Better?," *New York Times*, June 18, 2021, A12.

88. Eric C. Schneider, Arnav Shah, Pratha Sah, Seyed M. Moghadas, Thomas Vilches, and Alison P. Galvani, "The U.S. COVID-19 Vaccination Program at One Year: How Many Deaths and Hospitalizations Were Averted?," Commonwealth Fund, December 14, 2021, www.commonwealthfund.org/publications/issue-briefs/2021/dec/us -covid-19-vaccination-program-one-year-how-many-deaths-and.

89. Patricia Cohen and Alan Rappeport, "Supply Gridlock and Virus Hinder Global Recovery," *New York Times*, October 13, 2021, A1.

90. Nancy S. Jecker and Caesar A. Atuire, "What's Yours Is Ours: Waiving Intellectual Property Protections for COVID-19 Vaccines," *Journal of Medical Ethics* 47 (2021): 595–598.

91. Mervosh and Harmon, "US Vaccine Rollout Was Big."

92. Some said CDC officials should have targeted disadvantaged areas. See Muriel Jean-Jacques and Howard Bauchner, "Vaccine Distribution—Equity Left Behind?," *JAMA* 325, no. 9 (2021): 829–830. See also W. J. Hennigan, Alice Park, and Jamie

Ducharme, "The U.S. Fumbled Its Early Vaccine Rollout. Will the Biden Administration Put America Back on Track?," *Time*, January 21, 2021.

93. Akilah Johnson, "Lack of Health Services and Transportation Impede Access to Vaccine in Communities of Color," *Washington Post*, February 13, 2021.

94. Shingai Machingaidze and Charles Shey Wiysonge, "Understanding Covid-19 Vaccine Hesitancy," *Nature Medicine* 27 (August 2021): 1338–1344. See also Julio S. Solís Arce, Shana S. Warren, Niccolò F. Meriggi, Alexandra Scacco, Nina McMurry, Maarten Voors, Georgiy Syunyaev, et al., "COVID-19 Vaccine Acceptance and Hesitancy in Low- and Middle-Income Countries," *Nature Medicine* 27 (August 2021): 1385–1394. See also Mervosh and Harmon, "US Vaccine Rollout Was Big."

95. Noni MacDonald, "SAGE Working Group on Vaccine Hesitancy," *Vaccine* 33, no. 34 (2015): 4161–4164.

96. Melanie Schuster, Juhani Eskola, and Philippe Duclos, "Vaccine Hesitancy: Rationale, Remit and Methods," *Vaccine* 33 (2015): 4157–4160. See also Benjamin Hickler, Sherine Guirguis, and Rafael Obregon, "Special Issue on Vaccine Hesitancy," *Vaccine* 33 (2015): 4155–4156.

97. See Arce et al., "COVID-19 Vaccine Acceptance and Hesitancy in Low- and Middle-Income Countries." See also Machingaidze and Wiysonge, "Understanding Covid-19 Vaccine Hesitancy."

98. Apoorva Mandavilli, "Alarming Finding Drove CDC Mask Reversal," *New York Times*, July 30, 2021, A15.

99. Philippa Roxby and Jim Reed, "Covid Booster 88% Effective against Hospital Treatment with Omicron," BBC News, December 31, 2021, www.bbc.com/news/health-59840524.

100. Caroline Maslo, Richard Friedland, Mande Toubkin, Anchen Laubscher, Teshlin Akaloo, and Boniswa Kama, "Characteristics and Outcomes of Hospitalized Patients in South Africa during the COVID-19 Omicron Wave Compared with Previous Waves," *JAMA* 327 (December 30, 2021), https://doi.org/10.1001/jama.2021.24868.

101. The new approach allowed for the opening of schools, restaurants, and bars. It also required "vaccine passports" and rapid antibody tests before attending large gatherings. See "COVID Is Here to Stay: Countries Must Decide How to Adapt," *Nature* 601 (January 13, 2022): 165.

102. Nick Tate, "Vaccinated Americans Rage against Holdouts," WebMD Health News, August 10, 2021, www.webmd.com/vaccines/covid-19-vaccine/news/20210810/covid-resurges-vaccinated-americans-rage-against-holdouts.

103. "Ten Threats to Global Health in 2019," World Health Organization, accessed November 12, 2020, www.who.int/news-room/spotlight/ten-threats-to-global-health-in-2019.

104. Patricia Mazzei, "Mask Advisory Faces Defiance in Some States," *New York Times*, July 29, 2021, A1. See also Sharon LaFraniere and Noah Weiland, "Failings of CDC Prompt a Rebuke and an Overhaul," *New York Times*, August 18, 2022, A1 and A15.

105. Sheryl Gay Stolberg and Sharon Lafraniere, "Pfizer Pushes US Approval of 3rd Doses," *New York Times*, July 13, 2021, A1. See also Katherine Bennhold, "Germany Is Latest Rich Country to Offer Booster Shots for Covid Vaccine," *New York Times*, August 3, 2021, A8.

106. Alison Durkee, "Omicron So Far Isn't Persuading Most U.S. Adults to Get Vaccinated or Booster Shot, Poll Finds," *Forbes*, December 14, 2021, www.forbes.com/sites/alisondurkee/2021/12/14/omicron-so-far-isnt-persuading-most-us-adults-to-get-vaccinated-or-booster-shot-poll-finds/?sh=3633785b469e.

107. Jan Hoffman, "Rising Mistrust of Warp Speed Vaccine May Prolong Pandemic," *New York Times*, July 19, 2020, A1 and A9. See also Simon Romero and Miriam Jordan, "A Divided and Distrustful US Awaits Vaccines," *New York Times*, December 12, 2020.

108. Liz Hamel, Luna Lopes, Grace Spark, Ashley Kirzinger, Audrey Kearney, Mellisha Stokes, and Molyanne Brady, "KFF COVID-19 Vaccine Monitor: January 2022," January 28, 2022, https://www.kff.org/coronavirus-covid-19/poll-finding/kff-covid-19-vaccine-monitor-january-2022/.

109. Alba et al., "Misinformation Peddlers are Shifting Gears." See also Sheera Frenkel, "Disinformation Is Big Business for One Doctor," *New York Times*, July 25, 2021, A1.

110. Johnson Mayamba, "Low Supply and Public Mistrust Hinder COVID-19 Vaccine Roll-Out in Africa," *Global Campus of Human Rights* (blog), November, 11, 2021, https://gchumanrights.org/preparedness/article-on/low-supply-and-public-mistrust-hinder-covid-19-vaccine-roll-out-in-africa.html.

111. Michael Shear, Sheryl Gay Stolberg, and Annie Karni, "Biden Rekindles Vaccination Push with New Orders," *New York Times*, July 30, 2021.

112. Sharon Lafraniere and Noal Weiland, "Mandates on Way as Pfizer Vaccine Gets Full U.S. Nod," *New York Times*, August 24, 2021, A1.

113. *National Federation of Independent Businesses v. Department of Labor, Occupational Safety and Health Administration*, 595 U.S. ___ (2022).

114. "COVID Is Here to Stay."

115. Powel Kazanjian, interview with Peter Marks, director of Center for Biologics Evaluation and Research, U.S. FDA, January 14, 2022.

116. Emma G. Fitzsimmons, Shawn Hubler, and Jennifer Steinhauer, "2 Key Regions Give Workers Choice: Vaccines or Tests," *New York Times*, July 27, 2021, A1 and A15.

117. Derek Thompson, "How America Dropped to No. 36," *Atlantic*, September 26, 2021, www.theatlantic.com/ideas/archive/2021/09/how-america-lost-its-lead-vaccination/620201/.

118. Donald McNeil, "How Can We Achieve Herd Immunity? Experts Are Quietly Upping the Number," *New York Times*, December 27, 2020, A6.

119. Katie Thomas, Carl Zimmer, and Sharon Lafraniere, "A New Vaccine Shows Success, with a Caveat," *New York Times*, January 29, 2021, A1 and A6. See also Jacob E. Lemieux and Jonathan Z. Li, "Uncovering Ways That Emerging SARS-CoV-2 Lineages May Increase Transmissibility," *Journal of Infectious Diseases* 223, no. 10 (February 13, 2021): 1663–1665. See also Kathleen Neuzil, "Interplay between Emerging SARS-CoV-2 Variants and Pandemic Control," *NEJM* 348, no. 20 (May 20, 2021): 1952–1953.

120. David McKenzie, Ghazi Balkiz, Ivana Kottasova, and Laura Smith-Spark, "Omicron, a New Covid-19 Variant with High Number of Mutations, Sparks Travel Bans and Worries Scientists," CNN, November 26, 2021, www.cnn.com/2021/11/26/africa/new-covid-variant-discovered-south-africa-b11529-intl/index.html.

121. Katarina Zimmer, "A Guide to Emerging SARS-CoV-2 Variants," *The Scientist*, January 26, 2021, www.the-scientist.com/news-opinion/a-guide-to-emerging-sars-cov-2-variants-68387.

122. MacIntyre, "Case Isolation, Contact Tracing, and Physical Distancing Are Pillars." See also Laura Cornelissen and Emmanuel Andre, "Understanding the Drivers of Transmission of SARS-CoV-2," *Lancet Infectious Diseases* 21, no. 5 (May 2021): 580–581.

123. David Leonhardt, "When Do We Get Back to Normal? Maybe Now," *New York Times*, November 13, 2021, A14.

124. Sarah Zhang, "The Coronavirus Is Here Forever. This Is How We Live with It," *The Atlantic*, August 17, 2021, www.theatlantic.com/science/archive/2021/08/how-we -live-coronavirus-forever/619783.

125. See Mark Lipsitch and Natalie E. Dean, "Understanding Covid-19 Vaccine Effi-cacy," *Science* 370, no. 6518 (November 13, 2020): 763–765. See also Joseph Choi, "Health Experts Still Learning about Omicron Subvariant, Now Dominant in Northeast," *The Hill*, January 22, 2023, https://thehill.com/homenews/3821666 -health-experts-still-learning-about-omicron-subvariant-now-dominant-in -northeast/.

126. James Barron, "Coronovirus Update," *New York Times*, December 5, 2020, A4.

127. Anita E. Heywood and C. Raina Macintyre, "Elimination of Covid-19: What Would It Look Like and Is It Possible?," *Lancet Infectious Diseases* 20, no. 9 (2020): 1005–1007. See also Elisabeth Rosenthal, "When Will We Throw Our Masks Away?," *New York Times*, November 22, 2020.

128. J. Clinton, J. Cohen, J. Lapinski, and M. Trussler, "Partisan Pandemic: How Partisan-ship and Public Health Concerns Affect Individuals' Social Mobility during COVID-19," *Science Advances* 7, no. 2 (January 6, 2021), www.science.org/doi/10.1126 /sciadv.abd7204.

129. Powel Kazanjian, interview with Peter Marks.

130. Shana Kushner Gadarian, Sara Wallace Goodman, and Thomas B. Pepinsky, "Parti-sanship, Health Behavior, and Policy Attitudes in the Early Stages of the COVID-19 Pandemic," *PLOS ONE*, April 7, 2021, https://journals.plos.org/plosone/article?id=10 .1371/journal.pone.0249596.

131. William Galston, "For COVID-19 Vaccinations, Party Affiliation Matters More than Race and Ethnicity," Brookings Institution, October 1, 2021, www.brookings.edu/blog /fixgov/2021/10/01/for-covid-19-vaccinations-party-affiliation-matters-more-than -race-and-ethnicity/.

132. Vivian Wang, "Wary, Excited, and Uncertain How Far to Go. Chinese Unite in Anger over Covid Rules," *New York Times*, November 29, 2022, A1 and A7.

133. Patricia Cohen, "Unrest in China Is Latest to Test Global Economy," *New York Times*, November 29, 2022, A1 and A9.

134. "Omicron Omens: What Real-Time Indicators Suggest about Omicron's Economic Impact," *The Economist*, January 1, 2022, www.economist.com/finance-and -economics/2022/01/01/what-real-time-indicators-suggest-about-omicrons -economic-impact.

135. Apoorva Mandavilli, "Health Officials Warn of Rough Winter as Three Pathogens Swirl," *New York Times*, October 24, 2022, A1.

136. Jan Hoffman, "Many Rush to Get Boosters as Vaccine Refusers Dig In," *New York Times*, October 12, 2021, A1 and A15.

137. Jack Healy, Noah Weiland, and Richard Fausset, "Wily Virus Adds Fuel to Defiance of Unvaccinated," *New York Times*, December 26, 2021, A1 and A26.

138. Sheryl Gay Stolberg, "Scarred by Covid, Survivors and Victims' Families Aim to Be a Political Force," *New York Times*, July 21, 2021, A12.

139. "Long-COVID Advocates Join Together to Form Alliance to Make Policy Recommen-dations, Secure Research Funding, and Transform Understanding of Post-Viral Illnesses," Cision PR Newswire, February 25, 2021, www.prnewswire.com /news -releases/long-covid-advocates-join-together-to-form-alliance-to-make-policy -recommendations-secure-research-funding-and-transform-understanding-of -post-viral-illnesses-301235258.html. See also Peter Grant and Heather J. Smith,

"Activism in the Time of Covid," *Group Processes and Intergroup Relations* 24, no. 2 (2021): 297–305.

140. Apoorva Mandavilli, "Experts Seek More Data as They Weigh the Need for Another Virus Booster," *New York Times*, March 24, 2023, A20. See also Zhang, "The Coronavirus Is Here Forever."

141. Amy Gutmann and Jonathan Moreno, *Everybody Wants to Go to Heaven but Nobody Wants to Die* (New York City: Liveright Books, 2019).

142. Sian Beilock, "How to Live with Uncertainty," *Forbes*, September 30, 2021, www .forbes.com/sites/sianbeilock/2021/09/30/how-to-live-with-uncertainty/?sh =43197e1f3274.

143. Mandavilli, "Experts Seek More Data as They Weigh the Need for Another Virus Booster." See also Kimberly Drake, "COVID-19 Anxiety Syndrome: A Pandemic Phenomenon?," *Medical News Today*, May 7, 2021, www.medicalnewstoday.com /articles/covid-19-anxiety-syndrome-a-pandemic-phenomenon.

144. Emma Court and Josh Wingrove, "Biden Team to Use DPA for Vaccine Manufacturing, Testing," Bloomberg, February 5, 2021, www.bloomberg.com/news/articles/2021 -02-05/biden-team-to-use-dpa-for-vaccine-manufacturing-testing.

145. "Fact Sheet: Biden-Harris Administration Increases COVID-19 Testing in Schools to Keep Students Safe and Schools Open," The White House, January 12, 2022, www .whitehouse.gov/briefing-room/statements-releases/2022/01/12/fact-sheet-biden -harris-administration-increases-covid-19-testing-in-schools-to-keep-students-safe -and-schools-open/.

146. "Pfizer's Novel COVID-19 Oral Antiviral Treatment Candidate Reduced Risk of Hospitalization or Death by 89% in Interim Analysis of Phase 2/3 EPIC-HR Study," press release, Pfizer, accessed December 3, 2022, www.pfizer.com/news/press-release/press -release-detail/pfizers-novel-covid-19-oral-antiviral-treatment-candidate.

147. "Pfizer Announces Additional Phase 2/3 Study Results Confirming Robust Efficacy of Novel COVID-19 Oral Antiviral Treatment Candidate in Reducing Risk of Hospitalization or Death," press release, Pfizer, accessed January 11, 2023, www.pfizer.com /news/press-release/press-release-detail/pfizer-announces-additional-phase-23 -study-results. See also "Fact Sheet for Healthcare Providers: Emergency Use Authorization for Molnupiravir," FDA, accessed December 28, 2021, www.fda.gov/media /155054/download.

148. "World Coronavirus Deaths per Day for March 9, 2023," YCharts, accessed April 2, 2024, https://ycharts.com/indicators/world_coronavirus_deaths_per_day.

149. Talha Burki, "Global Covid 19 Vaccine Inequity," *Lancet Infectious Diseases* 21 (July 2021): 922–923.

150. Sharon LaFraniere, "FDA Tells J&J to Throw out 60 Million Doses Made at a Troubled Plant," *New York Times*, July 29, 2021.

151. S Jessica Glenza, "Coronavirus: How Wealthy Nations Are Creating a Vaccine Apartheid," *The Guardian*, March 31, 2021, www.theguardian.com/world/2021/mar/30 /coronavirus-vaccine-distribution-global-disparity.

152. Healy, Weiland, and Fausset, "Wily Virus Adds Fuel to Defiance of Unvaccinated."

153. H. K. Beecher, "Ethics and Clinical Research," *NEJM* 274, no. 24 (1966): 1354–1360.

154. Ralph Ellis, "Unvaccinated 14 Times More Likely to Die from COVID," Web MD, November 25, 2021, www.webmd.com/vaccines/covid-19-vaccine/news/20211124 /unvaccinated-14-times-more-likely-to-die-from-covid.

155. Charlie Savage, "US Urges Court Not to Block Vaccine Mandate on Big Employers," *New York Times*, November 9, 2021, A12.

156. See Steven Johnson, "Can Covid Lead to Progress? The Great Aftermath," *New York Times*, November 28, 2021, 34–35. See also Afifah Rahman-Sheperd, Charles Clift, Emma Ross, Lara Hollmann, Nina van der Mark, Benjamin Wakefield, Champa Patel, and Robert Yates, "Solidarity in Response to the COVID-19 Pandemic: Has the World Worked Together to Tackle the Coronavirus?," Chatham House, July 14, 2021, www.chathamhouse.org/2021/07/solidarity-response-covid-19-pandemic.

157. Bret Stevens, "Let's End the Covid Blame Games," *New York Times*, December 1, 2021, A22.

158. See Carolyn Crist, "COVID-19 Vaccine Mandates Are Working, Public Health Experts Say," WebMD, November 10, 2021, www.webmd.com/vaccines/covid-19-vaccine/news/20211110/covid-vaccine-mandates-working. See also Nina Totenberg, "Supreme Court Blocks Biden's Vaccine-or-Test Mandate for Large Private Companies," NPR, January 13, 2022, www.npr.org/2022/01/13/1072165393/supreme-court-blocks-bidens-vaccine-or-test-mandate-for-large-private-companies; Erin Mulvaney and Allie Reed, "Shot or No Shot: Workplaces in Limbo Split on Vaccine Mandates," Bloomberg Law, November 30, 2021, https://news.bloomberglaw.com/daily-labor-report/shot-or-not-workplaces-in-limbo-struggle-with-vaccine-mandates.

159. Tom Chang, Mireille Jacobson, Manisha Shah, Rajiv Pramanik, and Samir B. Shah, "Financial Incentives and Other Nudges Do Not Increase COVID-19 Vaccinations among the Vaccine Hesitant," NBER, October 2021, www.nber.org/papers/w29403.

160. Healy, Weiland, and Fausset, "Wily Virus Adds Fuel to Defiance of Unvaccinated." See also Stacy Wood and Kevin Schulman, "When Vaccine Apathy, Not Hesitancy, Drives Vaccine Disinterest," *JAMA* 325, no. 24 (June 22, 2021): 2435–2436.

161. Ata Uslu, David Lazer, Roy Perlis, Matthew Baum, Suji Kang, Alexi Quintana, Robin Xu Bayes, et al., "The COVID States Project #63: The Decision to Not Get Vaccinated, from the Perspective of the Unvaccinated," OSF Preprints, September 2021, https://osf.io/fazup/. See also David Leonhardt, "A Bigger Partisan Gap on Covid Divides," *New York Times*, November 9, 2021, A12; Lena Sun, "CDCs Credibility Is Eroded by Internal Blunders and External Attacks," *Washington Post*, September 28, 2020, www.washingtonpost.com/health/2020/09/28/cdc-under-attack/.

162. See "Governor Cuomo Announces Clinical Advisory Task Force and Vaccine Distribution and Implementation Task Force in Anticipation of Potential Federal Authorization of COVID-19 Vaccine This Fall," New York State, September 24, 2020, www.governor.ny.gov/news/governor-cuomo-announces-clinical-advisory-task-force-and-vaccine-distribution-and. See also Powel Kazanjian, interview with Peter Marks.

163. G. L. D'alo, E. Zorzoli, A. Capanna, G. Gervasi, E. Terracciano, L. Zaratti, and E. Franco, "Frequently Asked Questions on Seven Rare Adverse Events Following Immunization," *Journal of Preventive Medicine and Hygiene* 58 (2017): E13–E26. See also Brian Deer, *The Doctor Who Fooled the World: Science, Deception, and the War on Vaccines* (Baltimore, MD: Johns Hopkins University Press, 2020).

164. Jamie Reno, "Vaccine Side Effects vs. COVID-19 Damage? There's No Comparison," Healthline, July 6, 2021, www.healthline.com/health-news/vaccine-side-effects-vs-covid-19-damage-theres-no-comparison.

165. Bruce Yee, "As Covid-19 Vaccine Microchip Conspiracy Theories Spread, Here Are Responses on Twitter," *Forbes*, July 19, 2021, www.forbes.com/sites/brucelee/2021/05/09/as-covid-19-vaccine-microchip-conspiracy-theories-spread-here-are-some-responses/?sh=27d1eacb602d.

166. Nicoli Nattrass, "AIDS and the Scientific Governance of Medicine in Post-Apartheid South Africa," *African Affairs* 107, no. 427 (February 16, 2008): 157–176. See also Sarah Boseley, "Mbeki Insists Poverty Causes Aids," *The Guardian*, July 9, 2000.
167. Peter Duesberg, *Inventing the AIDS Virus* (Washington, DC: Regnery Publishing, 1996). Heneage Gibbs, a professor of pathology at the University of Michigan in the 1890s, believed that microbes found in diseased tissues were incidental findings and not related to disease. See also Wilfred B. Shaw, *The University of Michigan: An Encyclopedic Survey*. Part 5: *The Medical School, the University Hospital, the Law School, 1850–1940* (Ann Arbor: University of Michigan Press, 1951), 773–808, 821–827.
168. Pride Chigwedere, George R. Seage, Sofia Gruskin, Tun-Hou Lee, and M. Essex, "Estimating the Lost Benefits of Antiretroviral Drug Use in South Africa," *Journal of Acquired Immune Deficiency Syndromes* 49, no. 4 (December 1, 2008): 410–415.
169. Ronald Bayer and Gerald M. Oppenheimer, *AIDS Doctors: Voices from the Epidemic* (Oxford, UK: Oxford University Press, 2000), 63–118.
170. Elizabeth Fee and Daniel M. Fox, *AIDS: The Burdens of History* (Berkeley: University of California Press, 1988), 1–11. See also Virginia Berridge and Philip Strong, *AIDS and Contemporary History* (New York: Cambridge University Press, 1993), 1–14.
171. Henrik Ibsen, *An Enemy of the People* (London: Penguin, 1882, republished 1977).
172. Powel Kazanjian, "Frederick Novy and the 1901 San Francisco Plague Commission Investigation," *Clinical Infectious Diseases* 55, no. 10 (2012): 1373–1378.
173. Roni Caryn Rabin, "On Vaccines, 'He is Wrong' Family Says of Kennedy," *New York Times*, May 9, 2019, A13.
174. Rory Smith, Liliana Bounegru, and Jonathan Gray, "Anti-Vaccination Websites Employ Vast Configurations of Ad, Social Media and Analytics Trackers to Drive Traffic, Build Audiences and Monetize Misinformation," First Draft, August 12, 2021, https://firstdraftnews.org/articles/antivaccination-audiences-monetize/. See also Gregory A. Poland and Robert M. Jacobson, "The Age-Old Struggle against the Anti-vaccinationists," *NEJM* 364, no. 2 (2011): 97–99.
175. Donald McNeil, "Latest Tally: 880 Cases of Measles in 24 States," *New York Times*, May 21, 2019, A17.
176. "Chronic Traumatic Encephalopathy," Mayo Clinic, accessed December 12, 2022, www.mayoclinic.org/diseases-conditions/chronic-traumatic-encephalopathy/symptoms-causes/syc-20370921.
177. Mark Fainaru-Wada and Steve Fainaru, *League of Denial* (New York City: Three Rivers Press, 2013).
178. "NFL Official Acknowledges Link between Head Trauma and Brain Disease CTE," *The Guardian*, March 14, 2016, www.theguardian.com/sport/2016/mar/14/cte-nfl-link-football-brain-disease-senior-official-acknowledges.
179. Naomi Oereskes, *The Merchants of Doubt* (London: Bloomsbury Press, 2010).
180. Duesberg, *Inventing the AIDS Virus*. See also Edward Hooper, *The River: A Journey to the Source of HIV and AIDS* (Boston: Back Bay Books, 2000).
181. According to Hooper, a vaccine made in monkey cells would lead to human infection with HIV.
182. Kate Wong, "Controversial AIDS Theory Suffers Fatal Blow," *Scientific American*, April 27, 2001, www.scientificamerican.com/article/controversial-aids-theory/.
183. Radhika Gharpure, Candis M. Hunter, Amy H. Schnall, Catherine E. Barrett, Amy E. Kirby, Jasen Kunz, Kirsten Berling, et al., "Knowledge and Practices

Regarding Safe Household Cleaning and Disinfection for COVID-19 Prevention: United States, May 2020," *Morbidity and Mortality Weekly Report* 69, no. 23 (2020): 705–709.

184. See B. E. Bierer, S. A. White, J. M. Barnes, and L. Gelinas, "Ethical Challenges in Clinical Research during the COVID-19 Pandemic," *Journal of Bioethical Inquiry* (2020), www.ncbi.nlm.nih.gov/pmc/articles/PMC7651825/pdf/11673_2020_Article _10045.pdf. See also Kalil, "Treating Covid 19."

185. Kazanjian, "Polio, AIDS, and Ebola: A Recurrent Ethical Dilemma."

186. Clement Adebamowo, Oumou Bah-Sow, Fred Binka, Roberto Bruzzone, Arthur Caplan, Jean-Francois Delfraissy, David Heymann, et al., "Randomised Controlled Trials for Ebola: Practical and Ethical Issues," *Lancet* 384, no. 9952 (2014): 1423–1424. See also National Academics of Science, Engineering, and Medicine, *Integrating Clinical Research into Epidemic Response: The Ebola Experience* (Washington, DC: National Academies Press, 2017).

187. Benjamin Freedman, "Equipoise and the Ethics of Clinical Research," *NEJM* 317, no. 30 (1987): 141–145.

188. P. A. Singer, J. D. Lantos, P. F. Whitington, C. E. Broelsch, and M. Siegler, "Equipoise and the Ethics of Segmental Liver Transplantation," *Clinical Research* 36, no. 6 (1988): 539–545. See also Samuel Hellman, et al., "Of Mice but Not Men: Problems of the Randomized Clinical Trial," *NEJM* 324, no. 22 (1991): 1585–1589.

189. Samuel Hellman, "Randomized Clinical Trials and the Doctor-Patient Relationship: An Ethical Dilemma," *Cancer Clinical Trials* 2, no. 3 (1979): 189–193.

190. Robert J. Levine, *Ethics and Regulation of Clinical Research* (Baltimore, MD: Urban and Schwarzenberg, 1986).

191. Laura E. Bothwell and Scott H. Podolsky, "The Emergence of the Randomized, Controlled Trial," *NEJM* 275, no. 6 (2016): 501–504.

192. Bothwell and Podolsky, "The Emergence of the Randomized, Controlled Trial."

193. Eyler, "The State of Science, Microbiology and Vaccines circa 1918."

194. Abraham Lilenfield, "Ceteris Paribus: The Evolution of the Clinical Trial," *Bulletin of the History of Medicine* 56, no. 1 (1982): 1–18.

195. Robert Yarchoan, Kent J. Weinhold, H. Kim Lyerly, Edward Gelmann, Robert M. Blum, Gene M. Shearer, Hiroaki Mitsuya, et al., "Administration of 3'-azido-3'-deoxythymidine, an Inhibitor of HTLV-III/LAV Replication, to Patients with AIDS or AIDS-Related Complex," *Lancet* 327, no. 8481 (1986): 575–580.

196. Steven Epstein, *Impure Science: AIDS, Activism, and the Politics of Knowledge* (Berkeley: University of California Press, 1966). See also Dominique Lapierre, *Beyond Love* (New York: Warner Books, 1991), 369.

197. Margaret A. Fischl, Douglas D. Richman, Michael H. Grieco, Michael S. Gottlieb, Paul A. Volberding, Oscar L. Laskin, John M. Leedom, and Jerome E. Groopman, "The Efficacy of Azidothymidine (AZT) in the Treatment of Patients with AIDS and AIDS-Related Complex: A Double-Blind, Placebo-Controlled Trial," *NEJM* 317, no. 4 (1987): 1009–1014.

198. David France, *How to Survive a Plague: The Inside Story of How Citizens and Science Tamed AIDS* (New York: Knopf Press, 2016).

199. Concorde Coordinating Committee, "Concorde: MRC/ANRS Randomized Double-Blind Controlled Trial of Immediate and Deferred Zidovudine in Symptom-Free HIV Infection," *Lancet* 343, no. 8902 (1994): 871–881.

200. A. Novick, "Reflections on a Term of Public Service with the FDA Antivirals Advisory Committee," *AIDS and Public Policy Journal* 8 (1993): 55–61. See also Gregg

Gonsalves and Diana Zuckerman, "Commentary: Will 20th Century Patient Safeguards Be Reversed in the 21st Century?," *BMJ* 350 (2015): h1500.

201. Susan S. Ellenberg, Gerald T. Keusch, Abdel G. Babiker, Kathryn M. Edwards, Roger J. Lewis, Jens D. Lundgren, Charles D. Wells, et al., "Rigorous Clinical Trial Design in Public Health Emergencies Is Essential," *Clinical Infectious Diseases* 66, no. 9 (2018): 1467–1469.

202. Steven Joffe, "Evaluating Novel Therapies during the Ebola Epidemic," *JAMA* 312, no. 13 (2014): 1299–1300.

203. National Academics of Science, Engineering, and Medicine, *Integrating Clinical Research into Epidemic Response*.

204. Tony Gould, *A Summer Plague: Polio and Its Survivors* (New Haven, CT: Yale University Press, 1995), 18–19.

205. "Polio Vaccines," *NEJM* 213, no. 14 (1935): 687.

206. Thomas Francis Jr., R. F. Korns, R. B. Voight, M. Boisen, F. M. Hemphill, J. A. Napier, and E. Tolchinsky, "An Evaluation of the 1954 Poliomyelitis Vaccine Trials: Summary Report," *American Journal of Public Health* 45 (1955): S1–S50.

207. Thomas Francis Jr., *Evaluation of the 1954 Field Trial of Poliomyelitis Vaccine* (Ann Arbor, MI: Edwards Brothers/National Foundation for Infantile Paralysis, 1957).

208. K. Hemming, T. P. Haines, P. J. Chilton, A. J. Girling, and R. J. Lilford, "The Stepped Wedge Cluster Randomized Trial: Rationale, Design, Analysis, and Reporting," *BMJ* 350, no. 1 (2015): 1–7. See also Marc Lipsitch, Nir Eyal, M. Elizabeth Halloran, Miguel A. Hernan, Ira M. Longini, Eli N. Perencevich, and Rebecca F. Grais, "Obtaining Efficacy Data in an Environment of Variable and Uncertain Incidence: Ebola and Beyond," *Science* 348 (2015): 46–48.

209. Naomi Oreskes, *Why Trust Science?* (Princeton, NJ: Princeton University Press, 2019).

210. Ludwik Fleck, *Genesis of a Scientific Fact* (Chicago: University of Chicago Press, 1979).

211. Matthew Wills, "When America Incarcerated 'Promiscuous' Women," *JSTOR Daily*, November 1, 2018, https://daily.jstor.org/when-america-incarcerated-promiscuous-women/. See also Scott W. Stern, *The Trials of Nina McCall* (Boston: Beacon Press, 2018).

212. Eliseo J. Perez-Stable, "Cuba's Response to the HIV Epidemic," *American Journal of Public Health* 81, no. 5 (1991): 563–567. See also Jay Matthews, "LaRouche's Call to Quarantine AIDS Victims Trails in California," *Washington Post*, October 26, 1986; Richard Bernstein, "Fanning French Fears," *New York Times*, October 4, 1987, 50; Thomas Stoddard and Walter Rieman, "AIDS and the Rights of the Individual: Toward a More Sophisticated Understanding of Discrimination," *Milbank Quarterly* 68, no. 1 (1990): 143.

213. See Ronald Bayer, Carol Levine, and Susan M. Wolf, "HIV Antibody Screening: An Ethical Framework for Evaluating Proposed Programs," *JAMA* 256, no. 13 (1986): 1768–1774. See also *Jacobson v. Massachusetts*, 197 U.S. 11 (1905). This ruling by the U.S. Supreme Court upheld the authority of states to enforce compulsory vaccination laws.

214. Ronald Bayer, *Private Acts, Social Consequences: AIDS and the Politics of Public Health* (New Brunswick, NJ: Rutgers University Press, 1991).

215. Martin Holt, "Gay Men's HIV Risk-Reduction Practices," *AIDS Education and Prevention* 26, no. 3 (2014): 214–223.

216. Jonathan M. Mann and Daniel J. M. Tarantola, "HIV 1998: The Global Picture," *Scientific American* 279, no. 1 (1998).

217. "Advances on the AIDS Front," *New York Times*, December 3, 2010.
218. Laura Smock, Evan Caten, Katherine Hsu, and Alfred DeMaria Jr., "Economic Disparities and Syphilis Incidence in Massachusetts, 2001–2013," *Public Health Reports* 132, no. 3 (2017): 309–315. See also Cathy Cohen, *The Boundaries of Blackness: AIDS and the Breakdown of Black Politics* (Chicago: University of Chicago Press, 1999); James Jones, *Bad Blood: The Tuskegee Syphilis Experiment, a Tragedy of Race and Medicine* (New York: Free Press, 1981); Susan Reverby, "Ethical Failures and History Lessons: The U.S. Public Health Service Research Studies in Tuskegee and Guatemala," *Public Health Reviews* 34, no. 1 (2012): 1–19.
219. Charlie Warzel, "How to Actually Talk to Anti-Maskers," *New York Times*, July 26, 2020.
220. Roni Caryn Rabin, "Leading New Task Force, Yale Doctor Takes Aim at Racial Gaps in Care," *New York Times*, January 12, 2021.
221. Warzel, "How to Actually Talk to Anti-Maskers."
222. Rabin, "Leading New Task Force, Yale Doctor Takes Aim at Racial Gaps in Care."
223. Harald Schmidt, Parag Pathak, Tayfun Sonmez, and M. Utku Unver, "Covid-19: How to Prioritize Worse-off Populations in Allocating Safe and Effective Vaccines," *BMJ* 371 (2020): m3795.
224. Thomas Fuller, "Isolation Helps Homeless Who Avoid the Shelters," *New York Times*, December 24, 2020. See also Rebecca Robbins, Frances Robles, and Tim Arango, "Vaccines Lag as States Tackle Logistical Woes. Doses Wait on Shelves," *New York Times*, January 1, 2021; Adam Ferguson, "A City on the Edge: With Spiraling Cases and a Devastated Economy, Gallup, New Mexico, Is One of the Hardest-Hit Communities in the United States," *New York Times*, December 28, 2020; Nathaniel Kash, "The Coronavirus Found a Safe Harbor," *New York Times*, December 20, 2020, SR3; Julie Turkewitz and Isayen Herrera, "Empty Pockets and No Home after 1500 Miles," *New York Times*, November 27, 2020, A1 and A14.
225. Samantha Artiga and Bradley Corallo, "Racial Disparities in COVID-19: Key Findings from Available Data and Analysis," Kaiser Family Foundation, August 17, 2020, www.kff.org/racial-equity-and-health-policy/issue-brief/racial-disparities-covid-19-key-findings-available-data-analysis/. See also Abby Goodnough and Jan Hoffman, "Officials Agonize over Allotment of First Vaccines," *New York Times*, December 6, 2020; John Eligon, Audra D. S. Burch, Dionne Searcey, and Richard A. Oppel Jr., "Black Americans Bear the Brunt as Virus Spreads," *New York Times*, April 8, 2020; Gus Wezerek, "Racism's Hidden Toll," *New York Times*, August 16, 2020.
226. Eligon et al., "Black Americans Bear the Brunt."
227. Wezerek, "Racism's Hidden Toll."
228. Michael Evans, "Health Equity: Are We Finally on the Edge of a New Frontier?," *NEJM* 383, no. 11 (2020): 997–999. See also Jason DeParle, "Proximity Imperils Poor Americans Who Cannot Afford to Keep 6 Feet of Distance," *New York Times*, April 13, 2020, A1 and A15.
229. Dan Levin, "Pandemic Worsens Poverty's Ills for Families," *New York Times*, December 30, 2020, A6. See also Yaryna Serkez, "Who Is Most Likely to Die from Covid-19?," *New York Times*, June 7, 2020.
230. David Blumenthal, Elizabeth J. Fowler, Melinda Abrams, and Sara R. Collins, "Covid-19: Implications for the Health Care System," *NEJM* 383, no. 15 (2020): 1483–1488.
231. "Slow Progress," *The Economist*, June 6, 2020, 21. See also Robert Sellers, "Op-Ed: I Am So Tired," Office of Diversity, Equity, and Inclusion, University of Michigan, May 29, 2020, https://odei.umich.edu/2020/05/29/i-am-so-tired/.

232. Jeneen Interlandi, "The Coronavirus Race Gap Explained," *New York Times*, October 4, 2020, SR4.

233. Peter Goodman, "Poorer Nations at Back of Line for Vaccine. Unequal Distribution Is Increasing Disparity," *New York Times*, December 26, 2020, A1 and A8. See also Matt Apuzzo and Selam Gebrekidan, "Covid Vaccines Expose Gap in Global Allotment," *New York Times*, December 29, 2020, A1 and A6; Megan Twohey, Keith Collins, and Katie Thomas, "Rush by Rich Countries to Reserve Early Doses Leaves the Poor Behind," *New York Times*, December 16, 2020, A6.

234. "WHO Chief Warns against 'Catastrophic Moral Failure' in COVID-19 Vaccine Access," UN News, January 18, 2021, https://news.un.org/en/story/2021/01/1082362.

235. "A Vaccine for Everyone," *The Economist*, January 6, 2021, www.economist.com/the -world-in-2021. See also "WHO Says 184 Countries Have Now Joined COVAX Vaccine Program," VOA News, October 19, 2020, www.voanews.com/covid-19-pandemic /who-says-184-countries-have-now-joined-covax-vaccine-program#:~:text=The%20 World%20Health%20Organization%20says,ailment%20caused%20by%20the%20 coronavirus.

236. Tedros Adhanom Ghebreyesus, "Five Steps to Solving the Vaccine Inequity Crisis," *PLOS Global Public Health*, October 13, 2021, https://journals.plos.org/global publichealth/article?id=10.1371/journal.pgph.0000032.

237. "COVID Vaccines: Widening Inequality and Millions Vulnerable," U.N. News, September 19, 2021, https://news.un.org/en/story/2021/09/1100192.

238. Artiga and Corallo, "Racial Disparities in COVID-19."

239. Goodnough and Hoffman, "Officials Agonize over Allotment of First Vaccines."

240. Yingyi Ma and Ning Zhan, "To Mask or Not to Mask amid the COVID-19 Pandemic: How Chinese Students in America Experience and Cope with Stigma," *Chinese Sociological Review* (October 20, 2020), https://doi.org/10.1080/21620555.2020 .1833712.

241. Editorial Board, "Congress, Test Thyself," *New York Times*, August 3, 2020.

242. France, *How to Survive a Plague*, 472–474, 493–495.

243. Gutmann and Moreno, *Everybody Wants to Go to Heaven but Nobody Wants to Die.* In Denmark, high trust and a sense of community make policy implementation easier, allowing lockdowns without backlash and acceptance of limitations on social gatherings without the need for mandates or laws. See also Rebecca Adler-Nissen, Sune Lehmann, and Andreas Roepstorff, "Denmark's Hard Lessons about Trust and Covid," *New York Times*, November 17, 2021, A21.

244. Adler-Nissen, Lehmann, and Roepstorff, "Denmark's Hard Lessons about Trust and Covid."

245. Amy Roeder, "Social Solidarity and Widespread Public Trust Needed to Boost Vaccine Confidence during COVID-19," Harvard School of Public Health, July 20, 2020, www.hsph.harvard.edu/news/features/vaccine-confidence-social-solidarity -covid19/.

246. Emily Harrison and Julia W. Wu, "Vaccine Confidence in the Time of COVID-19," *European Journal of Epidemiology* 35, no. 4 (April 22, 2020): 1–6.

247. David Rosner, "Moral Virtue in the Time of Cholera," *Foreign Affairs*, November 18, 2020, www.foreignaffairs.com/articles/united-states/2020-11-18/moral-virtue-time -cholera.

248. See also George Rosen, *A History of Public Health* (Baltimore, MD: Johns Hopkins University Press, 1993 [1958]), 107–166. Not since the 1918 flu has the United States faced a disease outbreak that called for unelected health officials to impose

widespread mask mandates and business closures. See also David Rosner, "Vaccine Hesitancy and the Decline of the American Experiment?," *Milbank Quarterly*, September 8, 2021, www.milbank.org/quarterly/opinions/vaccine-hesitancy-and-the -decline-of-the-american-experiment/; David Rosner and Gerald Markowitz, "Building the World That Kills Us: The Politics of Lead, Science, and Polluted Homes, 1970 to 2000," *Journal of Urban History* 42, no. 2 (2016): 323–345.

249. Gift Trapence, Chris Collins, Sam Avrett, Robert Carr, and Hugo Sanchez, "From Personal Survival to Public Health: Community Leadership by Men Who Have Sex with Men in the Response to HIV," *Lancet* 380, no. 9839 (July 28, 2012): 400–410.

250. M. Shernoff, *The Changing Face of Gay Men's Sexuality in Response to AIDS* (Dubuque, IA: Kendall Hunt Publishing Co, 1990).

251. Richard Berkowitz, Michael Callen, and Richard Dworkin, *How to Have Sex in an Epidemic: One Approach* (New York: News from the Front Publications, 1983).

252. Advisory Committee of the People with AIDS, *The Denver Principles* (Denver: National Association of People with AIDS, 1983).

253. Michael Callen and Richard Dworkin, "We Know Who We Are: Two Gay Men Declare War on Promiscuity," *New York Native*, November 8, 1982.

254. Alfred Crosby, "The Early History of Syphilis: A Reappraisal," in *The Columbian Exchange* (Westport, CT: Praeger, 2003), 122–164.

255. J. Pepin, *The Origins of AIDS* (Cambridge, UK: Cambridge University Press, 2011).

256. R. McKay, *Patient Zero and the Making of the AIDS Epidemic* (Chicago: University of Chicago Press, 2017).

257. R. Dubos, *Mirage of Health: Utopias, Progress, and Biological Change* (Garden City, NY: Anchor Books, 1959), 182–211.

258. L. Garrett, *The Coming Plague* (New York: Penguin Books, 1994).

259. D. Quammen, *Spillover* (New York: W. W. Norton, 2012).

260. Daniel Engber, "The Lab-Leak Theory Meets Its Perfect Match," *The Atlantic*, November 24, 2011, www.theatlantic.com/ideas/archive/2021/11/lab-leak-covid-origin -coincidence-wet-market/620794/.

261. Janet T. Scott and Malcolm G. Semple, "Ebola Virus Disease Sequelae: A Challenge That Is Not Going Away," *Lancet Infection* 17 (2017): 470–471.

262. "Middle East Respiratory Syndrome (MERS)," CDC, accessed June 25, 2017, www .cdc.gov/coronavirus/mers/index.html.

263. Catharine I. Paules and Anthony S. Fauci, "Yellow Fever: Once Again on the Radar Screen in the Americas," *NEJM* 376, no. 15 (2017): 1397–1400.

264. Donald G. McNeil Jr., "Once Tamed, Measles Rears Its Ugly Head," *New York Times*, April 4, 2019, A1.

265. Morens, Daszak, and Taubenberger, "Escaping Pandora's Box."

266. Charles Rosenberg, "What Is an Epidemic? AIDS in Historical Perspective," *Daedalus* 118, no. 2 (1989): 2.

267. Guillaume Lachenal and Thomas Gaetan, "Epidemics Have Lost the Plot," *Bulletin of the History of Medicine* 94, no. 4 (Winter 2020): 670.

268. Samuel Cohn, "The Dramaturgy of Epidemics," *Bulletin of the History of Medicine* 94, no. 4 (Winter 2020): 578–589.

269. Selman Waksman, *The Conquest of Tuberculosis* (Berkeley: University of California Press, 1964), 4.

270. Alimuddin Zumla and John M. Grange, "Is the Eradication of Tuberculosis 'Yesterday's Ambition' or 'Tomorrow's Triumph'?," *Clinical Medicine* 10, no. 5 (2010): 450–453.

Chapter 6 Vulnerable Environments

1. Leona Baumgartner, Arthur C. Curtis, A. L. Gray, Benno E. Kuechle, and T. Lefoy Richman, *The Eradication of Syphilis: A Task Force Report to the Surgeon General, Public Health Service, on Syphilis Control in the United States* (Washington, DC: U.S. Government Printing Office, 1962), 1–30. See also Thomas Parran, *Shadow on the Land: Syphilis* (New York: Reynal and Hitchcock, 1937).
2. Laura J. McGough and H. Hunter Handsfield, "History of Behavioral Interventions in STD Control," in *Behavioral Interventions for Prevention and Control of Sexually Transmitted Diseases*, ed. Sevgi O. Aral and John M. Douglas Jr. (New York: Springer, 2007), 3–23.
3. H. Hunter Handsfield and Edward W. Hook III, "Foreword," in *Behavioral Interventions for Prevention and Control of Sexually Transmitted Diseases*, ed. Aral and Douglas, v, vi.
4. McGough and Handsfield, "History of Behavioral Interventions in STD Control."
5. Tony Barnett and Alan Whiteside, *AIDS in the Twenty-First Century: Disease and Globalization* (New York: Palgrave Macmillan, 2002), 182–221. See also Catherine Campbell, *Letting Them Die: Why HIV/AIDS Intervention Programmes Fail* (Bloomington: Indiana University Press, 2003), 132–196.
6. McGough and Handsfield, "History of Behavioral Interventions in STD Control," 33.
7. Campbell, *Letting Them Die*, 132–196.
8. Hung Y. Fan, Ross F. Conner, and Luis P. Villarreal, *AIDS: Science and Society* (Sudbury, MA: Jones and Bartlett, 2004), 140–182. See also Cathy Cohen, *The Boundaries of Blackness: AIDS and the Breakdown of Black Politics* (Chicago: University of Chicago Press, 1999); Jeffrey A. Kelly, Timothy G. Heckman, L. Yvonne Stevenson, Paul N. Williams, Thom Ertl, Robert B. Hays, Noelle R. Leonard, et al., "Transfer of Research-Based HIV Prevention Interventions to Community Service Providers: Fidelity and Adaptation," *AIDS Education and Prevention* 12, no. 5 (2000): 87–98; Richard A. Crosby and Ralph J. DiClemente, "Applying Behavioral and Social Science Theory to HIV Prevention: The Need for Structural Level Approaches," in *Structural Interventions for HIV Prevention*, ed. Richard Crosby and Ralph DiClemente (New York: Oxford University Press, 2019), 13–30.
9. Crosby and DiClemente, "Applying Behavioral and Social Science Theory to HIV Prevention," 18.
10. Ronald O. Valdiserri, "Mapping the Roots of HIV/AIDS Complacency: Implications for Program and Policy Development," *AIDS Education and Prevention* 16, no. 5 (2004): 426–439.
11. Handsfield and Hook, "Foreword," vi. See also Campbell, *Letting Them Die*, 132–196.
12. Crosby and DiClemente, "Applying Behavioral and Social Science Theory to HIV Prevention."
13. Mark Hunter, *Love in the Time of AIDS: Inequality, Gender, and Rights in South Africa* (Bloomington: Indiana University Press, 2010), 155–178.
14. Greg Szekeres, "The Next 5 Years of Global HIV/AIDS Policy: Critical Gaps and Strategies for Effective Responses," *AIDS* 22, no. S2 (2008): S9–S17.
15. Ezekiel Kalipeni, *HIV and AIDS in Africa: Beyond Epidemiology* (Malden, MA: Blackwell, 2004), 175–190.
16. Helen Epstein, *The Invisible Cure: Africa, the West and the Fight against AIDS* (New York: Farrar, Straus, and Giroux 2007), 141–152.

17. Jacob Levenson, *The Secret Epidemic: The Story of AIDS and Black America* (New York: Pantheon Books, 2004), 126–168. See also David McBride, *From TB to AIDS: Epidemics among Urban Blacks since 1900* (Albany: State University of New York Press, 1991), 159–172; Rodrick Wallace, Mindy Thompson Fullilove, and Alan J. Flisher, "AIDS, Violence and Behavioral Coding: Information Theory, Risk Behavior and Dynamic Process on Core-Group Sociogeographic Networks," *Social Science and Medicine* 43, no. 3 (1996): 339–352.

18. Chris Collins, Thomas J., and James Curran, "Moving beyond the Alphabet Soup of HIV Prevention," *AIDS* 22, no. 2 (2008): S5–S8.

19. Epstein, *The Invisible Cure*, 155–171.

20. McBride, *From TB to AIDS*, 159–172.

21. Geeta Rao Gupta, Justin O. Parkhurst, Jessica A. Ogden, Peter Aggleton, and Ajay Mahal, "Structural Approaches to HIV Prevention," *Lancet* 372, no. 9640 (2008): 764–775.

22. K. M. Blankenship, S. R. Friedman, S. Dworkin, and J. E. Mantell, "Structural Interventions: Concepts, Challenges and Opportunities for Research," *Journal of Urban Health* 83, no. 1 (2006): 59–72, esp. 20, 83.

23. David Dickinson, *Changing the Course of AIDS: Peer Education in South Africa and Its Lessons for the Global Crisis* (Ithaca, NY: ILR Press, 2009), 180–203.

24. Hans Peter Kohler and Rebecca L. Thornton, "Conditional Cash Transfers and HIV/AIDS Prevention: Unconditionally Promising?," *World Bank Economic Review* 26, no. 2 (2012): 1–26.

25. Cohen, *The Boundaries of Blackness*.

26. Thomas J. Coates, Linda Richter, and Carlos Caceres, "Behavioural Strategies to Reduce HIV Transmission: How to Make Them Work Better," *Lancet* 372, no. 9639 (2008): 669–684.

27. Susan Allen, Jeffrey Tice, Philippe Van de Perre, Antoine Serufilira, Esther Hudes, Francois Nsengumuremyi, Joseph Bogaerts, et al., "Effect of Serotesting with Counselling on Condom Use and Seroconversion among HIV Discordant Couples in Africa," *BMJ* 304, no. 6842 (1992): 1605–1609.

28. Coates, Richter, and Caceres, "Behavioural Strategies to Reduce HIV Transmission," 676.

29. Dickinson, *Changing the Course of AIDS*, 204–216.

30. Joep Lange, "Test and Treat: Is It Enough?," *Clinical Infectious Diseases* 52, no. 6 (2012): 801–802.

31. João Guilherme Biehl, *Will to Live: AIDS Therapies and the Politics of Survival* (Princeton, NJ: Princeton University Press, 2007), 105–336, esp. 148, 285.

32. Ethan B. Kapstein and Josh Busby, "Antiretrovirals as Merit Goods," in *Routledge Handbook in Global Public Health*, ed. Richard Parker and Marni Sommer (London: Routledge, 2011), 461–470.

33. Gupta et al., "Structural Approaches to HIV Prevention."

34. Barnett and Whiteside , *AIDS in the Twenty-First Century*, 316–346.

35. Donald McNeil, "An HIV Strategy Invites Addicts In: A Vancouver Injection Site Aimed to Show That Treatment Is Prevention. Now the City Is Driving Back the Disease," *New York Times*, February 8, 2011, D1.

36. Kevin Fenton, "Social and Structural Barriers to HIV Prevention" (Program and Abstract, 17th Conference on Retroviruses and Opportunistic Infections, San Francisco, CA, February 27–March 2, 2010). See also Kevin A. Fenton and Frederick R. Bloom, "STD Prevention with MSM: Examples of Structural Interventions," in

Behavioral Interventions for Prevention and Control of Sexually Transmitted Diseases, ed. Sevgi O. Aral, John M. Douglas, and Judith Lipshutz (New York: Springer, 2007), 325–354.

37. Sharon Friel and Michael Marmot, "Global Health Inequities," in *Routledge Handbook of Global Public Health*, ed. Richard Parker and Marni Sommer (London: Routledge, 2011), 65–79.

38. Richard Parker and Marni Sommer, "Introduction," in *Routledge Handbook in Global Public Health*, ed. Parker and Sommer, 1–8.

39. Kapstein and Busby, "Antiretrovirals as Merit Goods," 467.

40. Gupta et al., "Structural Approaches to HIV Prevention."

41. Theodore M. Brown and Elizabeth Fee, "Sidney Kark and John Cassel: Social Medicine Pioneers and South African Emigrés," *American Journal of Public Health* 92, no. 11 (2002): 1744–1745. See also J. Trostle, "Early Work in Anthropology and Epidemiology: From Social Medicine to the Germ Theory, 1840–1920," in *Anthropology and Epidemiology: Interdisciplinary Approaches to the Study of Health and Diseases*, ed. Craig R. Janes, Ron Stall, and Sandra Gifford (Dordrecht, Netherlands: Reidel, 1986), 35–57.

42. Sidney Kark, "The Social Pathology of Syphilis in Africans," *International Journal of Epidemiology* 32, no. 2 (2003): 181–186. See also Fitzhugh Mullan, "Community-Oriented Primary Care: An Agenda for the '80s," *NEJM* 307, no. 17 (1982): 1076–1078.

43. John Parascandola, *Sex, Sin, and Science: A History of Syphilis in America* (London: Praeger, 2008). See also "End of Syphilis Seen by Use of Penicillin: Health Agencies Must Give Free Treatment, Dr. Baehr Says," *New York Times*, May 26, 1944.

44. J. Dennis Mull, "The Primary Health Care Dialectic: History, Rhetoric, and Reality," in *Anthropology and Primary Health Care*, ed. Jeannine Coreil and J. Dennis Mull (Boulder, CO: Westview Press, 1990).

45. Carl Kendall, The Implementation of a Diarrheal Disease Control Program in Honduras: Is It 'Selective Primary Health Care' or 'Integrated Primary Health Care'?," *Social Science and Medicine* 27, no. 1 (1988): 17–23. See also "WHO Called to Return to the Declaration of Alma-Ata International Conference on Primary Health Care," WHO, accessed April 6, 2024, www.who.int/teams/social-determinants-of-health/declaration-of-alma-ata#:~:text=The%20Alma%2DAta%20Declaration%20of,goal%20of%20Health%20for%20.

46. Jeannine Coreil, "The Evolution of Anthropology in International Health," in *Anthropology and Primary Health Care*, ed. Coreil and Mull, 1–25.

47. Richard G. Parker, Delia Easton, and Charles H. Klein, "Structural Barriers and Facilitators in HIV Prevention: A Review of International Research," *AIDS* 14, no. S1 (2000): S22–S32.

48. Randy Shilts, *And the Band Played On: Politics, People, and the AIDS Epidemic* (New York: St. Martin's Press, 1987).

49. M. D. Sweat and J. A. Denison, "Reducing HIV Incidence in Developing Countries with Structural and Environmental Interventions," *AIDS* 9, no. SA (1995): S251–S257.

50. Kate Shannon, Steffanie A. Strathdee, Shira M. Goldenberg, Putu Duff, Peninah Mwangi, Maia Rusakova, Sushena Reza-Paul, et al., "Global Epidemiology of HIV among Female Sex Workers: Influence of Structural Determinants," *Lancet* 385, no. 9962 (2015): 55–71. See also Matthew Chersich, Stanley Luchters, Innocent Ntaganira, Antonio Gerbase, Ying-Ru Lo, Fiona Scorgie, and Richard Steen, "Priority Interventions to Reduce HIV Transmission in Sex Work Settings in Sub-Saharan

Africa and Delivery of These Services," *Journal of the International AIDS Society* 16, no. 1 (2013): 17980.

51. IOM, *Assessing the Social and Behavioral Science Base for Prevention and Intervention: Workshop Summary* (Washington, DC: National Academy Press, 1995).

52. K. M. Blankenship, Sarah J. Bray, and Michael H. Merson, "Structural Interventions in Public Health," *AIDS* 14, no. S1 (2000), https://pubmed.ncbi.nlm.nih.gov /10981470/.

53. Tim Rhodes, "The 'Risk Environment': A Framework for Understanding and Reducing Drug-Related Harm," *International Journal of Drug Policy* 13, no. 2 (2002): 85–94.

54. Susan Kippax, Niamh Stephenson, Richard G. Parker, and Peter Aggleton, "Between Individual Agency and Structure in HIV Prevention: Understanding the Middle Ground of Social Practice," *American Journal of Public Health* 103, no. 8 (2013): 1367–1375.

55. K. K. Holmes, "Human Ecology and Behavior and Sexually Transmitted Bacterial Infections," *Proceedings of the National Academy of Science* 91, no. 7 (1994): 2448–2455, esp. 2451.

56. Jennifer A. Taussig, Beth Weinstein, Scott Burris, and Stephen T. Jones, "Syringe Laws and Pharmacy Regulations Are Structural Constraints on HIV Prevention in the US," *AIDS* 14, no. S1 (2000): S47–S51.

57. William J. Woods, Diane Binson, Lance M. Pollack, Dan Wohlfeiler, Ronald D. Stall, and Joseph A. Catania, "Public Policy Regulating Private and Public Space in Gay Bathhouses," *Journal of AIDS* 32, no. 4 (2003): 417–423.

58. Sakina Z. Kudrati, Kamden Hayashi, and Tamara Taggart, "Social Media and PrEP: A Systematic Review of Social Media Campaigns to Increase PrEP Awareness and Uptake Among Young Black and Latinx MSM and Women," *AIDS and Behavior* 25, no. 12 (2021): 4225–4234.

59. Samuel L. Groseclose, Beth Weinstein, T. Stephen Jones, Linda A. Valleroy, Laura J. Fehrs, and William J. Kassler, "Impact of Increased Legal Access to Needles and Syringes on Practices of Injecting-Drug Users and Police Officers: Connecticut, 1992–1993," *Journal of AIDS* 10, no. 1 (1995): 82–89. See also Edward H. Kaplan and Robert Heimer, "A Model-Based Estimate of HIV Infectivity via Needle Sharing," *Journal of Acquired Immune Deficiency Syndromes* 5, no. 11 (1992): 1116–1118. See also Donald A. Calsyn, Andrew J. Saxon, George Freeman, and Stephen Whittaker, "Needle-Use Practices among Intravenous Drug Users in an Area Where Needle Purchase Is Legal," *AIDS* 5, no. 2 (1991): 187–193.

60. James G. Kahn, Susan M. Kegeles, Robert Hays, and Nathalie Beltzer, "Cost-Effectiveness of the Mpowerment Project, A Community-Level Intervention for Young Gay Men," *Journal of Acquired Immune Deficiency Syndromes* 27, no. 5 (2001): 482–491.

61. S. M. Kegeles, R. B. Hays, and T. J. Coates, "The Mpowerment Project: A Community-Level HIV Prevention Intervention for Young Gay Men," *American Journal of Public Health* 86, no. 8, pt. 1 (1996): 1129–1136.

62. Thomas Kerr, Evan Wood, Dan Small, Anita Palepu, and Mark W. Tyndall, "Potential Use of Safer Injecting Facilities among Injection Drug Users in Vancouver's Downtown Eastside," *CMAJ* 169, no. 8 (2003): 759–763. See also Evan Wood, Thomas Kerr, Patricia M. Spittal, Kathy Li, Will Small, Mark W. Tyndall, Robert S. Hogg, et al., "The Potential Public Health and Community Impacts of Safer Injecting Facilities: Evidence from a Cohort of Injection Drug Users," *Journal of Acquired Immune Deficiency Syndromes* 32, no. 1 (2003): 2–8.

63. James L. Chen, Dulmini Kodagoda, A. Michael Lawrence, and Peter R. Kerndt, "Rapid Public Health Interventions in Response to an Outbreak of Syphilis in Los Angeles," *Sexually Transmitted Diseases* 29, no. 5 (2002): 277–284. See also D. A. Calsyn, C. Meinecke, A. J. Saxon, and V. Stanton, "Risk Reduction in Sexual Behavior: A Condom Giveaway Program in a Drug Abuse Treatment Clinic," *American Journal of Public Health* 82, no. 11 (1992): 1536–1538.

64. Matt G. Mutchler, Trista Bingham, Miguel Chion, Richard A. Jenkins, Lee E. Klosinski, and Gina Secura, "Comparing Sexual Behavioral Patterns between Two Bathhouses: Implications for HIV Prevention Intervention Policy," *Journal of Homosexuality* 44, no. 3–4 (2003): 221–242.

65. J. A. Kelly, J. S. St. Lawrence, Y. E. Diaz, L. Y. Stevenson, A. C. Hauth, T. L. Brasfield, S. C. Kalichman, J. E. Smith, and M. E. Andrew, "HIV Risk Behavior Reduction Following Intervention with Key Opinion Leaders of a Population: An Experimental Analysis," *American Journal of Public Health* 81, no. 2 (1991): 168–171.

66. S. D. Pinkerton, "Cost Effectiveness of a Community-Level HIV Risk Reduction Intervention," *American Journal of Public Health* 88, no. 8 (1998): 1239–1242.

67. Kudrati, Hayashi, and Taggart, "Social Media and PrEP." See also Sarah K. Calabrese, Kristen Underhill, and Kenneth H. Mayer, "HIV Preexposure Prophylaxis and Condomless Sex: Disentangling Personal Values from Public Health Priorities," *American Journal of Public Health* 107, no. 10 (2017): 1572–1576.

68. Kamair Alaei, Christopher A. Paynter, Shao-Chiu Juan, and Arash Alaei, "Using Preexposure Prophylaxis, Losing Condoms? Preexposure Prophylaxis Promotion May Undermine Safe Sex," *AIDS* 30, no. 18 (2016): 2753–2756.

69. Will Nutland, "Getting to 40! Structural Approaches in England to Reducing HIV Incidence in Men Who Have Sex with Men," in *Structural Interventions for HIV Prevention*, ed. Crosby and DiClemente, 267–285, esp. 268–270.

70. Will Nutland, "The State of PrEP Activism in Europe and Worldwide" (presentation at PrEP in Europe 2018 Summit, Amsterdam, February 9, 2018). See also Nutland, "Getting to 40!," 280–282.

71. Gupta et al., "Structural Approaches to HIV Prevention."

72. Esther Sumartojo, Lynda Doll, David Holtgrave, Helene Gayle, and Michael Merson, "Enriching the Mix: Incorporating Structural Factors into HIV Prevention," *AIDS* 14, no. S1 (2000): S1.

73. Gupta et al., "Structural Approaches to HIV Prevention."

74. Rosa R. Cui, Ramon Lee, Harsha Thirumurthy, Kathryn E. Muessig, and Joseph D. Tucker, "Microenterprise Development Interventions for Sexual Risk Reduction: A Systematic Review," *AIDS and Behavior* 17, no. 9 (2013): 2864–2877.

75. Julia Dickson-Gomez and Katherine Quinn, "Enhancing Access to Safe and Secure Housing," in *Structural Interventions for HIV Prevention*, ed. Crosby and DiClemente, 105–142, esp. 105–108.

76. Mark S. Friedman, Michael P. Marshal, Ron Stall, Daniel P. Kidder, Kirk D. Henny, Cari Courtenay-Quirk, Angela Aidala, Scott Royal, and David R. Holtgrave, "Associations between Substance Use, Sexual Risk Taking and HIV Treatment Adherence among Homeless People Living with HIV," *AIDS Care* 21, no. 6 (2009): 692–700.

77. Brian W. Weir, "Uncovering Patterns of HIV Risk through Multiple Housing Measures," *AIDS and Behavior* 11, no. 6 (2007): 31–44. See also Scott W. Royal, Daniel P. Kidder, Satyendra Patrabansh, Richard J. Wolitski, David R. Holtgrave, Angela Aidala, Sherri Pals, and Ron Stall, "Factors Associated with Adherence to Highly Active Antiretroviral Therapy in Homeless or Unstably Housed Adults

Living with HIV," *AIDS Care* 21, no. 4 (2009): 448–455; Dickson-Gomez et al., "Enhancing Access to Safe and Secure Housing," 110–111.

78. Bridgette Brawner, Barbara Guthrie, Robin Stevens, Lynne Taylor, Michael Eberhart, and Jean J. Schensul, "Place Still Matters: Racial/Ethnic and Geographic Disparities in HIV Transmission and Disease Burden," *Journal of Urban Health* 94, no. 5 (2017): 716–727.

79. Katherine Alaimo, Thomas M. Reischl, and Julie Ober Allen, "Community Gardening, Neighborhood Meetings and Social Capital," *Journal of Community Psychology* 38, no. 4 (2010): 497–514.

80. Angelina Aidala, Maiko Yomogida, and Jennifer Leigh, "Food Insecurity and HIV/AIDS," in *Structural Interventions for HIV Prevention*, ed. Crosby and DiClemente, 143–177, esp. 168.

81. U.S. Health Resources and Services Administration, website of Ryan White HIV/AIDS Program: A Living History, accessed April 6, 2024, https://hab.hrsa.gov/livinghistory/.

82. Sheri D. Weiser, Abigail M. Hatcher, Lee L. Hufstedler, Elly Weke, Shari L. Dworkin, Elizabeth A. Bukusi, Rachel L. Burger, et al., "Changes in Health and Antiretroviral Adherence among HIV-Infected Adults in Kenya: Qualitative Longitudinal Findings from a Livelihood Intervention," *AIDS and Behavior* 21, no. 2 (2017): 415–427.

83. Divya Mehra, Saskia de Pee, and Martin W. Bloem, "Nutrition, Food Security, Social Protection, and Health Systems Strengthening for Ending AIDS," in *Food Insecurity and Public Health*, ed. Louise Ivers (Boca Raton, FL: CRC Press, 2015), 69–89.

84. Vandana Gurnani, Tara S. Beattie, Parinita Bhattacharjee, H. L. Mohan, Srinath Maddur, Reynold Washington, Shajy Isac, et al., "An Integrated Structural Intervention to Reduce Vulnerability to HIV and Sexually Transmitted Infections among Female Sex Workers in Karnataka State, South India," *BMC Public Health* 11, no. 1 (2011): 755.

85. Whitney Moret, "Economic Strengthening for Female Sex Workers: A Review of the Literature," ASPIRES, FHI 360, May 2014, accessed January 29, 2023, https://www.fhi360.org/wp-content/uploads/drupal/documents/Economic_Strengthening_for_Female_Sex_Workers.pdf. See also Adolfo Caldas, Fernando Arteaga, Maribel Munoz, Jhon Zeladita, Mayler Albujar, Jaime Bayona, and Sonya Shin, "Microfinance: A General Overview and Implications for Impoverished Individuals Living with HIV/AIDS," *Journal of Health Care for the Poor and Underserved* 21, no. 3 (2010): 986–1005; Shari Krishnaratne, Bernadette Hensen, Jillian Cordes, Joanne Enstone, and James R. Hargreaves, "Interventions to Strengthen the HIV Prevention Cascade: A Systematic Review of Reviews," *Lancet HIV* 3, no. 7 (2016): e307–e317.

86. Andrea Mantsios, Deanna Kerrigan, Jessie Mbwambo, Samuel Likindikoki, and Catherine Shembilu, "Economic Strengthening Approaches with Female Sex Workers," in *Structural Interventions for HIV Prevention*, ed. Crosby and DiClemente, 192. See also Shannon et al., "Global Epidemiology of HIV among Female Sex Workers"; Stefan Baral, Chris Beyrer, Kathryn Muessig, Tonia Poteat, Andrea Wirtz, Michele R. Decker, Susan G. Sherman, and Deanna Kerrigan, "Burden of HIV among Female Sex Workers in Low-Income and Middle-Income Countries: A Systematic Review and Meta-Analysis," *Lancet Infectious Diseases* 12, no .7 (2012): 538–549.

87. Deanna Kerrigan, Caitlin E. Kennedy, Ruth Morgan-Thomas, Sushena Reza-Paul, Peninah Mwangi, Kay Thi Win, Allison McFall, et al., "A Community Empowerment Approach to the HIV Response among Sex Workers: Effectiveness, Challenges,

and Considerations for Implementation and Scale-Up," *Lancet* 385, no. 9963 (2015): 172–175.

88. Caitlin Conrad, Heather M. Bradley, Dita Broz, Swamy Buddha, Erika L. Chapman, Romeo R. Galang, Daniel Hillman, et al., "Community Outbreak of HIV Infection Linked to Injection Drug Use of Oxymorphone—Indiana, 2015," *Morbidity and Mortality Weekly Report (MMWR)* 64, no. 16 (2015): 443–444.

89. Nabila El-Bassel, Phillip L. Marotta, Louisa Gilbert, Elwin Wu, Sandra Springer, Dawn A. Goddard-Eckrich, and Timothy Hunt, "Integrating Treatment for Opioid Use Disorders and HIV Services into Primary Care Solutions for the 21st Century," in *Structural Interventions for HIV Preventions*, ed. Crosby and DiClemente, 221–253. See also Debra L. Karch, Kristen Mahle Gray, Jing Shi, and H. Irene Hall, "HIV Infection Care and Viral Suppression among People who Inject Drugs, 28 US Jurisdictions, 2012–2013," *Open AIDS Journal* 10, no. 1 (2016), 127.

90. Frederick L. Altice, R. Douglas Bruce, Gregory M. Lucas, Paula J. Lum, Todd Korthuis, Timothy P. Flanigan, Chinazo O. Cunningham, et al., "HIV Treatment Outcomes among HIV-Infected, Opioid-Dependent Patients Receiving Buprenorphine/Naloxone Treatment within HIV Clinical Care Settings: Results from a Multisite Study," *Journal of Acquired Immune Deficiency Synromes* 56, no. S1 (2011): S22.

91. Richard Parker, Jonathan Garcia, Miguel Munoz-Laboy, Laura Rebecca Murray, and Fernando Seffner, "Community Mobilization as an HIV Prevention Strategy: The Political Challenges of Confronting the AIDS Epidemic in Brazil," in *Structural Interventions for HIV Prevention*, ed. Crosby and DiClemente, 285–310, esp. 289–290. See also National Coordination for STD and AIDS, *The Brazilian Response to HIV/ AIDS* (Brasilia: Ministry of Health 2000).

92. John Garrison and Jessica Rich, "Brazil's Virtuous Alliance: How the Grassroots and the Government Joined Forces against AIDS," *Grassroots Development Journal*, archive, Inter-American Foundation, accessed November 12, 2022, www.iaf.gov /resources/publications/grassroots-development-journal/2013-focus-the-iaf-s -investment-in-young-people/brazil-s-virtuous-alliance-how-the-grassroots-and-the -government-joined-forces-against-aids.

93. J. Galvao, "AIDS no Brasil," *Sao Paulo: Editora* 34 (2000): 7–105.

94. Agencia de Noticias de AIDS, "Estados Unidos cancelam grande programa de combate a AIDS no Brasil," accessed November 18, 2022, www.agenciaaids.com.br.

95. Blankenship, Bray, and Merson, "Structural Interventions in Public Health."

96. "UNAIDS Strategy Aligns HIV Priorities with Development Goals," *Lancet HIV* 8, no. 5 (2021): e245.

97. Roni Caryn Rabin, "Leading New Task Force, Yale Doctor Takes Aim at Racial Gaps in Cares," *New York Times*, January 12, 2021.

98. Charlie Warzel, "How to Actually Talk to Anti-Maskers," *New York Times*, July 26, 2020. See also Harald Schmidt, Parag Pathak, Tayfun Sonmez, and M. Utku Unver, "Covid-19: How to Prioritize Worse-off Populations in Allocating Safe and Effective Vaccines," *BMJ* 371 (2020): m3795.

99. Thomas Fuller, "Isolation Helps Homeless Who Avoid the Shelters," *New York Times*, December 24, 2020.

100. David Deming, "The Aqueducts and Water Supply of Ancient Rome," *Ground Water* 58, no. 1 (2020): 152–161.

101. "Ordinances against the Spread of Plague, Pistoia 1348," in *The Black Death*, trans. Rosemary Horrox (Manchester, UK: Manchester University Press, 1994), 194–203. See

also "Report of the Paris Medical Faculty, October 1348," in *The Black Death*, 158–163.

102. George Rosen, *A History of Public Health* (Baltimore, MD: Johns Hopkins University Press, 1993), 177.

103. Edwin Chadwick, *Report to Her Majesty's Principal Secretary of State for the Home Department from the Poor Law Commissioners, on an Inquiry into the Sanitary Condition of the Labouring Population of Great Britain, with Appendices* (London: Her Majesty's Stationary Office, 1842).

104. Rosen, *A History of Public Health*, 178, 186–191.

105. Daniel Pridan, "Rudolf Virchow and Social Medicine in Historical Perspective," *Medical History* 8, no. 3 (1964): 274–278.

106. P. E. Brown, "John Snow: The Autumn Loiterer," *Bulletin of the History of Medicine* 35, no. 6 (1961): 519–528.

107. Charles E. Rosenberg, "Florence Nightingale on Contagion: The Hospital as Moral Universe," in *Explaining Epidemics and Other Studies in the History of Medicine*, ed. Charles E. Rosenberg (New York: Cambridge University Press, 1992), 90–108.

108. Elizabeth Blackmar, "Accountability for Public Health: Regulating the Housing Market in Nineteenth-Century New York City," in *Hives of Sickness*, ed. David Rosner (New Brunswick, NJ: Rutgers University Press, 1995), 42–63.

109. John Duffy, *The Sanitarians: A History of American Public Health* (Urbana: University of Illinois Press, 1990), 138–192.

110. Barbara Gutmann Rosenkrantz, *Public Health and the State: Changing Views in Massachusetts, 1842–1936* (Cambridge, MA: Harvard University Press, 1972), 37–74, 171.

111. Rosenkrantz, *Public Health and the State*, 38, 44, 47–48, 66–71.

112. Crosby and DiClemente, eds., *Structural Interventions for HIV Preventions*.

113. Rosenkrantz, *Public Health and the State*, 94–96.

114. Rosen, *A History of Public Health*, 223. See also Rosenkrantz, *Public Health and the State*; Elizabeth Fee, *Disease and Discovery: A History of the Johns Hopkins School of Hygiene and Public Health, 1916–1939* (Baltimore, MD: Johns Hopkins University Press, 1987); Evelynn Hammonds, *Childhood's Deadly Scourge* (Baltimore, MD: John Hopkins University Press, 1999), 17–87; Bela Schick, "Die Diphtherietoxin-Hautreaktion des Menschen als Vorprobe der prophylaktischen Diphtherieheilserum-injection," *MMW* 60 (1913): 2608–2610.

115. Rosenkrantz, *Public Health and the State*, 7. See also Duffy, *The Sanitarians*; Judith Walzer Leavitt, *The Heathiest City: Milwaukee and the Politics of Health Reform* (Madison: University of Wisconsin Press, 1996).

116. Rosenkrantz, *Public Health and the State*, 37–96.

117. Bela Schick, "Die Diphtherietoxin-Hautreaktion des Menschen als Vorprobe der prophylaktischen Diphtherieheilserum-injection."

118. Charles V. Chapin, "Dirt, Disease and the Health Officer," *Public Health Papers and Reports* 28 (1902): 296–299. See also James H. Cassedy, *Charles V. Chapin and the Public Health Movement* (Cambridge, MA: Harvard University Press, 1962), 126–142.

119. Charles V. Chapin, *The Sources and Modes of Infection* (New York: John Wiley and Sons, 1910), 110–125.

120. Chapin, "Dirt, Disease and the Health Officer."

121. Milton J. Rosenau, *Preventive Medicine and Hygiene* (New York: D. Appleton, 1913).

122. Smith wrote, "Knowledge of disease transmission among individuals has superseded indiscriminate sanitary practices and superstition." See Stephen Smith, "The

History of Public Health, 1871–1921," in *A Half Century of Public Health: Jubilee Historical Volume of the American Public Health Association*, ed. Mazyck P. Ravenel (New York: American Public Health Association, 1921), 7–9.

123. Howard D. Kramer, "The Germ Theory and the Early Public Health Program in the United States," *Bulletin of the History of Medicine* 22, no. 3 (1948): 233–247.
124. Rosen, *A History of Public Health*, 270–319.
125. Duffy, *The Sanitarians*, 205–206.
126. Rosenkrantz, *Public Health and the State*, 97–127.
127. Robert U. Patterson, "The Work of Walter Reed and His Associates of the Medical Department of the United States Army," *American Journal of Public Health* 23, no. 11 (1933): 1127–1134.

Conclusion

1. Dubos maintained that new infectious threats would continue to arise unpredictably as microbes escape the ecologic niche within which they have co-evolved. See René Jules Dubos, *Mirage of Health: Utopias, Progress, and Biological Change* (New York: Harper and Brothers, 1959).
2. Elimination campaigns have been advocated by the WHO for malaria. Yet even when campaigns approach success, they become so logistically complex that maintaining them requires a growing number of resources from international health foundations. See Randall Packard, "The Origins of Antimalarial-Drug Resistance," *NEJM* 371, no. 5 (2014): 397–399.
3. Thucydides, *History of the Peloponnesian War*, book 2 (Oxford, UK: Clarendon Press, 1881), 135–140.
4. Giovanni Boccaccio, *The Decameron*, trans. G. H. McWilliam (London: Penguin Classics, 2003). See also Guy de Chuliac, "Bubonic Plague," in *Original Publications of the Black Death*, trans. Rosemary Horrox (Manchester, UK: Manchester University Press, 1994), 773–774.
5. Daniel Defoe, *A Journal of the Plague Year, London 1665* (New York: Penguin Books, 2003).
6. Albert Camus, *The Plague* (New York: Vintage Books, 1991).
7. Katherine Porter, *Pale Horse, Pale Rider* (Marrickville, NSW, Australia: Harcourt Publishers Group, 1990).
8. Sinclair Lewis, *Arrowsmith* (New York: Chelsea House Publishers, 1925).
9. In the twentieth century, public health departments upgraded water systems to limit typhoid and cholera, guaranteed food safety in restaurants, and protected the purity of milk from bacterial contamination. See *A History of Public Health*, ed. George Rosen (Baltimore, MD: Johns Hopkins University Press,1993).
10. John Barry, *The Great Influenza: The Epic Story of the Deadliest Plague in History* (New York: Penguin Books, 2004).
11. David Rosner, "Moral Virtue in the Time of Cholera," *Foreign Affairs*, November 18, 2020, www.foreignaffairs.com/articles/united-states/2020-11-18/moral-virtue-time -cholera.
12. Randy Shilts, *And the Band Played On: Politics, People, and the AIDS Epidemic* (New York: St. Martin's Press, 1987).
13. Tomes writes about how restraints were placed on everyday living by the encouragement of practices like washing foods, avoiding sharing cups, refraining from spitting, etc., to avoid the spread of contagion. Nancy Tomes, *The Gospel of Germs:*

Men, Women, and the Microbe in American Life (Cambridge, MA: Harvard University Press, 1998).

14. Thomas McKeown, *The Role of Medicine: Dream, Mirage or Nemesis?* (London: Nuffield Provincial Hospitals Trust, 1976).

15. Lewis Thomas, "Notes of a Biology-Watcher: Germs," *NEJM* 287, no. 11 (1972): 553–555.

16. Jacques Pépin, *The Origins of AIDS* (Cambridge, UK: Cambridge University Press, 2011).

17. Christopher Elias, John N. Nkengasong, and Firdausi Qadri, "Emerging Infectious Diseases: Learning from the Past and Looking to the Future," *NEJM* 384, no. 13 (2021): 1181–1184.

18. Marco Marani, Gabriel G. Katul, William K. Pan, and Anthony J. Parolari, "Intensity and Frequency of Extreme Novel Epidemics," *PNAS* 118, no. 35 (August 23, 2021), www.pnas.org/doi/10.1073/pnas.2105482118?cookieSet=1.

19. L. Madoff and J. Brownstein, "ProMED and HealthMap: Collaboration to Improve Emerging Disease Surveillance," *International Journal of Infectious Diseases* 14, no. 1, E184 (March 1, 2010), www.ijidonline.com/article/S1201-9712(10)01938-7/fulltext#%20.

20. See the website of EcoHealth Alliance, accessed June 23, 2017, www.ecohealthalliance.org/.

21. Yonatan H. Grad and Marc Lipsitch, "Epidemiologic Data and Pathogen Genome Sequences: A Powerful Synergy for Public Health," *Genome Biology* 15, no. 11 (2014): 538.

22. Liam Stack, "In Monkeypox, Gay Men Confront a Health Crisis with Echoes of the Past," *New York Times*, July 29, 2022.

23. Ezekiel J. Emanuel, David Michaels, Rick Bright, and Michael T. Osterholm, "We're Still Far from Ready for the Next Public Health Crisis," *New York Times*, October 21, 2022, A26.

24. The coalition's goals include developing next-generation vaccines and universal vaccines (e.g., for all coronaviruses, etc.), improving deliverability, shifting away from vaccines that require ultra-cold-chain storage, and improving the breadth of vaccines. See Udani Samarasekera, "CEPI Prepares for Future Pandemics and Epidemics," *Lancet ID* 21, no. 5 (May, 2021): 608.

25. Gina Kolata, "Fauci Advocates the Creation of Vaccines for the Next Pandemic before It Even Hits," *New York Times*, July 26, 2021, A14.

Index

Page numbers followed by the letter f denote figures.

About the Author

Powel H. Kazanjian, MD, PhD, is the chief of the Division of Infectious Diseases and a professor of history at the University of Michigan. He has published on the history of bacteriology, disease, and epidemiology in medical and historical journals. He is the author of *Frederick Novy and the Development of Bacteriology in Medicine* (Rutgers University Press).

Available titles in the Critical Issues in Health and Medicine series:

Rachel Grob, *Testing Baby: The Transformation of Newborn Screening, Parenting, and Policymaking*

Mark A. Hall and Sara Rosenbaum, eds., *The Health Care "Safety Net" in a Post-Reform World*

Laura L. Heinemann, *Transplanting Care: Shifting Commitments in Health and Care in the United States*

Rebecca J. Hester, *Embodied Politics: Indigenous Migrant Activism, Cultural Competency, and Health Promotion in California*

Laura D. Hirshbein, *American Melancholy: Constructions of Depression in the Twentieth Century*

Laura D. Hirshbein, *Smoking Privileges: Psychiatry, the Mentally Ill, and the Tobacco Industry in America*

Timothy Hoff, *Practice under Pressure: Primary Care Physicians and Their Medicine in the Twenty-first Century*

Beatrix Hoffman, Nancy Tomes, Rachel N. Grob, and Mark Schlesinger, eds., *Patients as Policy Actors*

Ruth Horowitz, *Deciding the Public Interest: Medical Licensing and Discipline*

Powel H. Kazanjian, *Frederick Novy and the Development of Bacteriology in Medicine*

Powel H. Kazanjian, *Persisting Pandemics: Syphilis, AIDS, and COVID*

Matthew Kelly, *The Sounds of Furious Living: Everyday Unorthodoxies in an Era of AIDS*

Claas Kirchhelle, *Pyrrhic Progress: The History of Antibiotics in Anglo-American Food Production*

Rebecca M. Kluchin, *Fit to Be Tied: Sterilization and Reproductive Rights in America, 1950–1980*

Jennifer Lisa Koslow, *Cultivating Health: Los Angeles Women and Public Health Reform*

Jennifer Lisa Koslow, *Exhibiting Health: Public Health Displays in the Progressive Era*

Susan C. Lawrence, *Privacy and the Past: Research, Law, Archives, Ethics*

Bonnie Lefkowitz, *Community Health Centers: A Movement and the People Who Made It Happen*

Ellen Leopold, *Under the Radar: Cancer and the Cold War*

Barbara L. Ley, *From Pink to Green: Disease Prevention and the Environmental Breast Cancer Movement*

Sonja Mackenzie, *Structural Intimacies: Sexual Stories in the Black AIDS Epidemic*

Stephen E. Mawdsley, *Selling Science: Polio and the Promise of Gamma Globulin*

Frank M. McClellan, *Healthcare and Human Dignity: Law Matters*

Michelle McClellan, *Lady Lushes: Gender, Alcohol, and Medicine in Modern America*

David Mechanic, *The Truth about Health Care: Why Reform Is Not Working in America*

Richard A. Meckel, *Classrooms and Clinics: Urban Schools and the Protection and Promotion of Child Health, 1870–1930*

Terry Mizrahi, *From Residency to Retirement: Physicians' Careers over a Professional Lifetime*

Manon Parry, *Broadcasting Birth Control: Mass Media and Family Planning*

Alyssa Picard, *Making the American Mouth: Dentists and Public Health in the Twentieth Century*

Heather Munro Prescott, *The Morning After: A History of Emergency Contraception in the United States*

Sarah B. Rodriguez, *The Love Surgeon: A Story of Trust, Harm, and the Limits of Medical Regulation*

David J. Rothman and David Blumenthal, eds., *Medical Professionalism in the New Information Age*

Andrew R. Ruis, *Eating to Learn, Learning to Eat: School Lunches and Nutrition Policy in the United States*

James A. Schafer Jr., *The Business of Private Medical Practice: Doctors, Specialization, and Urban Change in Philadelphia, 1900–1940*

Johanna Schoen, ed., *Abortion Care as Moral Work: Ethical Considerations of Maternal and Fetal Bodies*

David G. Schuster, *Neurasthenic Nation: America's Search for Health, Happiness, and Comfort, 1869–1920*

Karen Seccombe and Kim A. Hoffman, *Just Don't Get Sick: Access to Health Care in the Aftermath of Welfare Reform*

Leo B. Slater, *War and Disease: Biomedical Research on Malaria in the Twentieth Century*

Piper Sledge, *Bodies Unbound: Gender-Specific Cancer and Biolegitimacy*

Dena T. Smith, *Medicine over Mind: Mental Health Practice in the Biomedical Era*

Kylie M. Smith, *Talking Therapy: Knowledge and Power in American Psychiatric Nursing*

Matthew Smith, *An Alternative History of Hyperactivity: Food Additives and the Feingold Diet*

Paige Hall Smith, Bernice L. Hausman, and Miriam Labbok, *Beyond Health, Beyond Choice: Breastfeeding Constraints and Realities*

Susan L. Smith, *Toxic Exposures: Mustard Gas and the Health Consequences of World War II in the United States*

Rosemary A. Stevens, Charles E. Rosenberg, and Lawton R. Burns, eds., *History and Health Policy in the United States: Putting the Past Back In*

Marianne Sullivan, *Tainted Earth: Smelters, Public Health, and the Environment*

Courtney E. Thompson, *An Organ of Murder: Crime, Violence, and Phrenology in Nineteenth-Century America*

Barbra Mann Wall, *American Catholic Hospitals: A Century of Changing Markets and Missions*

Frances Ward, *The Door of Last Resort: Memoirs of a Nurse Practitioner*

Jean C. Whelan, *Nursing the Nation: Building the Nurse Labor Force*

Shannon Withycombe, *Lost: Miscarriage in Nineteenth-Century America*